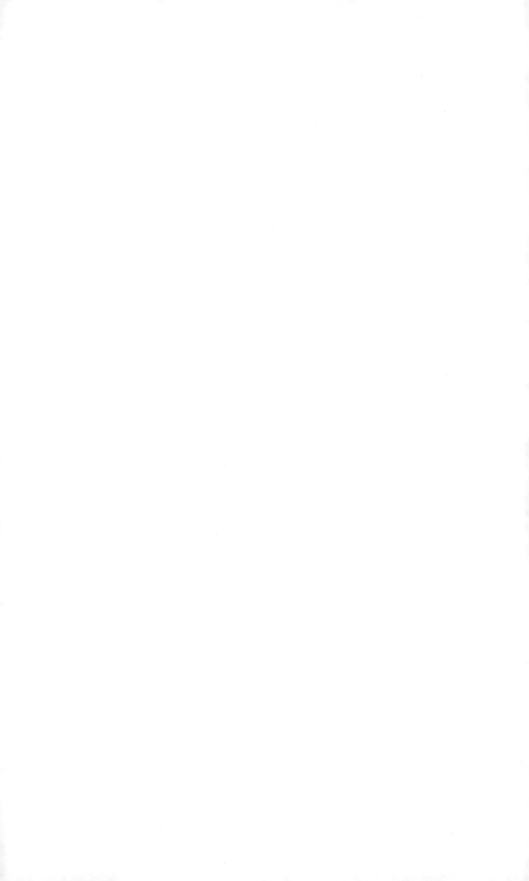

Obesity in Childhood
and Adolescence

Recent Titles in
Child Psychology and Mental Health

Children's Imaginative Play: A Visit to Wonderland
  Shlomo Ariel

Attachment Therapy on Trial: The Torture and Death of Candace Newmaker
  Jean Mercer, Larry Sarner, and Linda Ross

The Educated Parent: Recent Trends in Raising Children
  Joseph D. Sclafani

The Crisis in Youth Mental Health: Critical Issues and Effective Programs
Four Volumes
  Hiram E. Fitzgerald, Robert Zucker, and Kristine Freeark, editors

Learning from Behavior: How to Understand and Help "Challenging"
Children in School
  James E. Levine

OBESITY IN CHILDHOOD AND ADOLESCENCE

Volume 2
Understanding Development and Prevention

Hiram E. Fitzgerald and Vasiliki Mousouli
Volume Editors

H. Dele Davies and Hiram E. Fitzgerald
Set Editors

Forewords by Kimberlydawn Wisdom and Sheila Gahagan

PRAEGER PERSPECTIVES

Child Psychology and Mental Health
Hiram E. Fitzgerald and Susanne Ayres Denham, Series Editors

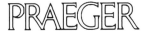

Westport, Connecticut
London

Library of Congress Cataloging-in-Publication Data

Obesity in childhood and adolescence / H. Dele Davies and Hiram E. Fitzgerald, set editors.
    v. ; cm. — (Child psychology and mental health, ISSN 1538–8883)
  Includes bibliographical references and index.
  Contents: v. 1. Medical, biological, and social issues / H. Dele Davies,
volume editor — v. 2. Understanding development and prevention /
Hiram E. Fitzgerald and Vasiliki Mousouli, volume editors.
  ISBN-13: 978–0–275–99615–4 (set : alk. paper)
  ISBN-13: 978–0–275–99617–8 (v. 1 : alk. paper)
  ISBN-13: 978–0–275–99619–2 (v. 2 : alk. paper)
1. Obesity in children—United States.   2. Obesity in adolescence—
United States.   3. Obesity in adolescence.
  [DNLM: 1. Obesity.   2. Adolescent.   3. Child. WD 210 O1205 2008]
I. Davies, H. Dele.   II. Fitzgerald, Hiram E.   III. Mousouli, Vasiliki.   IV. Series.
  RJ399.C6O3352 2008
  618.92'398—dc22   2007035295

British Library Cataloguing in Publication Data is available.

Library of Congress Catalog Card Number: 2007035295

ISBN-13: 978–0–275–99615–4 (set)
        978–0–275–99617–8 (vol. 1)
        978–0–275–99619–2 (vol. 2)
ISSN: 1538–8883

First published in 2008

Praeger Publishers, 88 Post Road West, Westport, CT 06881
An imprint of Greenwood Publishing Group, Inc.
www.praeger.com

Printed in the United States of America

The paper used in this book complies with the
Permanent Paper Standard issued by the National
Information Standards Organization (Z39.48–1984).

10 9 8 7 6 5 4 3 2 1

CONTENTS

Series Foreword   vii

Foreword *by Kimberlydawn Wisdom*   ix

Foreword: Special Commentary on Childhood Obesity
by Sheila Gahagan   xi

Preface   xvii

PART I: SOCIAL AND BEHAVIORAL DEVELOPMENT

1. Risk Factors for Obesity in Early Human Development   3
   John Worobey

2. The Role of Physical Activity in Obesity Prevention   25
   James M. Pivarnik

3. Childhood Overweight and Academic Achievement   49
   Sara Gable, Jennifer L. Krull, and Arathi Srikanta

4. Adiposity and Internalizing Problems: Infancy to
   Middle Childhood   73
   *Robert H. Bradley, Renate Houts, Phillip R. Nader,
   Marion O'Brien, Jay Belsky, and Robert Crosnoe*

5. Food Marketing Goes Online: A Content Analysis of
   Web Sites for Children   93
   Elizabeth S. Moore

6. Families and Obesity: A Family Process Approach to Obesity in Adolescents 117
Matthew P.Thorpe and Randal D. Day

PART II: INDIVIDUAL DIFFERENCES AND ETHNIC VARIATION

7. Responding to the Epidemic of American Indian and Alaska Native Childhood Obesity 143
Paul Spicer and Kelly Moore

8. Obesity in African Americans and Latino Americans 167
Helen D. Pratt, Manmohan Kamboj, and Robin Joseph

PART III: PREVENTION AND INTERVENTION

9. Managing the Overweight Child 191
Ihuoma Eneli and Karah Daniels Mantinan

10. Parents as the Primary Target for Healthy Eating among Young Children 227
Mildred A. Horodynski, Kami J. Silk, and Michelle Henry

11. Surgical Treatment of Obesity 251
Jeff M. Gauvin

12. Ethical Considerations Related to Obesity Intervention 271
Leonard M. Fleck and Karen A. Petersmarck

About the Editors and Contributors 305

Index 313

SERIES FOREWORD

The twentieth century closed with a decade devoted to the study of brain structure, function, and development that in parallel with studies of the human genome has revealed the extraordinary plasticity of biobehavioral organization and development. The twenty-first century opens with a decade focusing on behavior, but the linkages between brain and behavior are as dynamic as the linkages between parents and children, and children and the environment.

The Child Psychology and Mental Health series is designed to capture much of this dynamic interplay by advocating for strengthening the science of child development and linking that science to issues related to mental health, child care, parenting and public policy.

The series consists of individual monographs, each dealing with a subject that advanced knowledge related to the interplay between normal developmental process and developmental psychopathology. The books are intended to reflect the diverse methodologies and content areas encompassed by an age period ranging from conception to late adolescence. Topics of contemporary interest include studies of socioemotional development, behavioral undercontrol, aggression, attachment disorders and substance abuse.

Investigators involved with prospective longitudinal studies, large epidemiologic cross-sectional samples, intensely followed clinical cases or those wishing to report a systematic sequence of connected experiments are invited to submit manuscripts. Investigators from all fields in social and behavioral sciences, neurobiological sciences, medical and clinical sciences and education are invited to submit manuscripts with implications for child and adolescent mental health. In these volumes, investigators address many of the issues related to the "epidemic" of overweight and obese children in American society. Few topics rival obesity for the scope of systemic concerns about etiology. Genes! Fast foods! Television! Sedentary life! We are quick to place blame for America's obesity epidemic on single causal factors, but the point stressed in these volumes is that obesity, like many childhood disorders, has a multifaceted etiology and will require equally multifaceted solutions.

Hiram E. Fitzgerald
Susanne Ayres Denham
Series Editors

FOREWORD

Obesity has reached epidemic proportions among children and adults in the United States and around the world. Obese children are at high risk of becoming obese adults with all the associated complications of the condition including cardiovascular disease, diabetes, and premature deaths, among others.

Michigan has among the highest rates of adult obesity in the United States with 28.7 percent of the population considered obese and another 64.8 percent who are either obese or overweight. In 2003—as a direct result of this burgeoning epidemic—the Michigan Steps Up campaign was initiated to combat this epidemic, as well as to motivate our state population to adopt a healthier lifestyle in general.

Indeed, obesity reduction was one of the primary goals of our "Healthy Michigan 2010" health status report, which presented a "set of health objectives for the people of Michigan to achieve over the first decade of the new century to help them develop programs to improve health." In this report, we noted that the prevalence rates of diabetes had risen from 58 per 1,000 people in 1997 to 72 by 2001, an increase largely attributable to obesity. We also noted that the majority (53%) of all adults self-reported amounts of leisure time physical activity less than 30 minutes a day for five or more days a week. I am, therefore, delighted with the opportunity to write this foreword for *Obesity in Childhood and Adolescence*.

In this set, experts on obesity from Michigan and across the nation give one of the most comprehensive evidence-based reviews of the current state of knowledge about obesity among children. It is a set that is timely and that can be used by people from all walks of life including the general educated public seeking to be better informed, legislators needing information to guide policies related to obesity in children, or physicians looking to gain a better understanding of the complexities of how to manage the condition.

The authors have done an outstanding job of not only presenting the epidemiology of the disease and addressing traditional areas of concern such as nutrition and exercise, but also exploring other areas of importance in the obesity discussion including variations within different racial and ethnic groups. They have done this while highlighting the possible roles of individuals, communities, and governments in positively or negatively impacting the rates and outcomes of obesity,

They have articulated important concepts previously not fully elaborated on by previous authors on the topic, such as the relationship between the rates of obesity and the extent of obesity and social class. There is a clear delineation on how the built environment in which a person lives, the schools they attend, and their mode of transportation can significantly impact their ability to exercise or have access to nutritious diets and thus their body weight.

The authors also explore what role the media may play in creating a demand for healthy or unhealthy food choices or in portraying specific body images that influence our children and youth. The possible social and academic consequences of obesity are reviewed with associations of academic and financial disadvantages noted among obese children compared to their peers who are not obese. Finally, the authors present the current data on different medical and nonmedical interventions that may impact obesity, their efficacy, and some of the ethical challenges associated with them. Throughout the set, there are clearly identified research questions for the current and next generations of researchers to address to help us better understand how to tackle this growing epidemic.

This is a set that I strongly endorse and believe will help anyone who is truly interested in making a difference in the field—those in the medical profession as well as our policy makers.

Kimberlydawn Wisdom, MD, MS
Surgeon General State of Michigan
Vice President Community Health, Education and Wellness,
Henry Ford Health System

FOREWORD: SPECIAL COMMENTARY ON CHILDHOOD OBESITY

Obesity has dramatically increased in prevalence worldwide during the last half century, becoming an important health threat in developing as well as developed nations. The prevalence of obesity-related diseases, such as hypertension and type 2 diabetes, are rising at rates comparable to that of obesity. The expected direct and indirect cost of obesity-related disease is staggering and soon expected to exceed that of smoking-related morbidity expenditure in the United States. Addressing childhood obesity is particularly important, because most seriously obese adults (more than 100 pounds overweight) have been obese since childhood. Adolescent obesity is a strong precursor of adult obesity and related morbidity. The Institute of Medicine report on Preventing Childhood Obesity (Committee on Progress in Preventing Childhood Obesity, 2005) acknowledges that "a thorough understanding of the causes and determinants of the obesity epidemic is lacking" (p. 129). The term *overweight* is used by the Centers for Disease Control and Prevention for childhood body mass index (BMI) > 95th percentile. This BMI level corresponds to an adult BMI of 30, which is defined as "obese." The terms obese and overweight are used interchangeably in this commentary to refer to childhood BMI > 95th percentile and "risk for overweight" is not addressed. In the United States the prevalence of obesity (BMI > 95th percentile for age and gender) in 15-year-olds was 13.9 percent in boys and 15.1 percent in girls from 1998–1994 (Hedley, Ogden, Johnson, Carroll, Curtin, et al., 2004; Lissau, Overpeck, Ruan, Due, Holstein, et al., 2004). This represents a doubling of the adolescent obesity rate over 30 years. Ethnic disparities in obesity exist, such that African Americans, American Indians, and Hispanic Americans are at increased risk. Consequently, these groups also experience increased metabolic syndrome, type 2 diabetes and cardiovascular disease in adulthood.

Genetic determinants of height and weight act in concert with environmental influences on growth. In the United States, the food environment has changed during the past half century with increased availability of energy dense foods and drinks, larger portions, more marketing of food products, and increased consumption of food away from home. Other environmental changes, including urbanization, also create risks for obesity. Neighborhoods are less walkable and perceived as more dangerous than in the past. While work has become more sedentary and U.S. adults work longer hours, physical activity has decreased and sedentary activities have increased.

Culture—defined as socially transmitted patterns of beliefs, attitudes, and behaviors—may influence the risk for developing obesity. Group norms in eating and activity patterns, which may promote or protect against the development of obesity, are often dictated by culture. Cultural factors are likely to help explain why Hispanic boys and African American girls and women, in the United States, are at increased risk for obesity (Sundquist & Winkleby, 2000). These effects, attributed to race, are strongly influenced by the educational level of the mother (Gordon-Larsen, McMurray, & Popkin, 2000).

During development, sensitive periods are windows of time when an exposure causes a stronger effect than would occur outside of that time period. Infancy, adiposity rebound (when BMI is lowest at around age 5 years), and adolescence have been proposed as sensitive periods for the development of obesity (Dietz, 1994). Both fetal undernutrition and early postnatal malnutrition are associated with increased metabolic syndrome and cardiovascular risk. While there is increasing evidence that metabolic and hormonal systems may up- or down-regulate during fetal life, these systems are likely to be modified by subsequent exposures throughout life. Some studies suggest that very early infant feeding patterns and growth predict adult weight. Many studies have shown that breast feeding is associated with reduced risk for obesity later in life when compared to formula feeding. A recent meta-analysis of 17 studies showed that the duration of breast feeding was inversely associated with the risk of obesity in adolescence and adulthood (Harder, Bergmann, Kallischnigg, & Plagemann, 2005). Even after the nursing period, maternal feeding practices may relate to risk for childhood obesity. Nutrient intake of parents and children are correlated, suggesting that family eating patterns play a role. Portion size has also been associated with food intake in children as young as 5 years (Rolls, Engell, & Birch, 2006). Children who were taught to focus on feelings of hunger and satiety ate less than those who were encouraged to focus on the amount of food remaining on the plate or a reward. In a larger sample, 3- to 5-year-olds better regulated their energy intake if their parents took a less controlling approach to feeding (Birch, 1998).

Participating in regular physical activity helps control weight, builds lean muscle, reduces body fat, and also promotes psychological well-being. In the United States, physical activity decreases during the high school years, particularly for girls (Kimm, Glynn, Obarzanek, Kriska, Daniels, et al., 2005). The principal sedentary leisure time behavior in the United States is television viewing, which is related to obesity in young people. Social determinants of physical activity are clearly important. Lower educational level, minority race in women, low income, social isolation, depression, and low life satisfaction resulted in relative declines in physical activity during adulthood in a multi-decade longitudinal study (Kaplan, Lazarus, Cohen, & Leu, 1991). Parental obesity is associated with lower levels of child physical activity as early as preschool. Similarly, parental physical activity is associated with activity levels in their children and adolescents. Children with two active parents have been shown to have higher activity than those with only one or no physically active parents (Moore, Lombarda, White, Campbell, Oliveria, et al., 1991; DiLorenzo, Stucky-Ropp, Vander Wal, & Gotham, 1998). Adult encouragement and father involvement predict increased physical activity (Biddle & Goudas, 1996; Bungum & Vincent, 1997). Low maternal education is associated with more inactive leisure time (Gordon-Larsen, McMurray, & Popkin, 2000).

Many cross-sectional studies have focused on the relationship between psychological characteristics of youth and self-reported physical activity. Teen depression is associated with more sedentary leisure time. Living in a neighborhood with high crime is associated with lower physical activity in teens. Minority youth engage in less moderate to vigorous physical activity and are half as likely to participate in daily school physical education compared to whites. A recent study, found that this racial disparity was explained largely by school of attendance (Richmond, Hayward, Gahagan, & Heisler, 2006). Minority students who attended predominantly white schools were more likely to be physically active than those who attended predominantly minority schools. School of attendance could represent the school environment, neighborhood environment, or both; average household income by school was also associated with minority attendance.

Sleep is believed to play an important role in energy balance. In rodents total sleep deprivation leads to hyperphagia. Some studies show that human adults who sleep less are more likely to be overweight or obese compared to those with higher levels of sleep. According to self report, sleep duration for adults in the United States has decreased by 1 to 2 hours during the past 40 years. More than one third of young adults report sleeping fewer than 7 hours per night, double the proportion reported in 1960 (National Sleep Foundation, 2002). A small randomized 2-period, 2-condition crossover trial in young, healthy, lean men found that short sleep duration was associated with increased hunger, appetite, and ghrelin levels and decreased leptin levels, even when calories were delivered by intravenous infusion and exactly equivalent (Van der Lely, Tschop, Heiman, & Ghigo, 2004; Muccioli, Tschop, Papotti, Deghenghi, Heiman, et al., 2002).

Fitness and fatness are both related to risk for metabolic syndrome and cardiovascular disease. Randomized controlled trials in children show that even small changes in physical activity can improve body composition, fitness, and insulin levels (Nemet, Barkan, Epstein, Friedland, Kowen, et al., 2005) and, when combined with good nutrition, improve lipid levels as well (Jones & Campbell, 2004). Regular moderate to vigorous physical activity appears to explain decreased risk for obesity in some groups of adolescents. Reduction of sedentary behaviors can also result in significant reductions in BMI (Epstein, Paluch, Kilanowski, & Raynor, 2004).

There is an epidemic, but we don't have cost-effective prevention or treatment strategies yet. Healthcare professionals and others who interact with children can help to educate families about nutrition with a focus on what to eat (grains, fruits, and vegetables) and what to limit (fats, and low-nutrition, high-caloric foods and drinks) from the time that infants begin eating infant foods at six months. Professionals can encourage families to allow their children to take breaks from eating and drinking. It is not necessary to always have a drink or snack in hand. Equally important is a focus on physical activity. Developing strategies that work for families in each community is critical. Parental nutrition and physical activity may be equally important as they predict the child's current and future caloric intake and physical activity. Making sure that primary care physicians monitor BMI and growth velocity will improve early identification and intervention strategies. Advocacy should be for more: (1) physical education (PE) in schools and more active time while in PE; (2) sports for *all* kids even those who are not destined to be elite athletes; (3) safe neighborhoods for walking to school; and (4) places for safe active recreation. While the "cure" for obesity in children is not yet evident, accurate information about physical activity and healthy eating can point children, families, and communities toward healthier weight and fitness.

Sheila Gahagan, M.D. M.P.H.
President, Michigan Chapter—American Academy of Pediatrics

REFERENCES

Biddle, S. & Goudas, M. (1996). Analysis of children's physical activity and its association with adult encouragement and social cognitive variables. *Journal of School Health, 66,* 75–78.

Birch, L. L. (1998). Psychological influences on the childhood diet. *Journal of Nutrition, 128,* 407S–410S.

Bungum, T. J. & Vincent, M. L. (1997). Determinants of physical activity among female adolescents. *American Journal of Preventive Medicine, 13,* 115–122.

Committee on Progress in Preventing Childhood Obesity. (2005). Institute of Medicine Regional Symposium. *Progress in preventing childhood obesity: Focus on schools.* Washington DC: The National Academies Press.

Dietz, W. H. (1994). Critical Periods in childhood for the development of obesity. *American Journal of Clinical Nutrition, 59,* 955–959.

DiLorenzo, T. M., Stucky-Ropp, R. C., Vander Wal, J. S., & Gotham, H. J. (1998). Determinants of exercise among children, II: A longitudinal analysis. *Preventive Medicine,27*(3), 470–477.

Epstein, L. H., Paluch, R. A., Kilanowski, C. K., & Raynor, H. A. (2004). The effect of reinforcement or stimulus control to reduce sedentary behavior in the treatment of pediatric obesity. *Health Psychology, 23,* 371–380.

Gordon-Larsen, P., McMurray, R. G., & Popkin, B. M. (2000). Determinants of adolescent physical activity and inactivity patterns. *Pediatrics, 105*(6), E83.

Harder, T., Bergmann, R., Kallischnigg, G., & Plagemann, A. (2005). Duration of breastfeeding and risk of overweight: a meta-analysis. *American Journal of Epidemiology, 162,* 397–403.

Hedley, A. A., Ogden, C. L., Johnson, C. L., Carroll, M. D., Curtin, L. R., & Flegal, K. M. (2004). Prevalence of overweight and obesity among U.S. children, adolescents, and adults, 1999–2002. *Journal of the American Medical Association, 291,* 2847–2850.

Jones, A.M. & Campbell, I. G. (2004). Lipid-lipoproteins in children: An exercise dose-response study. *Medicine & Science in Sports & Exercise, 36*(3), 418–427.

Kaplan, G. A., Lazarus, N. B., Cohen, R. D., & Leu, D. J. (1991). Psychosocial factors in the natural history of physical activity. *American Journal of Preventive Medicine, 7,* 12–17.

Kimm, S. Y., Glynn, N. W., Obarzanek, E., Kriska, A. M., Daniels, S. R., Barton, B. A., et al. (2005). Relation between the changes in physical activity and body-mass index during adolescence: A multicentre longitudinal study. *Lancet,366*(9482), 301–307.

Lissau, I., Overpeck, M. D., Ruan, W. J., Due, P., Holstein, B. E., & Hediger, M. L. (2004). Health behaviour in school-aged children obesity working group. Body mass index and overweight in adolescents in 13 European countries, Israel, and the United States. *Archives of Pediatrics & Adolescent Medicine, 158*, 27–33.

Moore, L. L., Lombarda, D. A., White, M. J., Campbell, J. L., Oliveria, S. A., & Ellison, R. C. (1991). Influence of parents' physical activity levels on activity levels of young children. *Journal of Pediatrics, 118*, 215–219.

Muccioli, G., Tschop, M., Papotti, M., Deghenghi, R., Heiman, M., & Ghigo, E. (2002). Neuroendocrine and peripheral activities of ghrelin: implications in metabolism and obesity. *European Journal of Pharmacology, 440*, 235–254.

National Sleep Foundation. (2002). "Sleep in America" poll. Washington, DC: National Sleep Foundation.

Nemet, D., Barkan, S., Epstein, Y., Friedland, O., Kowen, G., & Eliakim, A. (2005). Short- and long-term beneficial effects of a combined dietary-behavioral-physical activity intervention for the treatment of childhood obesity. *Pediatrics,115*, e443–449.

Richmond, T. K., Hayward, R. A., Gahagan, S., & Heisler, M. (2006). Can school income and racial composition explain the ethnic disparity in adolescent physical activity participation? *Pediatrics, 17*, 2158–2166.

Rolls, B. J., Engell, D., & Birch, L. L. (2006). Serving portion size influences 5-year-old but not 3-year-old children's food intakes. *Journal of the American Dietetic Association, 100*(2), 232–234.

Sundquist, J., & Winkleby, M. (2000). Country of birth, acculturation status and abdominal obesity in a national sample of Mexican-American women and men. *International Journal of Epidemiology,29*(3), 470–477.

Van der Lely, A. J., Tschop, M., Heiman, M. L., & Ghigo, E. (2004). Biological, physiological, pathophysiological, and pharmacological aspects of ghrelin. *Endocrine Reviews,25*, 426–457.

PREFACE

Obesity is now widely acknowledged as the number one public health threat to the health of Americans. Childhood obesity has increased dramatically during the past generation, with significant increases in prevalence rates during the past decade. Obesity has clear linkages to mental health. Obesity rates are higher among children with behavior problems, depression, and who live in chronic stress related to poverty and under-stimulating environments. Moreover, there is strong evidence for continuity when factors contributing to obesity provide maintenance structures. For example, obese adolescents are 15 times more likely to be obese when adults than are adolescents who are not obese. The significance of the problem is clear: 15 percent of all children in the United States are obese.

Although there are clear health disparities, the rise in obesity cuts across all age groups, both genders, and all cultural and racial groups. Lack of physical activity and poor nutritional habits are the leading causes of the rise in obesity. Contributing to these two causes are a myriad of factors including genetics, the built environment in which increasing numbers of Americans are living, lack of access to nutritious food choices, more eating out behavior with supersized portions and higher fat content, the ubiquitous influence of the media on eating habits and choices, and sedentary lifestyles associated with the rise in proportion of time spent watching television, playing video games, and surfing the Internet.

There are clear adverse consequences to the increasing rates of obesity. Rising rates of hypertension, type 2 diabetes, and hypercholesterolemia have all been associated with obesity and obesity is an independent risk factor for cardiovascular disease. Obese children are more likely to be victims of low self-esteem and bullying targets. Recent studies suggest that obesity causes a reduction in life span of about nine months. There are major personal and societal financial costs to obesity as well, with the World Bank estimating that obesity and related complications are responsible for 12 percent of the American health care costs.

This two-volume set presents to the public the problem of obesity, the consequences of obesity in American society, as well as the potential primary, secondary, and tertiary preventative practices available to limit its impact. We hope that this book will be a strong tool for advocating for strong personal and public health practices within local communities, legislatures, and health care settings, and for policy makers in general. We have tried to connect the dots for the readers in terms of the multidimensional complex nature of obesity in America. For example, a poor teenaged African American male living in a dangerous part of a metropolitan city who is overweight has very different challenges to his white male counterpart living in a more suburban part of the same city and will need very different counseling and intervention in order to reduce weight. For the poor urban teenager, the simple advice of "you need to exercise more and eat more nutritious meals" is complicated by the lack of access to any green spaces, and immediate access to proper nutritious foods. Even walking outside one's home could be a dangerous activity wrought with crossing paths with gangs and dealers. Eating more vegetables is complicated by the lack of immediate access to supermarkets, as well as a possible lack of access to a motorized vehicle. Oftentimes the only consistent source of nutrition in poor urban neighborhoods is a local corner store that primarily sells processed foods.

Obesity, therefore, has multiple determinants stemming from genetic inheritance to a range of environment influences, including behavioral dysregulation, familial cultural practices, media influences, built and stressful environments, and poor nutritional choices. The study of obesity as well as programs designed to prevent or interfere with the development of obesity in children require multidisciplinary perspectives.

In these two volumes, the chapters reflect the disciplines of epidemiology, genetics, geography, environmental science, nutrition, landscape architecture, clinical and developmental psychology, pediatrics, kinesiology, anthropology, family science, nursing, communications, advertising, community health, and surgery, scanning the full range of issues related to child and adolescent obesity. The life-span approach gives perspective to both the long-term effects of early overweight and obesity, as well as familial contributors to its etiology.

H. Dele Davies
Hiram E. Fitzgerald
Editors

Part I

SOCIAL AND BEHAVIORAL DEVELOPMENT

Chapter 1

RISK FACTORS FOR OBESITY IN EARLY HUMAN DEVELOPMENT

John Worobey

In a study that appeared over 30 years ago, Charney and his colleagues (1976) posed the tongue-in-cheek question, "Do chubby infants become obese adults?" At a time when the incidence of adult obesity may have been of little concern to anyone besides those directly affected, they found that 36 percent of infants who exceeded the 90th percentile became overweight adults (relative to only 14 percent who were of light- or average-weight). These results raised few eyebrows back then. Today, however, with obesity levels having reached epidemic—indeed, some would say pandemic—proportions, an examination of the early antecedents of obesity certainly warrants a closer inspection. As with adult and even child obesity, the determinants are many. From this perspective, recent research on overweight in infancy as well as correlates of excessive weight gain that are traceable to the first postpartum years make an analysis of how factors in early development contribute to later obesity extremely worthwhile. The purpose of this chapter is to identify and describe the risk factors that may serve to predict obesity. While some factors may be immutable, others may be seen as being within familial or societal control, and may spur future research and intervention efforts that can help to slow, if not reverse, what may be *the* public health problem of the twenty-first century.

The author wishes to thank Isabel Martin for her assistance in identifying some of the recent research articles described herein.

THE PROBLEM

Current estimates place the number of obese individuals at more than a billion worldwide. Obesity in adults is often determined using a mathematical proxy, that is, body mass index or BMI, which is computed using the formula: weight in kilograms divided by the square of height in meters. Normal weight is defined as a BMI of approximately 19–24, with overweight being any number above 25. Such a criterion score is inappropriate for children, however, whose BMIs run much lower. Indeed, the Centers for Disease Control and Prevention (CDC) have sex-specific, percentile-based growth charts for plotting BMI by age in children ages 2–20 (http://www.cdc.gov/growthcharts). Under these guidelines, a BMI for age at or above the 85th percentile places a child at risk for overweight, and a BMI for age at or above the 95th percentile indicates a child who *is* overweight. With infants under age two, length- and weight-for-age charts are used with similar percentile cutoffs.

While the health risks for adults are well-documented, numerous, and will engender sizeable health care costs, the incidence of overweight in children is no less serious a concern, since as many as one-third of children in the United States are presently affected, with European estimates not far below this amount (Livingstone, 2001). Among 6 to 11 year-olds, the most recent prevalence estimate for overweight children in the United States is around 19 percent, with a similar estimate reported for low-income children ages two to four (Ogden et al., 2002; Sherry et al., 2004). The prevalence of overweight in the United States for low-income Hispanic children younger than age five is significantly higher than for non-Hispanic blacks, which in turn is higher than for non-Hispanic whites (Mei et al., 1998). From the mid-1980s to mid-1990s, non-Hispanic black children had the largest absolute increase in prevalence of overweight among two- to five-year-olds, while low-income non-Hispanic white infants less than two years of age had the largest absolute increase in prevalence of overweight. Though not nationally representative, a recent study based on 22 years of records from a Massachusetts health maintenance organization reported that the percentage of infants under six-months who were overweight or at risk for overweight increased from approximately 10 percent in 1980–1981 to 17 percent in 2000–2001, with Hispanic greater than black, who in turn were greater than white infants in prevalence as well as relative increase in overweight (Kimm et al., 2006). Such trends for infants strongly argue for increased attention to the factors that may contribute to excess weight gain in early human development.

THE ENERGY BALANCE EQUATION

Differential patterns of infant obesity by race and ethnicity are informative, but merely descriptive. To understand why more infants may be growing at a faster rate than ever before, it is necessary to examine the causal mechanisms that may be contributing to this phenomenon. As in childhood, obesity in infancy is ostensibly due to a variety of complex factors. For example, genetic predisposition, excessive feeding, low activity, poor intake regulation, maternal attitudes toward feeding, and mother-infant interactions have all been mentioned as likely antecedents of infant obesity. Indeed, even feeding on demand has been reported as promoting weight gain (Saxon & Gollipalli, 2000). Aside from this array of factors, however, excessive weight gain in infancy may be explained by a rather straightforward mechanism, that is, the principle of energy balance. To put it simply, weight gain in humans results from an extended period wherein energy intake exceeds energy expenditure (Goran et al., 1999). Applying this principle to early development, for an infant to become overweight, either excessive energy intake, reduced energy expenditure, or both of these phenomena must occur.

In an oft-cited study, Roberts and her colleagues (1988) examined the energy balance equation in 18 infants—6 born to lean mothers and 12 infants to obese mothers—tracking the babies from birth through one year. No advice concerning infant diets was given to the mothers, nor were they told that their own body weights had determined their eligibility for the study. At three and six months the mothers kept a 24-hour record of all the food and drink consumed by their infants. Also at three months, infants' energy expenditure was measured over a period of seven days using the doubly labeled water method (DLW). (DLW is a well-validated technique for estimating energy expenditure in infants, by measuring the disappearance rates of non-toxic isotopes of water). Standard anthropometric measures were made on the infants at 3 days, and 3, 6, 9, and 12 months. By 12 months, 6 of the 12 infants born to obese mothers became overweight (or, in other words, above the 90 percentile of weight for length), while none of the infants born to lean mothers did so. Despite equivalence across groups in terms of metabolizable energy intake, the six infants who became overweight consumed 42 percent more energy at six months than the 12 infants who remained lean (Roberts, 1991). However, these six infants also had reduced total energy expenditure at three months of age, as measured with the DLW procedure. This finding led the authors to argue that energy spent on activity played a more important role in the development of infant obesity than energy intake, but was not the last word.

One study, for example, found that energy intake at 6 months predicted body fatness at 12 months (Dewey et al., 1993). However, others have reported that energy intake at three months is not an important determinant of body fatness at two years (Wells et al., 1998). A number of subsequent investigations have attempted to replicate the Roberts study with larger samples. Surprisingly, none have shown an association between energy expenditure via the DLW in three-month-old infants and later fat mass (Wells et al., 1996). As neither of those studies included overweight mothers, the findings of Roberts may point to a regulatory system in infants that may be differentially expressed depending on inherited genetic susceptibility.

In a study similar to Roberts that used the DLW method with infants born to 40 obese mothers and 38 lean mothers, Stunkard and his research team (1999) reported that energy intake at 3 months accounted for 8 percent of the variability in five measures of body size and composition at 12 months. However, they failed to demonstrate an association between total and sleeping energy expenditure in 3-month-old infants and their measures of body size at 12 months, regardless of maternal BMI. Hence, in their interpretation, energy intake was actually found to be more important than energy expenditure. Quite emphatically, they concluded that energy intake predicted weight, weight-for-length, body fat, fat-free mass, and skin fold thickness at 12-months; and that neither energy expenditure nor maternal obesity predicted any of these measures.

The energy balance equation may therefore be useful in theory to explain excess weight gain, but is too simplistic to capture the complex interactions between feeding, activity, and the variety of behavioral and psychosocial factors that relate to overweight in infancy. In the following sections the factors that have been suggested, validated, or even dismissed as contributors to infant overweight will be addressed. As will be seen, despite the limited age span for the period in question, the correlates of early weight gain are many and in some ways inextricably linked. Their definitive role in later obesity is even less certain, but may provide the earliest clues to the phenomenon of overweight and thus merit our attention.

AN ECOLOGICAL MODEL OF INFANT EXCESS WEIGHT GAIN

As just seen, the simplistic model of energy intake versus energy expenditure falls short in explaining infant weight gain and early obesity. While both are necessary to the equation, they must be examined simultaneously but with consideration of other factors, as their interaction and measurable levels depend on variables that go well beyond amount of milk and movement. The human ecology model of psychologist Urie Bronfenbrenner (1979) suggests that early development can be best understood by considering the infant in context—of caregiver, of family, of community—and the condition of overweight lends itself well to this approach. The *microsystem* views the infant as an active partner with the caregiver; the *mesosystem* places the caregiver-infant interaction in the context of the home and extended family; the *exosytem* adds the impact of the mother's workplace, for example; and the *macrosystem* may be defined as the culture in which the preceding systems operate. Using this framework, the recently formulated concept of the *obesigenic* environment, where highly palatable foods are readily and cheaply available may be construed as a macrosystemic influence on excess energy intake. The obesigenic environment will be further discussed later in this chapter. For present purposes and ease of explication, the myriad factors that contribute to early weight gain will be addressed under the headings of infant, maternal, and environmental, but the reader is reminded that they assuredly interact within this ecological perspective.

INFANT FACTORS: THE INFANT IN THE MICROSYSTEM

Birth Weight and Later BMI

As the individual's own biology is considered to be part of the microsystem, it may be useful to start with the infant's contribution to his or her weight trajectory. Some two dozen studies have addressed the association between birth weight and BMI in childhood or adulthood, with nearly all reporting a direct association, that is, that higher birth weight is associated with higher attained BMI. Some studies have found no association, but none have found an inverse association. As Oken and Gillman (2003) note in their review of this work, however, most of these studies suffer from the limitations of incomplete or missing data on gestational age, birth length, parental BMI, socioeconomic factors, and cigarette smoking—the last important because of its association with prematurity.

Interestingly enough, a number of studies have demonstrated that *reduced* size at birth is also related to later measures of fatness (e.g., Loos et al., 2002). That is, low-birth-weight is inversely associated with insulin resistance, the metabolic syndrome, and central adiposity, suggesting a

U-shaped relationship between birth weight and later BMI, as well as with other comorbidities such as type 2 diabetes. An emerging literature on the fetal origins of adult diseases suggests that the quality of the intra-uterine environment may serve to program the developing human, with fetal insulin hypersecretion, for example, resulting from diabetes during pregnancy (Barker, 1998). With large infants at risk for eventual obesity and type 2 diabetes, and small infants at risk for higher central adiposity, insulin resistance, and metabolic syndrome, it is hypothesized that insulin may mediate both these outcomes (Oken & Gillman, 2003). The mother's weight, nutrition, and health status during pregnancy are obviously impor-tant in determining birth weight, and will be further examined under a subsequent heading.

Rapid Growth and Later BMI

There is also evidence that the rate of infant growth may directly bear on childhood obesity. A recent review identified ten studies that assessed the relation between infant growth and subsequent obesity (Baird et al., 2006). Seven of them found more rapid growth in infancy to be associated with greater risk of obesity at ages ranging from 5 to 20 years, with three failing to show a relationship. Stettler and his associates (2002), for exam-ple, in a cohort of nearly 20,000 seven-year-old children with BMIs above the 95th percentile born from 1985 to 1990, reported an adjusted odds ratio of 1.17 for those who exhibited rapid weight gain from birth to four months. More recently, Dennison and colleagues (2006) reported that the rate of weight gain during the first six months of life was associated with a significantly increased risk of overweight at four years, in a 1999 to 2000 multiethnic cohort of WIC children. (WIC is the Special Supplemental Nutrition Program for Women, Infants and Children, funded by Congress to promote and ensure good nutrition in early development.)

Temperament and Early Weight Gain

Apart from birth weight and its rate of increase over the first postpartum months, the infant's *temperament* has also been hypothesized as a contrib-uting factor to overweight in the early years. For instance, activity level, an element of behavioral style, is believed to be inborn and is observable from birth (Groome et al., 1999). A dimension of many temperament frameworks (e.g., Rothbart, 1981; Thomas et al., 1968), it is generally considered to be the dimension that shows the greatest continuity from infancy through childhood (Hubert et al., 1982). Research has provided some support for its being a useful proxy for energy expenditure, as activity level has been inversely related to weight gain in infants. In an early report, Rose and Mayer (1968) showed that both qualitative and quantitative assessments of activity (as measured by actometers) were better predictors of body size at five months than was caloric intake. Mack and Kleinhenz (1974) also used actometers in a small sample of infants at high risk for obesity given their obese mothers and low-income status. They found that over the first two months of life, the two least active of their five infants stayed the least active, consumed the most calories, and gained weight faster than the other three infants did. In contrast, some have found no consistent associations between the energy intake, weight, or ratings of activity level of breast-fed infants over the first year. But with infants who had been formula-fed, Li and colleagues (1995) showed that percentage of body fat was inversely related to infant activity level (as scored by observers), and the correlations became stronger with increasing age.

A difficult infant is defined as fussing, crying, or exhibiting general irritability. DeVries (1984) made the observation that difficult Masai infants had higher survival rates than their easier peers under famine conditions in Africa, presumably because they were likelier to make their needs known. Finding that infants who gained the most weight from 6 to 12 months were also perceived by their mothers as more difficult, Carey (1985) suggested that such infants might have been fed more often in order to quiet them. From an easy perspective, it has been reported that infants rated by their mothers as easier to soothe at 12 weeks were leaner and displayed more activity when seen again at two-and-a-half years (Wells et al., 1997). This author found that mothers' perceptions of higher difficulty were correlated with higher weight in 3-month-old infants, although the association held only for males, who interestingly enough were rated less difficult than the females (Worobey, 2001). Conversely, activity was negatively correlated with weight for the female infants, who were rated as less active than the males. It was more recently reported that temperament as a whole related significantly to weight gain by 8-week-old infants, explaining 11 percent of the variance (Darlington & Wright, 2006). Specifically, rapid weight gain was related to higher scores on distress to limitations, a temperament dimension reflecting irritability in response to everyday situations like waiting for food or being dressed. These reports are intriguing, but in none of these investigations was maternal feeding behavior actually observed. Rather, the researchers relied on the inference that difficulty might be eliciting more feeding, supporting their hypotheses with statistical correlations between maternal ratings of difficulty and infant weight.

Using diary records of feeding, crying, and sleeping with a cohort of 60 low-income minority mother-infant pairs, Worobey and Islas (2004) have presented some preliminary data that suggests that this process may actually be at work. That is, formula-feeding mothers who perceived their infants as more difficult at one month reported one more feeding per day on the average at three months. In turn, perceptions of difficulty at three months predicted the number of feeds at six months, and the number of feeds at both three and six months correlated with infant weight gain from three to six months. Not incidentally, over half of the infants at six months in this study were at or above the 85th percentile of weight for age by sex.

MATERNAL FACTORS: THE CAREGIVER IN THE MICROSYSTEM

Maternal BMI and Infant Overweight

Recent research has shown that maternal concurrent obesity is more highly correlated with childhood obesity than factors such as infant birth weight (Frisancho, 2000). However, this may reflect the mother's post-pregnancy weight gain concomitant with her child's postpartum growth. Maternal prepregnancy obesity may be a more reliable indicator of the mother's impact on her child's overweight status, as this would represent both shared genes and shared prenatal and postnatal environmental factors within families. Over 30 years ago, it was first reported that mothers of obese children tended to be obese before their pregnancy (Fisch et al., 1975). More recently, Baker and colleagues (2004) found that maternal prepregnant BMI was strongly associated with infant birth weight and infant weight gain from birth to one year. Compared with infants of normal weight women, infants of women with a BMI above 30 were generally born heavier and over the first year grew an average of 135 grams more.

It is worth noting that a number of studies find maternal overweight and obesity to interact with breastfeeding as a choice as well as with its duration. Women who are overweight or obese prior to becoming pregnant are less likely to initiate breastfeeding and discontinue it earlier than do normal weight women (Donath & Amir, 2000). Using data on more than 120,000 mother-infant pairs from the from the Pediatric Nutrition Surveillance System and the Pregnancy Nutrition Surveillance System, Li and associates (2003) recently found that regardless of gestational weight gain, women who were obese before pregnancy were less likely to initiate breastfeeding than were women with a normal BMI before pregnancy.

Furthermore, women who were obese before pregnancy and chose to breastfeed, breastfed their infants approximately two weeks less than the normal weight comparison mothers. This pattern is not inconsequential, given some evidence that prepregnant maternal obesity and a lack of breastfeeding may act in combination to increase the risk of childhood overweight (Li et al., 2005). As discussed next, however, maternal feeding method has been investigated in and of itself as to its role in early weight gain.

Feeding Method and Subsequent Fatness

Breastfeeding is the preferred method for feeding infants, recommended by pediatricians and dietitians, and increasing its prevalence is one of the stated goals of Healthy People 2010. Breastfeeding has been shown to reduce the incidence of gastrointestinal, respiratory, and ear infections, as well as allergies, diarrhea, and bacteria meningitis. Numerous studies also indicate its association with reduced risk of type 2 diabetes (Owen et al., 2006). However, in a review of the literature prior to the year 2000, Parsons and colleagues (1999) concluded that no consistent pattern emerged as to a relationship between mode of infant feeding or duration of breastfeeding and later risk of obesity. For example, of the six studies that investigated breast versus formula feeding, four found no influence on fatness at two to seven years, and one found a small but significant association between breastfeeding and fatness in 32-year-old men. The sixth reported that formula feeding, breastfeeding, or *neither* was associated with greater fatness at two years, depending on the specific outcome variable examined (Heinig et al., 1993). The conclusions for the work on duration of breastfeeding, while based on six other studies, showed remarkably similar results, as one study indicated longer breastfeeding to be associated with less risk of obesity in early childhood, one indicated the reverse association, and four indicated no relationship. Since that review, and likely due to the increased interest in scrutinizing all possible factors that may be contributing to the obesity crisis, a number of investigations have re-opened the question of feeding method.

In a study that garnered much attention, von Kries and colleagues (1999) examined the impact of breastfeeding on the risk of children being overweight. With a sample of 9,357 children aged 5–6 years participating in a health examination at the time of school entry in Bavaria, parental responses to a questionnaire assessing early feeding, diet, and lifestyle factors were analyzed based on never breastfeeding or its duration if breastfeeding. The prevalence of what they termed obesity in children

(BMI > 97th percentile) was 4.5 percent as compared to 2.8 percent in breastfed children. Moreover, a dose response effect for duration of breastfeeding was apparent, as the prevalence rates for 2, 3–5, 6–12, and more than 12 months of exclusive breastfeeding were 3.8 percent, 2.3 percent, 1.7 percent, and 0.8 percent respectively. Similarly, Gillman et al. (2001), using data on 14,297 9- to 14-year-olds participating in the Growing Up Today Study, a U.S. nationwide cohort study of diet, activity, and growth, found that infants who were fed breast milk more than infant formula, or who were breastfed for longer periods, had a lower risk of being overweight when reaching childhood or adolescence.

Although at first glance these two studies, with relatively large sample sizes, make a persuasive case for breastfeeding as a deterrent to later obesity, the limitations of these investigations must be acknowledged. The primary criticism is the reliance on retrospective reports of the duration of breastfeeding or its proportionate use when formula was also fed to the infants. When their target children were five or six years old, or even older, mothers were asked to recall not only the number of months they had breastfed this child, but to estimate the ratio of breast milk feeds to formula feeds. While some mothers may have kept baby diaries they could have consulted, the Bavarian mothers, for example, were asked to recall this information on the spot and could have had fuzzy recollections, especially if they had other children. Hediger et al. (2001) confined their sample to three- to five-year-olds, which at least reduced the temporal distance from infancy for the feeding information the mothers had to recall. Interestingly, with the 2,685 children they drew from the National Health and Nutrition Examination Survey III, they found a reduced risk of being *at risk* for overweight for children ever breastfed as infants, but no reduced risk for being overweight.

A more recent exhaustive review of mostly European studies, published since 1966, on the effect of feeding on the risk of obesity across the life course identified 61 reports on this issue, 28 of which provided odds ratio estimates (Owen et al., 2005). In their analysis, breastfeeding was associated with a reduced risk of obesity, compared with formula feeding (odds ratio: 0.87). Sensitive to confounding factors, especially since mothers can not be randomly assigned to breast- versus formula-feeding conditions for experimental purposes, the investigators isolated 6 of the 28 studies that adjusted for parental obesity, maternal smoking, and social class. Following this procedure, the odds ratio was reduced to 0.93. While less impressive, this still suggests that breastfeeding may provide some protection from later obesity, and should encourage public health workers to join their pediatric and dietetics colleagues in endorsing this practice.

THE DYNAMICS OF INFANT FEEDING

Infant Formula and Overfeeding

The question may be posed, if breastfeeding does deter the likelihood of obesity, what may account for this effect? Conceivably, the composition of breast milk may be of influence. While cow's milk-based infant formulas are suitable substitutes for breast milk in terms of ensuring adequate infant growth by virtue of their macronutrient composition and added vitamins, minerals, and (in recent years) some essential fatty acids, there may be bioactive substances in human milk that play a role yet undiscovered. Miralles et al. (2006), for example, recently reported that leptin, a hormone that regulates food intake and metabolism and is present in breast milk, may have a role in the body weight control of developing infants. In their study of 28 normal weight mothers and their infants, moderate amounts of leptin in breast milk at one month seemed to provide moderate protection to the infants from an excess of weight gain through 24 months.

In contrast to a bioactive hypothesis, the results of many reports suggest that overfeeding may be a more apt explanation. A vigorous feeding style, where high-energy intake results, has been correlated with greater adiposity in early childhood—even for breast fed infants (Agras et al., 1987). But overfeeding can likelier occur when infants are formula-fed, where the mother may persist in presenting the bottle in order for the infant to finish what she may perceive as a nutrition expert's recommended amount. The real possibility of overconsumption of calories may induce adipose tissue hyper-cellularity, and the formula-fed infant may self-regulate its energy intake at a higher level, with either process resulting in more body fat. Indeed, formula-fed infants begin to surpass breast-fed infants in terms of weight gain by two to three months (Dewey et al., 1993).

In an effort to bridge the temperament and formula studies described above, the author has conducted some research that assessed motor activity by feeding method in low-risk, non-Hispanic, middle-class white infants (Worobey, 1993; 1998). In an investigation with a convenience sample of three-month-olds, 13 formula-fed infants demonstrated lower arm activity relative to 33 breastfed infants as measured with a custom-built actometer apparatus. In a second study, with a sample of 40 breastfed and 40 formula-fed three-month-old infants carefully matched for weight and sex, total motor activity was lower for the formula-fed infants relative to the breast-fed infants. More research is warranted to replicate these findings, but these results tentatively suggest that formula-feeding may additionally place the developing infant at increased risk for excess weight gain by virtue of reduced activity levels.

Introduction of Solid Foods

Since mothers who formula feed tend to introduce solid foods to their infants sooner than mothers who breastfeed (Worobey, 1992), it has been assumed that this practice may also promote early overweight. Baranowski et al. (1990) cited four studies suggesting that the earlier introduction of solid foods to formula-fed infants promoted more rapid weight gain relative to breastfed infants, but noted four other studies that found no such differences. Their own investigation also found no differences in children who were seen once at about four years of age, and is laudable for including what they termed "Anglo-," Mexican, and African American subjects. In truth, the role of weaning and its timing is, at best, equivocal. For example, Quandt (1986) found that the early introduction of *beikost* led to reduced fatness, while Agras and his colleagues (1990) found that prolonged breastfeeding, coupled with *later* weaning, predicted greater adiposity at three years of age. They posited that earlier weaning might better satiate infants who displayed a vigorous sucking style as newborns, and thereby reduce their appetite. Similarly, others have shown early weaning to be associated with a minor *reduction* in fatness at two-and-a-half years (Wells et al., 1998). These authors suggested that either milk may be better metabolized than baby foods, so weight gain would be slowed, or that weaning reduces infant fussing, so that the infant becomes less demanding. With a sample of merely 20 infants, however, they correctly acknowledged that their provocative hypotheses should be further investigated.

Maternal Control During Feeding

In recent years, a growing literature has identified the possible role of maternal feeding style as a factor in explaining certain risks for childhood obesity. For example, it has been shown that mothers who tend to control their preschool-age daughters' eating by the use of restrictive techniques, have daughters who become less adept at regulating energy intake and tend to be heavier in later childhood (Birch & Fisher, 1998). Little research on this phenomenon exists on mothers of infants. However, Farrow and Blissett (2006) observed 69 women feeding their infants solid foods at six months. Maternal control was scored by rating mothers on a range from one (allowing the infant free autonomy during feeding) to nine (continuously offering, forcing, or positioning the infant to eat). When maternal control was low, infants seemed to regulate their own weight gain across the first year, with those with rapid early weight gain slowing down and those with slow early weight gain accelerating from 6 to 12 months. However, when maternal control at six months was high, infants followed the opposite pattern and maintained consistency in their weight gain. This provocative finding suggests that the relevance of assessing maternal control in child weight gain may indeed extend to infancy.

ENVIRONMENTAL FACTORS: THE MOTHER-INFANT DYAD IN THE MACROSYSTEM

As stated earlier, the macrosystem has been defined as the culture in which the caregiver–infant and other systems operate. As also noted above, demographic differences are apparent when estimating the prevalence of early overweight across income, race, and ethnicity. To recapitulate, early overweight is associated with lower income levels relative to higher, with Hispanic infants greater than black who are greater than white infants in prevalence as well as relative increases in overweight. Low-income mothers often introduce their infants to solid foods earlier than is professionally recommended, stating their belief that a heavy infant is a healthy infant (Baughcum et al., 1998). Although the data do not support this practice as ensuring rapid weight gain, it would nevertheless seem to reflect the mothers' desire for that outcome.

Breastfeeding Patterns by Race and Ethnicity

If breastfeeding is revealed to ward off early obesity, it is worth noting that breastfeeding rates show a direct linear relationship to income levels. Only 32 percent of mothers living below the poverty level, for example, exclusively breastfeed at three months, as compared to 46 percent of mothers at or above 350 percent of the poverty-income ratio (CDC's National Center for Health Statistics, 2005). Breastfeeding rates by race and ethnicity also reflect demographic differences, but they do not cleanly support the pattern shown for early overweight. That is, non-Hispanic white infants are likelier to be ever breastfed than non-Hispanic black infants (approximately 75% vs. 57%, respectively), but Hispanic infants, who by some accounts currently display the highest prevalence of overweight, also boast the highest rate of ever being breastfed at 79 percent

(CDC's National Center for Health Statistics, 2005). This pattern by race and ethnicity also holds for exclusive breastfeeding at three months.

The adding of cereal to infant formula has also been hypothesized as increasing the risk of overnutrition in the first three months of the infant's life. Within the WIC population of low-income mothers, adding other foods to formula does not significantly differ by infant birth order, birth weight, or poverty level, and somewhat surprisingly is more commonly practiced by high school graduates than dropouts (Baydar et al., 1997). However, as with the pattern for formula feeding inferred above, non-Hispanic blacks are likelier to add supplemental foods to formula than non-Hispanic whites, who in turn are likelier to add than Hispanics.

Culture and Maternal Attitudes Toward Infant Weight

As mentioned above, among low-income mothers at least, the fat baby, healthy baby myth—the idea that fatness connotes a happy, healthy infant—would seem to persist. Studies with Mexican-American samples have demonstrated the selection of chubby infants as ideal by mothers of obese preschoolers, relative to mothers of non-obese children (Alexander et al., 1991). However, these attitudes could be a reaction to having raised an obese child. Among mothers of infants, a recent report by Worobey and Lopez (2005) is illuminating. These investigators asked a multi-racial, low-income sample of WIC mothers to indicate where they perceived their one-month-old infants to fall on a pictorial continuum of babies who differed by size, what size they would like their infants to be, and their attitudes toward feeding under different circumstances. Although the Mexican- and other Latino-infants were of average weight when recruited, the mothers in both these sub-groups estimated their infants as leaner, and indicated a fatter infant as desirable, relative to white mothers. They also reported a greater level of pushiness relative to white mothers. Black mothers' estimates were generally in between these groups. The Mexican infants, in particular, were found to be the only sub-group whose weights were above what would have been expected given their reported birth weights, suggesting that their mothers may have been overfeeding them to actually produce a heavier baby.

The Obesigenic Environment of Today

Hill and Peters (1998) have succinctly defined the energy intake aspect of the current obesigenic environment as one that surrounds the consumer with large amounts of readily available, inexpensive, palatable, and energy-dense foods. In such an environment, all individuals would appear to be at risk. To see that our youngest citizens are no exception, one need only consider some of the results of the recent report sponsored by the Gerber baby food company. The Feeding Infants and Toddlers Study [FITS] (2004) was commissioned by Gerber in response to the growing epidemic of childhood obesity, in order to better understand the eating habits of America's infants. Single day dietary recalls were completed by parents or primary caregivers of 3,022 infants and toddlers between 4- and 24-months of age. The predominantly middle-class sample was stratified by race and ethnicity and geography, with the majority of respondents offspring identified as white (80%), followed by Hispanic/Latino (12.1%) and black (7.4%). While the reported energy intakes in FITS, particularly of toddlers, were higher than the recommended estimated energy requirements (EER), what stands out as particularly noteworthy is the degree to which the diets of infants are already mimicking those of their parents. For example, at 7–8 months, approximately 24 of the infants did not consume any fruit, and approximately 33 percent consumed no vegetables. More sobering, perhaps, were the findings that approximately 46 percent of 7–8-month-olds were consuming some type of sugary dessert, and that by 15–18-months, French fries were the most common vegetable.

As the obesity crisis has garnered increased attention, much has also been made of the apparent reduction in physical activity by children and adults, whether due to the elimination of physical education classes, more and more sedentary jobs, or a reliance on automobiles instead of walking to our destinations. The obesigenic environment undoubtedly includes an energy expenditure side. Leisure time pursuits, such as video games, surfing the Internet, or watching television have come under fire as further promoting sedentary behavior. Although the importance of motor activity in infants as a buffer against excess weight gain remains to be quantified, patterns of inactivity, much like patterns of eating, may nevertheless be established through parental modeling or negligence. In this vein, the present author would volunteer an unpublished finding from our current longitudinal investigation of the precursors of excess weight gain. The Rutgers Infant Nutrition and Growth Project has enrolled well over 200 low-income minority infants and mothers to date, and in conducting home visits to observe feedings, interview mothers, and measure the infants for growth and activity level, we make notes on the home environment from an infant-friendly perspective. Of the 240 home visits our staff has conducted since the study's inception, the television has been on at our arrival, most often with the infant placed on the floor in an infant seat facing the screen, a remarkable 238 times. This is anecdotal data, to be sure, but nonetheless good evidence that infancy is not too young an age to examine for factors contributing to childhood overweight.

CONCLUSION

The present chapter has summarized recent research on the factors in infancy that may bear on early overweight and later obesity. Two conclusions should now be obvious. First, the determinants of overweight and obesity are many, with some that may have direct effects but most acting in combination. The list of suspected factors in infancy is no shorter in length, but because of the malleable nature of the human organism, may have at best, only a tenuous relationship to child overweight, let alone adult obesity. This leads us to the second conclusion. Obesity tracks more certainly from adolescence to adulthood, with weaker associations from childhood to adolescence, and weaker still when linking from infancy. However, recent data strongly suggests that being overweight as early as toddler-hood may predict overweight some 10 years later. Growth data from the National Institute of Child Health and Human Development Early Care Research Network indicate that children who were ever categorized as overweight (defined as BMI above 85th percentile) just once at 24, 36, or 54 months were more than five times as likely to be overweight at 12 years than those who were under the 85th percentile at all three measurement points (Nader et al., 2006). Indeed, two in five children whose BMIs were over the 50th percentile by three-years-old were overweight at 12-years-old.

From this perspective, an understanding of the myriad factors that relate to early overweight in infants must continue to be explored. In now answering the question, "Do chubby infants become obese adults?", we can say probably not, or at least not necessarily. But 24-month-old toddlers do not suddenly balloon when simply renamed two-year-olds—the foundation is laid in the preceding months. The unsettling conclusion must be that many risk factors for overweight are already apparent in infancy, and their ultimate predictive ability can not yet be gauged. The optimistic slant is that we have identified many of the possible risk factors. How they interact in the world of the developing infant and how we may best provide advice and intervene with caregivers becomes our next challenge.

REFERENCES

Agras, W. S, Kraemer, H. C., Berkowitz, R. I., & Hammer, L. D. (1990). Influence of early feeding style on adiposity at 6 years of age. *Journal of Pediatrics, 116*(5), 805–809.

Agras, W. S, Kraemer, H. C., Berkowitz, R. I., Korner, A. F., & Hammer, L. D. (1987). Does a vigorous feeding style influence early development of adiposity. *Journal of Pediatrics, 110,* 799–804.

Alexander, M. A., Sherman, J. B., & Clark, L. (1991). Obesity in Mexican-American preschool children—A population group at risk. *Public Health Nursing, 8*(1), 53–58.

Baird, J., Fisher, D., Lucas, P., Kleijnen, J., Roberts, H., & Law, C. (2006). Being fat or growing fast: Systematic review of size and growth in infancy and later obesity. *BMJ Online First.* doi:10.1136/bmj.38586.411273.EO.

Baker, J. L., Michaelsen, K. F., Rasmusssen, K. M, & Sorenson, T. I. A. (2004). Maternal prepregnant body mass index, duration of breastfeeding, and timing of complementary food introduction are associated with infant weight gain. *American Journal of Clinical Nutrition, 80,* 1579–1588.

Baranowski, T., Bryan, G. T. Rassin, D. K., Harrison, J. A., & Henske, J. C. (1990). Ethnicity, feeding practices, and childhood adiposity. *Developmental and Behavioral Pediatrics, 11,* 234–239.

Barker, D. (1998). *Mothers, babies and health in later life.* Edinburgh: Harcourt Brace.

Baughcum, A. E., Burklow, K. A., Deeks, C. M., Powers, S. W., & Whitaker, R. C. (1998). Maternal feeding practices and childhood obesity. A focus group study of low-income mothers. *Archives of Pediatrics and Adolescent Medicine, 152*(10), 1010–1014.

Baydar, N., McCann, M., Williams, R., & Vesper, E. (1997). *Final report: WIC infant feeding practices study.* Alexandria, VA: USDA Food and Consumer Service, Office of Analysis and Evaluation.

Birch, L. L., & Fisher, J. O. (1998). Development of eating behaviors among children and adolescents. *Pediatrics, 101,* 539–549.

Bronfenbrenner, U. (1979). *The ecology of human development: Experiments by nature and design.* Cambridge, MA: Harvard University Press.

Carey, W. B. (1985). Temperament and increased weight gain in infants. *Developmental and Behavioral Pediatrics, 6*(3), 128–131.

Centers for Disease Control's National Center for Health Statistics (2005). Breastfeeding: Data and statistics: Breastfeeding practices—Results from the 2005 National Immunization Survey. http://www.cdc.gov/breastfeeding/data/NIS_data/data_2005.htm.

Charney, E., Goodman, H. C., McBride, M., Lyon, B., & Pratt, R. (1976). Childhood antecedents of adult obesity: Do chubby infants become obese adults? *New England Journal of Medicine, 295*(1), 6–9.

Darlington, A. S. E., & Wright, C. M. (2006). Their influence of temperament on weight gain in early infancy. *Developmental and Behavioral Pediatrics, 27*(4), 329–335.

Dennison, B. A. Edmunds, L. S., Stratton, H. H., & Pruzek, R. M. (2006). Rapid infant weight gain predicts childhood overweight. *Obesity, 14*(3), 491–499.

DeVries, M. W. (1984). Temperament and mortality among the Masai of east Africa. *American Journal of Psychiatry, 11*(10), 1189–1194.

Dewey, K. G., Heinig, M. J., Nommsen, L. A., Peerson, J. M., & Lonnerdal, B. (1993). Breast-fed infants are leaner than formula-fed infants at 1-year of age: The DARLING Study. *American Journal of Clinical Nutrition, 57,* 140–145.

Donath, S. M., & Amir, L. H. (2000). Does maternal obesity adversely affect breastfeeding initiation and duration? *Journal of Paediatric Child Health, 36,* 482–486.

Farrow, C., & Blissett, J. (2006). Does maternal control during feeding moderate early weight gain? *Pediatrics, 118*(2), e293–e298.

Feeding Infants and Toddlers Study (2004). *Journal of the American Dietetic Association, 104*(1) (Suppl.1).

Fisch, R. O., Bilek, M. K., & Ulstrom, R. (1975). Obesity and leanness at birth and their relationship to body habitus in later childhood. *Pediatrics, 56,* 521–528.

Frisancho, A. R. (2000). Prenatal compared with parental origins of adolescent fatness. *American Journal of Clinical Nutrition, 72,* 1186–1190.

Gillman, M. W., Rifas-Shiman, S. L., Camargo, C. A., Berkey, C. S., Frazier, A. L., Rockett, H. R. H., Field, A. F., & Colditz, G. A. (2001). Risk of overweight among adolescents who were breastfed as infants. *Journal of American Medical Association, 285*(19), 2461–2467.

Goran, M. I., Reynolds, K. D. & Lindquist, C. H. (1999). Role of physical activity in the prevention of obesity in children. *International Journal of Obesity, 23*(Suppl.), S18–S33.

Groome, L. J., Swiber, M. J., Holland, S. B., Bentz, J. L., Atterbury, J. L., & Trimm, R. F. (1999). Spontaneous motor activity in the perinatal infant before and after birth: Stability of individual differences. *Developmental Psychobiology, 32,* 15–24.

Hediger, M. L., Overpeck, M. D., Kuczmarski, R. J., & Ruan, W. J. (2001). Association between infant breastfeeding and overweight in young children. Risk of overweight among adolescents who were breastfed as infants. *Journal of the American Medical Association, 285*(19), 2453–2460.

Heinig, M. J., Nommsen, L. A., Peerson, J. M., Lonnerdal, B., & Dewey, K. G. (1993). Intake and growth of breast-fed and formula-fed infants in relation to the timing of introduction of complementary foods: The DARLING Study. *Acta Paediatrica, 82,* 999–1006.

Hill, J. O., & Peters, J. C. (1998). Environmental contributions to the obesity epidemic. *Science, 280,* 1371–1374.

Hubert, N. C., Wachs, T. D., Peters-Martin, P., & Gandour, M. (1982). The study of early temperament: Measurement and conceptual issues. *Child Development, 53,* 571–600.

Kimm, J., Peterson, K. E., Sxcanlon, K. S., Fitzmaurice, G. M., Must, A., Oken, E., Rifas-Shiman, S. L., Rich-Edwards, J. W., & Gillmam, M. W. (2006). Trends in overweight from 1980–2001 among preschool-aged children enrolled in a health maintenance organization. *Obesity, 14*(7), 1107–1112.

Li, C., Kaur, H., Choi, W. S., Huang, T. T. K., Lee, R. E, & Ahluwalia, J. S. (2005). Additive interaction of maternal prepregnancy BMI and breastfeeding on childhood overweight. *Obesity Research, 13*(2), 362–371.

Li, R., Jewell, S., & Grummer-Strawn, L. (2003). Maternal obesity and breast-feeding practices. *American Journal of Clinical Nutrition, 77,* 931–936.

Li, R., O'Connor, L., Buckley, D., & Specker, B. (1995). Relation of activity levels to body fat in infants 6 to 12 months of age. *Journal of Pediatrics, 126*(3), 353–357.

Livingstone, M. B. (2001). Childhood obesity in Europe: A growing concern. *Public Health Nutrition, 4,* 109–116.

Loos, R. J., Bennen, G., Fagard, R., Derom, C., & Vlietinck, R. (2002). Birth weight and body composition in young adult women—A prospective twin study. *American Journal of Clinical Nutrition, 75,* 676–682..

Mack, R. W., & Kleinhenz, M. E. (1974). Growth, caloric intake, and activity levels in early infancy: A preliminary report. *Human Biology, 46,* 345–354.

Mei, Z., Scanlon, K. S., Grummer-Strawn, L. M., Freedman, D. S., Yip, R., & Trowbridge, F. L. (1998). Increasing prevalence of overweight among US low-income preschool children: The Centers for Disease Control and Prevention Pediatric Nutrition Surveillance, 1983–1995. *Pediatrics, 101,* www.pediatrics.org/cgi/content/full/101/1/e12.

Miralles, O., Sanchez, J., Palou, A., & Pico, C. (2006). A physiological role of breast milk leptin in body weight control in developing infants. *Obesity, 14*(8), 1371–1377.

Nader, P. R., O'Brien, M., Houts, R., Bradley, R., Belsky, J., Crosnoe, R., Friedman, S., Mei, Z., & Susman, E. J. (2006). Identifying risk for obesity in early childhood. *Pediatrics, 118*(3), e594–e601.

Ogden, C. L., Flegal, K. M., Carroll, M. D., & Johnson, C. L. (2002). Prevalence and trends in overweight among US children and adolescents, 1999–2000. *Journal of the American Medical Association, 288,* 1728–1732.

Oken, E., & Gillman, M. W. (2003). Fetal origins of obesity. *Obesity Research, 11*(4), 496–506.

Owen, C. G., Martin, R. M., Whincup, P. H., Smith, G. D., & Cook, D. G. (2005). Effect of infant feeding on the risk of obesity across the life course: A quantitative review of published evidence. *Pediatrics, 115*(5), 1367–1376.

Owen, C. G., Martin, R. M., Whincup, P. H., Smith, G. D., & Cook, D. G. (2006). Does breastfeeding influence risk of type 2 diabetes in later life? A quantitative analysis of published evidence. *American Journal of Clinical Nutrition, 84,* 1043–1054.

Parsons, T. J., Power, C., Logan, S., & Summerbell, C. D. (1999). Childhood predictors of adult obesity: A systematic review. *International Journal of Obesity, 23* (Suppl. B), S1–S107.

Parsons, T. J., Power C., & Manor, O. (2001). Fetal and early life growth and body mass index from birth to early adulthood in 1958 British cohort: Longitudinal study. *British Medical Journal, 323,* 1331–1335.

Quandt, S. A. (1986). The effect of beikost on the diet of breast fed infants. *Journal of the American Dietetic Association, 84,* 47–51.

Roberts, S. B. (1991). Early diet and obesity. In W. Heird (ed.), *Nutritional needs of the six to twelve month old infant* (vol. 2, pp. 303–316). New York: Raven Press.

Roberts, S. B., Savage, J., Coward, W. A., Chew, B., & Lucas. A. (1988). Energy expenditure and intake in infants born to lean and overweight mothers. *New England Journal of Medicine, 318*(8), 461–466.

Rose, H. E., & Mayer, J. (1968). Activity, caloric intake, fat storage, and the energy balance of infants. *Pediatrics, 41*(1), 18–29.

Rothbart, M. K. (1981). Measurement of temperament in infancy. *Child Development, 52,* 569–578.

Saxon, T. F, & Gollipalli, A. (2000, July). *Feed-on-demand or feed-on-schedule: Infant weight gain from birth to six months.* Paper presented at the International Conference on Infant Studies, Brighton, England.

Sherry, B., Mei, Z., Scanlon, K. S., Mokdad, A. H., & Grummer-Strawn, L. M. (2004). Trends in the state-specific prevalence of overweight and underweight in 2 thru 4 year-old children from low-income families from 1989 through 2000. *Archives of Pediatric and Adolescent Medicine, 158*(12), 1116–1124.

Stettler, N., Zemel, B. S., Kumanyika, S., & Stallings, V. (2002). Infant weight gain and childhood overweight status in a multicenter cohort study. *Pediatrics, 109,* 194–199.

Stunkard, A. J., Berkowitz, R. I., Stallings, V. A., & Schoeller, D. A. (1999). Energy intake, not energy output, is a determinant of body size in infants. *American Journal of Clinical Nutrition, 69,* 524–530.

Thomas, A., Chess, S., & Birch, H. G. (1968). *Temperament and behavior disorders in children.* New York: New York University Press.

von Kries, R., Koletzko, B., Sauerwald, T., von Mutius, E., Barnert, D., Grunert, V., & von Voss, H. (1999). Breast feeding and obesity: Cross sectional study. *British Medical Journal, 319,* 147–150.

Wells, J. C. K., Stanley, M., Laidlaw, A. S., Day, J. M., & Davies, P. S. W. (1996). The relationship between components of infant energy expenditure and childhood body fatness. *International Journal of Obesity, 20,* 848–853.

Wells, J. C. K., Stanley, M., Laidlaw, A. S., Day, J. M., & Davies, P. S. W. (1998). Energy intake in early infancy and childhood fatness. *International Journal of Obesity, 22,* 387–392.

Wells, J. C. K., Stanley, M., Laidlaw, A. S., Day, J. M., Stafford, M., & Davies, P. S. W. (1997). Investigation of the relationship between infant temperament and later body composition. *International Journal of Obesity, 21,* 400–406.

Worobey, J. (1992). Development milestones related to feeding status: Evidence from the Child Health Supplement to the 1981 National Health Interview Survey. *Journal of Human Nutrition and Dietetics, 5*, 363–399.

Worobey, J. (1993). Effects of feeding method on infant temperament. In H. W. Reese (Ed.), *Advances in child development and behavior* (Vol. 24, pp. 37–61). New York: Academic Press.

Worobey, J. (1998). Feeding method and motor activity in 3-month-old human infants. *Perceptual and Motor Skills, 86*, 883–895.

Worobey, J. (2001). Temperamental activity and fussiness: Implications for weight of 3-month-old infants. *Perceptual and Motor Skills, 92*, 1211–1212.

Worobey, J. & Islas, M. (2004, May). *Perceived difficulty and overfeeding in low-income infants: A risk factor for excess weight gain.* Paper presented at the International Conference on Infant Studies, Chicago.

Worobey, J. & Lopez, M. I. (2005). Perceptions and preferences for infant body size by low-income mothers. *Journal of Reproductive and Infant Psychology, 23*(4), 303–308.

Chapter 2

THE ROLE OF PHYSICAL ACTIVITY IN OBESITY PREVENTION

James M. Pivarnik

In 2000, Healthy People 2010 was unveiled as an ambitious program designed to positively impact the health of the citizens residing in the United States. Spearheaded by the Department of Health and Human Services, Healthy People 2010 is the latest of health promotion efforts that began in the last half of the twentieth century. The two main goals of Healthy People 2010 focus on increasing the quality and years of healthy life, and eliminating health disparities in the United States. To help meet the 28 focus areas included in Healthy People 2010, a set of leading health indicators was developed to help measure the health of the nation during the first 10 years of the twenty-first century: physical activity, overweight and obesity, tobacco use, substance abuse, responsible sexual behavior, mental health, injury and violence, environmental quality, immunization, access to health care (United States Department of Health and Human Services [USDHHS], 2001).

The leading health indicators were developed by various agencies within the Department of Health and Human Services, as well as from input from other scientific groups such as the Institute of Medicine and the National Academy of Sciences. The leading health indicators reflect major health concerns in the United States today, and their relationships with the primary chronic diseases that plague our citizens. It is no coincidence that physical activity is first on the list, and overweight/obesity is second. These health indicators were placed at the top of the list due to the fact that (a) they are related to many chronic disease states, and (b) it is believed that, emphasizing the importance of physical activity and weight control in overall health could result in significant health improvements for a large percentage of the population.

It is acknowledged that the obesity epidemic cannot be eliminated completely by claiming that the cause is simply a function of eating too much or exercising too little. There are other, more subtle issues involved, including hormonal imbalances, environmental factors, and genetic factors that have their origins in utero (Eisenmann, 2006). However, it is beyond the scope of this chapter to focus on these multi-component processes that will be discussed in other sections of this book. The purpose of this chapter is to discuss the various factors involved in physical activity as it relates to energy expenditure, and hopefully, weight control and obesity prevention.

WHAT IS THE COST OF PHYSICAL INACTIVITY?

The costs of physical inactivity, both direct and indirect, are considered large, and have been calculated in various ways in the past several years (Chenowith, Hollander, & Bortz, 2006). Using data obtained from the National Library of Medicine, Colditz (1999) estimated that the direct cost of physical inactivity was approximately 24 billion dollars (in 1995 dollars) and represented 2.4 percent of all health care expenditures. Considering the potential effect of physical activity on obesity and obesity-related illnesses, indirect costs were closer to 10 percent of all health care expenditures. Pratt, Macera, and Wang (2000) analyzed the costs of physical inactivity on a per person basis using data from the 1987 National Medical Expenditures Survey. They estimated that average annual direct medical costs for individual adults who performed leisure time physical activity on a regular basis were just over $1,000 per year, compared to over $1,300 for individuals who reported being sedentary. This cost discrepancy was not significantly affected by gender, age, or smoking status. More recently, Pratt, Macera, Sallis, O'Donnell, and Frank (2004) used data from the 1995 National Health Interview Survey and the 1996 Medical Expenditure Panel Survey to determine costs of physical inactivity related to cardiovascular disease in 2001. The authors calculated that over $23 billion of cardiovascular disease related costs were associated with physical inactivity.

Several individual states have also estimated the cost of physical inactivity for their citizens (Chenowith, Hollander, & Bortz, 2006). State health departments can use these data when they lobby legislators for funding directed at physical activity programs, and to evaluate cost effectiveness. For example, in Michigan, the cost of physical inactivity was estimated to be nearly $9 billion in 2002. Moreover, estimates have indicated that if 1 in 20 Michigan adults who were currently sedentary became physically active on a regular basis, the savings could exceed $500 million per year (Chenowith, 2003). Other states have performed similar calculations, and the message is the same (Chenowith et al., 2006). In summary, the costs of practicing a sedentary lifestyle are very high, and comparable to the health care costs associated with smoking.

WHAT IS THE PROBLEM?

Historically, there has been an inverse and strong relationship between the work performed by humans to hunt, gather, or grow food necessary to maintain life, and body size (Prentice, 1998). Except in the case of the few wealthy landowners who paid others to do their work for them, the result was very tight control between energy spent and energy consumed, and little chance for most individuals to gain excess body weight. However, the energy balance equation has shifted with the advent of modern conveniences designed to help reduce manual labor, electronic inventions and gadgets that keep us occupied (and sedentary) in our leisure time, and our ability to produce energy dense foods in mass quantity. The result has been that our technologically advanced society has seen a steady rise in body weight and fatness over the past few decades (Flegal, Carroll, Kuczmarski, & Johnson, 1998). This occurrence, coupled with the eradication of most infectious diseases in industrialized nations, means that chronic disease has become the major health threat. Thus, behavioral lifestyle changes and interventions must occur to counteract the otherwise inevitable gains in body weight that technology and affluence has provided us.

Increased availability of energy dense foods has been particularly problematic, especially when coupled with a lifestyle that includes little naturally occurring physical activity. Studies have shown that humans have limited ability to recognize when energy content of food has been altered (Stubbs, Ritz, Coward, & Prentice, 1995), and they do not decrease intake when feeding ad libitum, or according to desire. Even in laboratory studies where physical activity was tightly regulated, individuals placed under sedentary conditions did not reduce food intake accordingly (Murgatroyd, Goldberg, Leahy, Gilsenan, & Prentice, 1999). In fact, the combination of low physical activity and high caloric diet eaten ad libitum appeared to have a synergistic effect; that is, study volunteers chose to eat more, not less, of the high energy foods compared to those who performed greater amounts of physical activity (Stubbs, Harbron, Murgatroyd, & Prentice, 1995; Stubbs, Ritz, Coward & Prentice, 1995). In summary, cost effective ways to increase daily physical activity and curb excess energy intake must be designed and implemented for the majority of U.S. citizens. Unfortunately, what has occurred is pharmacological, medical, and surgical interventions are implemented in place of more basic and natural strategies designed to help individuals achieve energy balance (Prentice, 1998).

ENERGY BALANCE AND METABOLISM

In its simplest terms, energy balance refers to the body's state when the amount of energy intake equals the amount expended over a given period of time. With energy balance, body weight remains relatively stable over time, allowing for periodic changes in hydration status. Any imbalance in energy stores will mean that over the short or long term, body weight will tend to increase or decrease accordingly. Positive energy balance occurs when intake exceeds output. Muscle and liver glycogen stores are full, and blood glucose is set at an optimal level. Unless there is significant alteration in muscle mass, which occurs as a result of high intensity weight training, most excess energy will be converted to fat and stored in the adipocytes. In contrast, negative energy balance occurs when there is greater expenditure than intake. Metabolic pathways are altered in an effort to maintain glycogen and blood glucose levels as much as possible. Thus, primary fuel oxidation occurs in the fat, and to some extent muscle (protein) stores.

Most research has shown that unless protein intake is compromised for extended periods of time, the body is able to maintain nitrogen reserves adequately. In addition, protein typically makes up only a small fraction of the daily diet, averaging 10–15 percent of total caloric intake. Thus, most energy metabolism results from burning fat and carbohydrate stores for fuel. The percentage of either substrate used depends on a number of factors including, but not limited to, available glycogen stores, and intensity of the activity being performed.

Although it is essential for the body to maintain blood glucose for nervous system activity, glucose and glycogen stores are relatively limited, totaling no more than one to two pounds of body weight. Unless an individual is in a state where a great deal of muscle anabolism is occurring, such as high intensity weight lifting, or normal growth of a child, any excess energy intake is stored as fat.

Triglycerides stored in the adipocytes are the main source of daily energy expenditure from fat. Triglycerides are under the control of lipase enzymes that help maintain a balance between stored, and circulating levels available for metabolism. Lipase enzymes are regulated by insulin and catecholamine levels. The ability to mobilize fat stores for energy metabolism is down regulated in some obese individuals, while many who exercise have more sensitivity to hormonal stimuli. The result is that at any level of exertion, chronic exercisers will metabolize more fat than sedentary individuals (Horowitz, 2001). This effect has been shown in both lean and obese individuals, but the independent role of weight loss has not always been accounted for when overweight individuals have been studied.

A few comments about alcohol consumption are warranted. In general, alcohol ingestion does not account for a larger percentage of the daily diet (Block, Dresser, Hartman, & Carroll, 1985). However, any alcohol that is not metabolized for energy will eventually be stored as fat and can contribute significantly to weight gain in adults (Wannamethee & Shaper, 2003). The high energy content of many alcoholic beverages associated with either participating in, or watching sporting events is surprising to many. Indeed, there are many anecdotal success stories about individuals who have decreased body weight simply by giving up or cutting way back on alcoholic beverages.

Considering the amount of food that is eaten over an individual's life-time, and the amount of physical activity performed, it is remarkable that most individuals show such controlled energy balance, allowing their weight to creep up only slowly over time.

Research has shown that several factors can work to modulate basic energy balance. These may play a significant role for individuals who struggle with weight maintenance or loss. For instance, individuals who are successful at losing large amounts of body mass, particularly through diet restriction, often lower their basal metabolic rate as a way for the body to conserve energy (Astrup et al., 1999). This metabolic adjustment can make the last bit of weight loss more difficult. Recent recognition of a genetic predisposition to obesity (as evidenced by low leptin levels and other biomarkers) helps explain why some individuals tend to overeat or accrue more body fat for a given diet (Boghossian, Lecklin, Torto, Kalra, & Kalra, 2005; Farooqi, 2005). These and other hormonal imbalances may result in significant variability in a given individual's ability to maintain weight. However, in general it appears that individuals who are successful at losing weight (and keeping it off) use the same strategies as have been used historically (Phelan, Wyatt, Hill & Wing, 2006). Successful weight losers consume low-calorie diets with low fat content, and perform high levels of physical activity on a regular basis.

Most research suggests that the energy gap between normal weight and overweight/obesity is not large. Hill, Wyatt, Reed, and Peters (2003) estimate it to be approximately 100–200 kilocalories per day in adults. This estimate is based on data from the Coronary Artery Risk Development in Young Adults (CARDIA) study where individuals were followed for weight gain over eight years. In children, the energy gap may be larger (approximately 263 kilocalories per day), based on carefully measured body weight and fatness changes in Hispanic children. If these data are correct, then a careful and consistent intervention of reduced caloric intake and increased caloric output totaling approximately 250 kilocalories per day might prove effective for many overweight or obese individuals.

PHYSICAL ACTIVITY, EXERCISE, AND FITNESS: IS THERE A DIFFERENCE?

From a biological perspective, there is no difference between physical activity and exercise. The physiological stress and resulting caloric expenditure associated with performing any type of physical exertion is not affected by whether the activity is planned or unplanned. For instance, the same amount of energy is used when walking 30 minutes each way to work and back as during a 60 minute planned walking session performed at lunchtime in a local health club. However, there are both real and somewhat cosmetic reasons why physical activity and exercise should not be used interchangeably.

Physical activity is usually defined as any bodily movement produced by skeletal muscles, which results in energy expenditure (Casperson, Powell, & Christenson, 1985). Exercise is a type of physical activity, but it is different in that it is a planned and structured activity, often sport related. Repetitive bodily movement during sports is performed to enhance athletic skill and improve or maintain one or more of the components of physical fitness (Casperson et al., 1985). In contrast, physical fitness is a set of attributes that people have or achieve that relates to and enhances their ability to perform physical activity (Casperson et al., 1985).

Physical fitness is sometimes (incorrectly) used interchangeably with physical activity and exercise by laypersons and even some researchers. Historically, investigators have used physical activity as a surrogate for fitness, and vice-versa. While the two are correlated, there is a significant genetic component to physical fitness (Fagard, Bielen, & Amery, 1991; Gaskill et al., 2001). In other words, improvements in fitness will not be the same in a group of individuals, even if they perform the same physical activity or exercise program. Some individuals can adapt physiologically to chronic physical activity rather quickly and distinctly, while others may take much longer or become injured or ill in the process, as a result of overtraining. In addition, physical fitness should not be considered an all or nothing proposition. Physical fitness attributes most related to health status are appropriately termed health-related fitness attributes (Bouchard & Shephard, 1994). These include cardiorespiratory fitness, body composition, musculoskeletal strength, endurance, and flexibility. While all health-related components are important, most evidence relating fitness to disease prevention is found in studies where individuals possess or obtain (through physical activity) optimal levels of cardiorespiratory fitness and body composition (USDHHS, 1996).

ENERGY EXPENDITURE

Resting energy expenditure accounts for approximately 60 percent of daily energy expenditure. In simple terms, resting energy expenditure is the amount of energy needed to sustain life by maintaining basic metabolism and whole body homeostasis when someone is awake, and in a seated or lying position. Resting energy expenditure is slightly more than true basal metabolic rate, which is more coincident with minimal energy required to sustain life during a restful sleep. Resting energy expenditure is positively related to body size; that is, the larger the person, the more energy needed to maintain life. Thus, when indexed by body weight, much of the difference in resting energy expenditure that exists among individuals is eliminated.

Precise values for resting energy expenditure can be measured using a technique known as indirect calorimetry. Expired respiratory gases are collected while the individual lies supine. Tests are usually performed in the early morning before daily activities begin. These respiratory gases are analyzed to determine the volume of oxygen consumed and carbon dioxide produced in a given period of time. From these values, caloric expenditure can be calculated mathematically (hence the term, *indirect calorimetry*). Expired respiratory gases can be obtained when an individual is at rest, or performing moderate or vigorous physical activity.

Resting energy expenditure measures via indirect calorimetry are not commonplace, but rather, they usually occur only in research or clinical laboratories. More often, resting energy expenditure is estimated at one kilocalorie per kilogram of body weight, per hour (1 kcal.kg^{-1}. hr^{-1}). Using standard units that reflect indirect calorimetry measures, this value is equivalent to 3.5 ml O$_2$ per kg body weight, per minute (3.5 ml. kg^{-1}·min). This value is commonly referred to as *one metabolic equivalent*, or *1 MET*. The term *MET* refers to the fact that resting energy expenditure is equivalent to one's daily metabolic rate. A 1 MET value for a child corresponds to a greater resting energy expenditure value (~4–5 ml. kg^{-1}. min^{-1}) due to higher energy expenditure associated with normal growth and development.

According to data from the 2000 Behavioral Risk Factor Survey, the standard adult man weighs approximately 85.4 kg (188 pounds), and the standard woman weighs 67.7 kg (149 pounds). Therefore, resting energy expenditure could be estimated at approximately 2050 kcals per day for men (85.4 kg × 24 hours) and approximately 1625 kcals per day for women. Since up to 10 percent variability in resting energy expenditure among adults is still considered normal, individuals of a given body weight on opposite ends of the normal range could differ by several hundred kcals per day. For example, our standard man described above, who has an expected resting energy expenditure of 2050 kcals per day, could be as low as 1845 kcals per day or as high as 2255 kcals per day and still be considered to have normal resting energy expenditure. However, it is clear that weight gains or losses would occur if two individuals with identical physical characteristics, and dietary and physical activity patterns were on opposite ends of the normal range.

A small, yet consistent source of daily energy expenditure is called the thermic effect of food. The thermic effect of food accounts for less than 10 percent of daily energy expenditure, but is ever present since it is a result of the body's daily requirements to digest and assimilate food. It can be estimated using indirect calorimetry, by combining a meal of known caloric value and measuring the resulting change in resting energy expenditure (Reed & Hill, 1996). There have been several studies examining the role of the thermic effect of food on obesity. At this time, there does not appear to be consensus on whether the thermic effect of food is compromised in obese individuals, and if so, the effect appears to be modest (Granata & Brandon, 2002).

Spontaneous physical activity appears to be a significant component of energy expenditure in laboratory animals, and closely tied to their body size. In humans, spontaneous physical activity is typically represented by the kilocalories utilized through the subconscious process of fidgeting during activities considered to be restful such as standing, sitting, and lying down. The contribution of spontaneous physical activity on total daily energy expenditure can vary greatly among individuals. For example, studies of fidgeting behavior have shown that energy spent during sitting and standing can increase from 50–90 percent compared to lying, in individuals who fidget (Levine, Schleusner, & Jensen, 2000). More recently, the role of spontaneous or lifestyle physical activity has been termed non-exercise activity thermogenesis, or NEAT (Levine, 2004). It has been estimated that NEAT values may range from 10–50 percent of total daily energy expenditure in sedentary and active individuals, respectively (Blundell & King, 1999; Jakicic, Wing, Butler, & Robertson, 1995). At present, it is difficult to reconcile precisely the energy expenditure contribution of NEAT versus that of actual planned physical activity sessions, since the two are tightly related. However, it is clear that some individuals have a propensity to be in a continual state of motion, even when doing apparently sedentary or light activities. This NEAT caloric expenditure may be small compared to exercise in a given period of time such as 20 or 30 minutes. However, if continued throughout the day, small energy contributions may contribute significantly to an individual's ability to maintain a steady body weight.

Although the effect of resting energy expenditure, thermic effect of food, and NEAT on the incidence of obesity are important research topics, the variable most under control of the individual is voluntary physical activity. Regardless of body size or fitness level, extended or multiple bouts of leisure-time physical activity added to an individual's daily energy expenditure could have a significant impact on body weight.

WHAT IS THE ENERGY COST OF PHYSICAL ACTIVITY?

Physical activity, whether planned or unplanned, is usually divided into moderate and vigorous intensities for both accounting and research purposes. Moderate activities are those that can be performed by most individuals, and are coincident with little to no sweating, and little noticeable change in respiration and heart rate. Moderate activities range from 3–6 METs in intensity; that is, any activity that increases an individual's resting energy expenditure from three to six times would qualify. Brisk walking is typically used as a benchmark moderate physical activity for most individuals, and usually equates to a 4 MET intensity. In contrast, vigorous activities are those with MET levels at 7 and above, usually coincident with sweating, significant increases in respiration and elevated heart rate. A modest jog is a vigorous activity performed at approximately 8–9 METS. Obviously, other vigorous activities such as fast running, swimming, and cycling can equate to greater caloric expenditure compared to modest jogging.

Recommendations from the American College of Sports Medicine (ACSM) and the Centers for Disease Control and Prevention (CDC) indicate that all adults should perform at least 30 minutes of moderate (e.g., brisk walking) physical activity, five days per week, or 20 minutes of vigorous (e.g., running) activity, three days per week (Pate et al., 1995). While more activity is recommended for those who can do it, recent data from the Behavioral Risk Factor Surveillance System indicates that these minimum recommendations are being met by only 28 percent of all adults (CDC, 2000).

A reasonable question to ask is, "How many kilocalories will be used by an average individual who meets the minimal ACSM/CDC recommendations for physical activity?" Our previously described average 188 pound man and 149 pound woman would utilize 641 and 508 kcals per week, respectively, when fulfilling the ACSM/CDC minimum recommendations for moderate physical activity. If minimum recommended levels of vigorous physical activity were performed, the kcal totals would be slightly lower at 513 and 406 kcals per week for men and women, respectively. This assumes that moderate activity is performed at a 4–5 MET intensity, or vigorous activity is performed at 7–8 METs.

Assuming that an individual must expend approximately 3500 kcals to lose one pound of body weight that is mostly fat, an individual who changes from no leisure time physical activity to meeting minimal weekly recommendations would have a yearly weight loss of 10–12 (men) or 8–10 (women) pounds. This weight loss projection assumes that eating habits, resting energy expenditure, and all other activities of daily living stay the same.

The Institute of Medicine, a private highly regarded scientific organization, also has recommendations for physical activity, which are a bit more ambitious than those of the ACSM/CDC. The Institute of Medicine calls for all adults to perform 60 minutes of moderate physical activity during their leisure-time, per day (Brooks, Butte, Rand, Flatt, & Caballero, 2004). These recommendations were developed based on data indicating that individuals with a BMI that is less than 25 routinely perform this much physical activity. An average man would expend nearly 1800 kilocalories per week if he met these recommendations, and a woman would use just over 1400 kilocalories per week. This would require an individual to walk between 3–4 miles per day, every day of the week. While this activity level is laudable and might be doable for many healthy individuals seeking to maintain current weight, recent U.S. population data indicate that less than 7 percent of adults who perform any leisure-time physical activity are exercising at this level (Mudd, Pivarnik, Ode, Rafferty, & Reeves, 2006).

PHYSICAL ACTIVITY AND WEIGHT GAIN

Several studies have been published demonstrating the relationship between physical activity level and body weight change over time. In a cross sectional study, Rissanen, Heliovaara, Knekt, Reunanen, and Aromaa (1991) found that physical activity was inversely related to prevalence of obesity in adult Finns and their tendency to gain weight over time. This was particularly true with less educated individuals. However, in this cross sectional study it is not possible to determine whether lack of activity led to weight gain, or if those who gained a great deal of weight over time tended to subsequently decrease their physical activity levels. The Amsterdam Growth and Health study also showed a relationship between body fatness (skinfold thickness) and physical activity in young adults (Kemper, Post, Twisk, & van Mechelen, 1999).

In the United States, data from the first National Health and Nutrition Examination Survey indicated that recreational physical activity was inversely related to body weight (Williamson, Madans, Anda, Kleinman, Kahn, & Byers, 1993). However, the investigators found that weight gain over the following 10-year period was not related to initial physical activity levels. Thus, it is possible that lack of physical activity led to weight gain, or that individuals who gained a great deal of weight over the 10-year period tended to decrease their physical activity levels as a result of the weight gain.

Results obtained from research involving young adults participating in the Coronary Artery Risk Development in Young Adults (CARDIA) study (Schmitz, Jacobs, Leon, Schreiner, & Sternfeld, 2000) showed an inverse relationship between physical activity and weight gain. The authors followed 18–30 year-olds for 10 years, and found that weight gain was reduced in those who were active for at least two hours per week. Weight gain attenuation was particularly effective in the larger CARDIA participants. Similar findings have come from the U.S. Health Professionals study of middle-aged adults. Results indicated that, during a four-year period, adults who increased their physical activity levels in place of sedentary activities (e.g., television viewing) decreased their body weights (Coakley, Rimm, Colditz, Kawachi, & Willett, 1998). Those who did not change their physical activity habits gained weight over the same four-year period. Most recently, Littman, Kristal, and White (2005) provided further evidence for the link between physical activity and weight gain in middle-aged adults. While most groups who participated in regular aerobic physical activities tended to lose or maintain weight, obese individuals who participated in 75–100 minutes of fast walking per week appeared to have realized the most benefit.

ROLE OF PHYSICAL ACTIVITY INTERVENTION IN WEIGHT LOSS PROGRAMS

Several studies have shown that exercise alone does not appear to be an effective mechanism for weight loss (Garrow & Summerbell, 1995), but combined with diet modification, is effective in reducing body weight in many adults. Although the mechanism of the weight loss is not clear, it may be related to changes in resting metabolic rate in some individuals. Stiegler and Cunliffe (2006) have found that resting metabolic rate may increase or decrease in obese individuals involved in exercise intervention programs. Byrne and Wilmore (2001) found that resting metabolic rate increased slightly, yet significantly in obese, sedentary women who performed strength-training activities for 20 weeks. In contrast, women who added walking to a strength-training program showed a significant decrease in resting metabolism.

In their classic study, Pavlou, Krey, and Steffee (1989) showed that during strict dietary intervention, exercise did not contribute significantly to weight loss efforts. However, exercise proved critical in keeping the weight off over a year later. This makes intuitive sense since the ability to restrict energy intake exceeds the ability to increase energy expenditure in most individuals on a weight loss program. However, exercise provides an excellent means of helping to reshape an individual in terms of the ratio of fat to fat-free mass, regardless of body weight.

High intensity, supervised weight loss programs have shown some short-term success. Grodstein et al. (1996) surveyed 192 individuals after they participated in a commercial weight loss program. The authors found that individuals who did not regain their weight three years after the intervention were more likely to have maintained their exercise programs during the same time period. Recently, investigators evaluated the results from over 60,000 individuals who participated in a commercial weight loss program (Finley et al., 2007). As part of the program, participants were encouraged to perform at least 30 minutes of moderate physical activity at least five days per week, as recommended by the ACSM/CDC. Results showed that the program was effective for those who remained with it for the duration of the intervention, which was 52 weeks. While these results are encouraging, the real test comes several years later if the individuals involved in such programs maintain their post-intervention body weights.

CHILDREN AND ADOLESCENTS

Average body weight of children has increased in recent years, resulting in a higher prevalence of youth with type II diabetes and many chronic disease risk factors (Hardy, Harrell, & Bell, 2004; Rodriquez et al., 2006). Prevalence of overweight in children and adolescents has increased from approximately 13–17 percent from 1999–2004 (Ogden et al., 2006). Therefore the importance of physical activity for weight control is as important in children as it is in adults. But defining important terms correctly should precede discussion of this subject. Currently there are no universally accepted definitions for obesity in children and adolescents. Rather, the terms *at risk of overweight,* and *overweight* are used. By definition, children and adolescents are at risk of overweight if their BMI falls between the 85th and 95th percentile for their age and gender. They are considered overweight if they exceed the 95th percentile. The Expert Committee on Clinical Guidelines for Overweight in Adolescent Services developed these definitions (Himes & Dietz, 1994). The committee chose to use relative (percentile) standards, rather than absolute BMI values, because weight for height is very unstable during childhood and adolescence. Rapid changes may not be associated with increased body fatness, but rather, with overall growth and development. In addition, the panel felt that the term *obesity* was not appropriate, even for youth at the high end of the norm charts, since body fatness may be poorly related to BMI during childhood and adolescence. Regardless of terminology used, there is little debate that youth at the upper ends of their respective percentiles for BMI are at risk for future health problems (Schiel, Beltschikow, Kramer, & Stein, 2006). There is great concern that school-based physical activity opportunities for youth are becoming restricted because of reductions in physical education classes, and a growing tendency to require additional fees to participate in school sponsored sports programs.

Overall, it appears that boys are more physically active than girls, even at young ages. Unless the girls are involved in organized sports, this disparity tends to increase during the teenage years (Pate, Long, & Heath, 1994). In addition to lower physical activity values, differences can also be seen in cardiorespiratory fitness, where girls' values typically decrease as they achieve menarche and puberty (Krahenbuhl, Skinner, & Kohrt, 1985). While there is good evidence that some fitness difference is due to gender related differences in cardiovascular system development associated with puberty, it is likely that decreased physical activity by girls plays a role as well.

The reasons why childhood overweight is increasing in recent years are not known with certainty. However, many nutrition experts believe it is only partially due to increased caloric intake resulting from fast food supersizing, increased school vending machine usage, and fewer sit-down family meals with adequate portion control (Malecka-Tendera & Mazur, 2006). Decreased energy expenditure is also a likely cause of increased childhood overweight. Although resting metabolic rate represents a major component of daily energy expenditure, there is little evidence to suggest that this has changed in recent years in children. While resting metabolism has been shown to be less in children born to obese parents, this does not appear to affect their own body weights as they mature (Griffiths, Payne, Stunkard, Rivers, & Cox, 1990). Therefore, it appears that decreased daily physical activity in children could be a major contributing factor to excess weight gain.

Anecdotal evidence suggests that children and adolescents are less physically active than previously, with television, video games, and non-school-related computer use as replacement activities. There is finite leisure-time available, and these modern entertainment opportunities may lead to less spontaneous physical activity by today's youth (Motl, McAuley, Birnbaum, & Lytle, 2006). However, there are not sufficient data available from large sample studies to show this conclusively (Adams, 2006). In addition, it is plausible that with less physical education available in schools, children have less opportunity to learn motor skills (running, jumping, kicking) that are involved in most physical activities. Thus, their success and ultimate enjoyment of playing sports is limited. This could lead to less activity, which promotes greater weight gain, leading to even less success at sports and exercise, and the cycle continues.

Recently, the Center for Disease Control gathered an expert panel to develop evidence-based physical activity recommendations for children (Strong et al., 2005). Cross sectional studies examined for the recommendations clearly showed the link between physical inactivity and childhood overweight. The consensus was that youth ages 8–18 should participate in at least 60 min of moderate to vigorous physical activity on a daily basis. However, this amount of physical activity may not be sufficient to effect a healthy change in body weight in children who are already overweight.

IS BMI THE BEST MEASURE OF BODY FATNESS AND OBESITY?

As stated previously, overweight and obesity are related to a myriad of chronic conditions, resulting in elevated morbidity and early mortality of U.S. adult citizens. In 1998, the Executive Summary of the Clinical Guidelines on the Identification, Evaluation, and Treatment of Overweight and Obesity in Adults established the most recent definitions available for adult overweight and obesity (1998). The panel indicated that a BMI of 25.0–29.9 is considered overweight, and a BMI above 30.0 is considered obese. In addition to overall weight for height index, waist circumference is considered a good way to classify individuals with respect to their health risk (Han, van Leer, Seidell, & Lean, 1995; Lean, Han, & Seidell, 1998).

BMI is thought to be a good index of health status because of the assumption that increased weight for height (i.e., BMI) is coincident with greater body fat storage. Research suggests that the correlation may range between 0.60–0.80 in most populations (Smalley, Knerr, Kendrick, Colliver, & Owen, 1990). There is significant biological plausibility linking increased body fatness to increased health risk. Excess fat storage means more body weight, which increases strain on the musculoskeletal system, resulting in orthopedic ailments. Further, the extra blood supply and circulatory demands of excess body fat can result in high blood pressure and significant cardiac strain. Excess fatness is also associated with plasma lipid and lipoprotein levels, as well as insulin resistance.

Because individuals with larger waist circumferences tend to store fat centrally, they have greater disease risk than those with fat that is more evenly distributed throughout the body (Cassells & Haffner, 2006). The waist circumference value indicating increased risk is usually considered to be above 102 cm for men and 88 cm for women. Data from a cross section of nationally representative adults using National Health and Nutrition Examination Study data indicates support for both BMI and waist circumference cut points being indicative of increased health risk (Janssen, Katzmarzyk, & Ross, 2002).

Currently, there are no universally accepted body fat ranges that predict specific disease risk because sufficient prospective data are not available. While it is clear that the two are positively related in most populations, the relationship is not always straightforward and linear. Gallagher and colleagues (2000) evaluated the relationship between BMI and percent of body fat in over 1,600 adults of all ages. The authors developed body fat ranges that corresponded to overweight and obese BMI categories. The authors acknowledged that while this is one of the largest studies to date, it marks only the beginning of ongoing efforts to reconcile the role that actual measured body fatness has on disease risk.

Despite the excellent study performed by Gallagher et al. (2006) a disconnect may exist between BMI and body fatness, particularly in individuals whose body mass is high due to unusually large muscle mass (Ode, Pivarnik, Reeves, & Knous, 2007). The study found that many college athletes, both male and females, as well as college men, would be classified as overweight, and even obese, using BMI cutoffs. However, these same individuals were found to have healthy levels of body fatness for their size, likely due to their normal exercise regimens.

The issue of BMI being an appropriate surrogate for body fatness is not only related to the small percentage of adults who are heavy exercisers. The issue may become increasingly problematic if we are campaigning for individuals to be more physically active, and they heed these messages. We are encouraging both strength and resistance training, and aerobic activities. If these programs are successful, some individuals may not see large decreases in body mass and their BMI values might show little or no change after initiating and maintaining a regular physical activity program. However, these individuals may achieve significant increases in muscle mass, and decreases in body fat. For instance, Schmitz, Jensen, Kugler, Jeffery, and Leon (2003) found that 30–50 year-old sedentary women were able to show significant increases in fat-free mass after 15 weeks of resistance training. However, their body weights remained unchanged. Exactly how much risk for chronic disease is associated with this new, yet unchanged BMI is not known. It is possible that we may eventually have to stratify BMI risk categories according to percent body fat levels. However, there currently are not sufficient data to warrant this approach.

WHAT IF A PERSON IS PHYSICALLY FIT AND ACTIVE BUT STILL OVERWEIGHT OR OBESE?

The previous section showed that the relationship between BMI and body fatness could be influenced by physical activity level. Thus, it is possible that not all individuals of a given BMI, even if it is high, have the same risk for chronic disease. Studies published over the past 20 years provide evidence to support this hypothesis. Researchers with the Harvard Alumni Health Study gathered self-reported physical activity data from nearly 17,000 alumni (Paffenbarger, Hyde, Wing, & Hsieh, 1986). Results showed a significant inverse trend between physical activity and all-cause mortality. This relationship held up at any BMI level. Researchers of the Aerobics Center Longitudinal Study provide even more compelling evidence for the importance of fitness at any body size on health. Investigators have followed over 25,000 men and 7,000 women for over 30 years. They found that at any level of BMI, death rates were significantly lower in those with high, and even moderate levels of fitness (Barlow, Kohl, Gibbons, & Blair, 1995). Moreover, this fitness protection was greater in overweight individuals, compared to unfit participants of normal body weight. The authors suggest that standards for body weight should take aerobic fitness into account (Lee, Blair, & Jackson, 1999). In support of our previous discussion of a possible disconnect between BMI and percent fat in some individuals, the Aerobics Institute researchers also present data to suggest that body fatness is a better predictor of cardiovascular disease risk than weight alone (Lee, Blair, & Jackson, 1999). These findings should be good news for those who are not seeing the results they had hoped for (in terms of weight loss) from an exercise program. Perhaps knowing that at any given body weight level, gains in aerobic fitness resulting from regular physical activity result in significant health effects.

SUMMARY

Obesity is a condition that has increased in prevalence in recent years, and it is related to many of the major chronic diseases and all-cause mortality. It appears that this condition is caused by many factors, both genetic and environmental. Treatment, particularly on a population basis, is difficult. Given it's significant role in daily energy expenditure, physical activity is certainly related to weight control. While a regular physical activity program does not guarantee obesity prevention, or even reduction, it has been shown to be an integral part of nearly every successful obesity intervention program. Moreover, the health benefits gained from regular physical activity, independent of body weight or other chronic disease risk factors, provide clear evidence that it should be included as a part of every individual's daily activities.

REFERENCES

Adams, J. (2006). Trends in physical activity and inactivity amongst U.S. 14–18 year olds by gender, school grade and race, 1993–2003: Evidence from the youth risk behavior survey. *BMC Public Health,* (March 7); 6, 57.

Astrup, A., Gotzsche, P. C., van de Werken, K., Ranneries, C., Toubro, S., Raben, A., et al. (1999). Meta-analysis of resting metabolic rate in formerly obese subjects. *American Journal of Clinical Nutrition, 69,* 1117–1122.

Barlow, C. E., Kohl III, H. W., Gibbons, L. W., & Blair, S. N. (1995). Physical fitness, mortality and obesity. *International Journal of Obesity and Related Metabolic Disorders,19*(Suppl.), S41–S44.

Block, G., Dresser, C. M., Hartman, A. M., & Carroll, M. D. (1985). Nutrient sources in the American diet: Quantitative data from the NHANES II survey. Macronutrients and fats. *American Journal of Epidemiology, 122,* 27–40.

Blundell, J. E., & King, N. A. (1999). Physical activity and regulation of food intake: Current evidence. *Medicine and Science in Sports and Exercise, 31,* S573–S583.

Boghossian, S., Lecklin, A., Torto, R., Kalra, P. S., & Kalra, S .P. (2005). Suppression of fat deposition for the life time with gene therapy. *Peptides, 26,* 1512–1519.

Bouchard, C., & Shephard, R. J. (1994). Physical activity, fitness, and health: The model and key concepts. In C. Bouchard, R. J. Shephard, and T. Stephens (Eds.), *Physical Activity, Fitness, and Health: International Proceedings and Consensus Statement* (Champaign, IL: Human Kinetics), 78.

Brooks, G. A, Butte, N. F., Rand, W. M., Flatt, J. P., & Caballero B. (2004). Chronicle of the Institute of Medicine physical activity recommendation: How a physical activity recommendation came to be among dietary recommendations. *American Journal of Clinical Nutrition, 79,* 921S–930S.

Byrne, H. K., & Wilmore, J. H. (2001). The effects of a 20-week exercise training program on resting metabolic rate in previously sedentary, moderately obese women. *International Journal of Sport Nutrition and Exercise Metabolism, 11,* 15–31.

Casperson, C. J., Powell, K. E., & Christenson, G. M. (1985). Physical activity, exercise, and physical fitness: Definitions and distinctions for health-related research. *Public Health Reports, 100,* 128–131.

Cassells, H. B., & Haffner, S. M. (2006). The metabolic syndrome: Risk factors and management. *Journal of Cardiovascular Nursing, 21,* 306–313.

Centers for Disease Control and Prevention (2000). *Behavioral Risk Factor Surveillance System Survey Data.* Atlanta, GA: U.S. Department of Health and Human Services.

Chenowith, D. (2003). *The economic cost of physical inactivity in Michigan.* From Michigan Fitness Foundation Web site: http://www.michiganfitness.org/indexpagedownloads/CostofInactivity.pdf.

Chenowith, D., Hollander, M., & Bortz II, W. M. (2006). The cost of sloth: Using a tool to measure the cost of physical inactivity. *ACSM's Health & Fitness Journal, 10*(2), 8–13.

Coakley, E. H., Rimm, E. B., Colditz, G., Kawachi, I., & Willett, W. (1998). Predictors of weight change in men: Results from the Health Professionals. *International Journal of Obesity and Related Metabolic Disorders, 22,* 89–96.

Colditz, G. A. (1999). Economic costs of obesity and inactivity. *Medicine and Science in Sports and Exercise, 31,* S663–S667.

Eisenmann, J. C. (2006). Insight into the causes of the recent secular trend in pediatric obesity: Common sense does not always prevail for complex, multifactorial phenotypes. *Preventive Medicine, 42,* 329–335.

Executive Summary of the Clinical Guidelines on the Identification, Evaluation, and Treatment of Overweight and Obesity in Adults. (1998). *Archives of Internal Medicine, 158,* 1855–1867.

Fagard, R., Bielen, E., & Amery, A. (1991). Heritability of aerobic power and anaerobic energy generation during exercise. *Journal of Applied Physiology, 70,* 357–362.

Farooqi, I. S. (2005). Genetic and heredity aspects of childhood obesity. *Best Practices in Research on Clinical Endocrinology and Metabolism, 19,* 359, 374.

Finley, C. E., Barlow, C. E., Greenway, F. L., Rock, C. L., Rolls, B. J., & Blair, S. N. (2007). Retention rates and weight loss in a commercial weight loss program. *International Journal of Obesity, 31,* 292–298

Flegal, K. M., Carroll, M. D., Kuczmarski, R. J., & Johnson, C. L. (1998). Overweight and obesity in the United States: Prevalence and trends, 1960–1994. *International Journal of Obesity and Related Metabolic Disorders, 22,* 39–47.

Gallagher, D., Heymsfield, S. B., Heo, M., Jebb, S. A., Murgatroyd, P. R., & Sakamoto, Y. (2006). Healthy percentage body fat ranges: An approach for developing guidelines based on body mass index. *American Journal of Clinical Nutrition, 72,* 694–701.

Garrow, J. S., & Summerbell, C. D. (1995). Meta-analysis: Effect of exercise, with or without dieting, on the body composition of overweight subjects. *European Journal of Clinical Nutrition, 49,* 1–10.

Gaskill, S. E., Rice, T., Bouchard, C., Gagnon, J., Rao, D. C., Skinner, J. S., et al. (2001). Familial resemblance in ventilatory threshold: The HERITAGE Family Study. *Medicine and Science in Sports and Exercise, 33,* 1832–1840.

Granata, G. P., & Brandon, L. J. (2002). The thermic effect of food and obesity: Discrepant results and methodological variations. *Nutrition Reviews, 60,* 223–233.

Griffiths, M., Payne, P. R., Stunkard, A. J., Rivers, J. P. W., & Cox, M. (1990). Metabolic rate and physical development in children at risk of obesity. *Lancet, 336,* 76–78.

Grodstein, F., Levine, R, Troy, L., Spencer, T., Colditz, G. A., & Stampfer, M. J. (1996). Three-year follow-up of participants in a commercial weight loss program: Can you keep it off? *Archives of Internal Medicine, 156,* 1302–1306.

Han, T. S., van Leer, E. M., Seidell, J. C., & Lean, M. E. J. (1995). Waist circumference action levels in the identification of cardiovascular risk factors: Prevalence study in a random sample. *British Medical Journal, 311,* 1401–1405.

Hardy, L. R., Harrell, J. S., & Bell, R. A. (2004). Overweight in children: Definitions, measurements, confounding factors, and health consequences. *Journal of Pediatric Nursing,19,* 376–382.

Hill, J. O., Wyatt, H. R., Reed, G. W., & Peters, J. C. (2003). Obesity and the environment: Where do we go from here? *Science, 299,* 853–855.

Himes, J. H., & Dietz, W. H. (1994). Guidelines for overweight in adolescent preventive service: Recommendations from an expert committee. *American Journal of Clinical Nutrition, 59,* 307–316.

Horowitz, J. F. (2001). Regulation of lipid mobilization and oxidation during exercise in obesity. *Exercise and Sport Sciences Reviews, 29,* 42–46.

Jakicic, J. M., Wing, R. R., Butler, B. A., & Robertson, R. J. (1995). Prescribing exercise in multiple short bouts versus one continuous bout: Effects on adherence, cardiorespiratory fitness, and weight loss in overweight women. *International Journal of Obesity and Related Metabolic Disorders, 19,* 893–901.

Janssen, I., Katzmarzyk, P. T., & Ross, R. (2002). Body mass index, waist circumference, and health risk: Evidence in support of current National Institutes of Health guidelines. *Archives of Internal Medicine, 162,* 2074–2079.

Kemper, H. C., Post, G. B., Twisk, J. W., & van Mechelen, W. (1999). Lifestyle and obesity in adolescence in young adulthood: Results from the Amsterdam Growth And Health Longitudinal Study (AGAHLS). *International Journal of Obesity and Related Metabolic Disorders, 23*(Suppl. 3), S34–S40.

Krahenbuhl, G. S., Skinner, J. S., & Kohrt, W. M. (1985). Developmental aspects of maximal aerobic power in children. *Exercise and Sport Sciences Reviews, 13,* 503–538.

Lean, M.E.J., Han, T. S., & Seidell, J. C. (1998). Impairment of health and quality of life in men and women with a large waist. *Lancet, 351,* 853–856.

Lee, C. D., Blair, S. N. & Jackson, A. S. (1999). Cardiorespiratory fitness, body composition, and all-cause and cardiovascular disease mortality in men. *American Journal of Clinical Nutrition, 691,* 373–380.

Levine, J. A. (2004) Non-exercise activity thermogenesis (NEAT). *Nutrition Reviews, 2,* S82–S87.

Levine, J. A., Schleusner, S. J., & Jensen, M. D. (2000). Energy expenditure of nonexercise activity. *American Journal of Clinical Nutrition, 72,* 1451–1454.

Littman, A. J., Kristal, A. R., & White, E. (2005). Effects of physical activity intensity, frequency, and activity type on 10-y weight chance in middle-aged men and women. *International Journal of Obesity (London), 29,* 524–533.

Malecka-Tendera, E., & Mazur, A. (2006). Childhood obesity: a pandemic of the twenty-first century. *International Journal of Obesity(London), 30*(Suppl.), S1–S3.

Motl, R. W., McAuley, E., Birnbaum, A. S., & Lytle, L. A. (2006). Naturally occurring changes in time spent watching television are inversely related to frequency of physical activity during early adolescence. *Journal of Adolescence, 29,* 19–32.

Mudd, L. M., Pivarnik, J. M., Ode, J. J., Rafferty, A. P., & Reeves, M. J. (2006). Energy expenditure and compliance with physical activity recommendations: What should we believe? *Medicine and Science in Sports and Exercise, 38*(Suppl.), S377.

Murgatroyd, P. R., Goldberg, G. R., Leahy, F. E., Gilsenan, M. B., & Prentice, A. M. (1999) Effects of inactivity and diet composition on human energy balance. *International Journal of Obesity and Related Metabolic Disorders, 23,* 1269–1275.

Ode, J. J., Pivarnik, J. M., Reeves, M. J., & Knous, J. L. (2007). Body mass index as a predictor of percent fat in college athletes and non-athletes. *Medicine and Science in Sports and Exercise, 39,* 403–409.

Ogden, C. L., Carroll, M. D., Curtin, L. R., McDowell, M. A., Tabak, C. J., & Flegal, K. M. (2006). Prevalence of overweight and obesity in the United States, 1999–2004. *Journal of the American Medical Association, 295,* 1549–1555.

Paffenbarger, R. S., Jr., Hyde, R. T., Wing, A. L., & Hsieh, C. C. (1986). Physical activity, all-cause mortality, and longevity of college alumni. *New England Journal of Medicine, 314,* 605–613.

Pate, R. R., Long, B. J., & Heath, G. (1994). Descriptive epidemiology of physical activity in adolescents. *Pediatric Exercise Science, 6,* 434–447.

Pate, R. R., Pratt, M., Blair, S. N., Haskell, W. L., Macera, C. A., Bouchard, C., et al. (1995). Physical activity and public health: A recommendation from the Centers for Disease Control and Prevention and the American College of Sports Medicine. *Journal of the American Medical Association, 273*(5), 402–407.

Pavlou, K. N., Krey, S., & Steffee, W. P. (1989). Exercise as an adjunct to weight loss and maintenance in moderately obese subjects. *American Journal of Clinical Nutrition, 49,* 1115–1123.

Phelan, S., Wyatt, H. R., Hill, J. O., & Wing, R. R. (2006). Are the eating and exercise habits of successful weight losers changing? *Obesity, 14,* 710–716.

Pratt, M., Macera, C. A., Sallis, J. F., O'Donnell, M., & Frank, L. D. (2004). Economic interventions to promote physical activity: application of the SLOTH model. *American Journal of Preventive Medicine, 27*(Suppl. 3), 136–145.

Pratt, M., Macera, C. A., & Wang, G. (2000). Higher direct medical costs associated with physical inactivity. *The Physician and Sportsmedicine, 28*(10), 63.

Prentice, A. M. (1998). Manipulation of dietary fat and energy density and subsequent effects on substrate flux and food intake. *American Journal of Clinical Nutrition, 67,* 535S–541S.

Reed, G. W., & Hill, J. O. (1996). Measuring the thermic effect of food. *American Journal of Clinical Nutrition, 63,* 164–169.

Rissanen, A. M., Heliovaara, M., Knekt, P., Reunanen, A., & Aromaa, A. (1991). Determinants of weight gain and overweight in adult Finns. *European Journal of Clinical Nutrition, 45,* 419–430.

Rodriguez, B. L., Fujimoto, W. Y., Mayer-Davis, E. J., Imerpatore, G., Williams, D. E., Bell, R. A., et al. (2006). Prevalence of cardiovascular disease risk factors in U.S. children and adolescents with diabetes: The SEARCH for diabetes in youth study. *Diabetes Care, 29,* 1891–1896.

Schiel, R., Beltschikow, W., Kramer, G. & Stein, G. (2006). Overweight, obesity and elevated blood pressure in children and adolescents. *European Journal of Medical Research, 27,* 97–101.

Schmitz, K. H., Jacobs, D. R., Jr., Leon, A. S., Schreiner, P. J., & Sternfeld, B. (2000). Physical activity and body weight: Associations over ten years in the CARDIA study. Coronary Artery Risk Development in Young Adults. *International Journal of Obesity and Metabolic Disorders, 24,* 1475–1487.

Schmitz, K. H., Jensen, M. D., Kugler, K. C., Jeffery, R. W., & Leon, A. S. (2003). Strength training for obesity prevention in midlife women. *International Journal of Obesity, 27,* 326–333.

Smalley, K. J., Knerr A. N., Kendrick Z. V., Colliver, J. A., & Owen, O. E. (1990). Reassessment of body mass indices. *American Journal of Clinical Nutrition, 52,* 405–408.

Stiegler, P., & Cunliffe, A. (2006). The role of diet and exercise for the maintenance of fat-free mass and resting metabolic rate during weight loss. *Sports Medicine, 36,* 239–262.

Strong, W. B., Malina, R. M., Blimkie, C. J. R., Daniels, S. R., Dishman, R. K., et al. (2005). Evidence based physical activity for school-age youth. *Journal of Pediatrics, 146,* 732–737.

Stubbs, R. J., Harbron, C. G., Murgatroyd, P. R., & Prentice, A. M. (1995). Covert manipulation of dietary fat and energy density: Effect on substrate flux and food intake in men eating ad libitum. *American Journal of Clinical Nutrition, 62,* 316–329.

Stubbs, R. J., Ritz, P., Coward, W. A., & Prentice, A. M. (1995). Covert manipulation of the ratio of dietary fat to carbohydrate and energy density: Effect on food intake and energy balance in free-living men eating ad libitum. *American Journal of Clinical Nutrition, 62,* 330–337.

U.S. Department of Health and Human Services (1996). *Physical activity and health: A report of the Surgeon General.* Atlanta, GA: U.S. Department of

Health and Human Services, Centers for Disease Control and Prevention, National Center for Chronic Disease Prevention and Health Promotion.

U.S. Department of Health and Human Services. (2001). *The Surgeon General's Call to Action to Prevent and Decrease Overweight and Obesity.* Rockville, MD: U.S. Department of Health and Human Services, Public Health Service, Office of the Surgeon General. Available from: US GPO, Washington. http://www.surgeon general.gov/topics/obesity/calltoaction/toc.htm.

Wannamethee, S. G., & Shaper, A. G. (2003). Alcohol, body weight, and weight gain in middle-aged men. *American Journal of Clinical Nutrition, 77,* 1312–1317.

Williamson, D. F., Madans, J., Anda, R. F., Kleinman, J. C., Kahn, H. S., & Byers, T. (1993). *International Journal of Obesity and Related Metabolic Disorders, 17,* 279–286.

Chapter 3

CHILDHOOD OVERWEIGHT AND ACADEMIC ACHIEVEMENT

Sara Gable, Jennifer L. Krull, and Arathi Srikanta

Experts agree that overweight is the most serious health threat facing today's children and that despite increased prevention efforts, the threat is not subsiding. A recent analysis of the National Health and Nutrition Examination Survey showed that from 1999–2000 to 2003–2004, *overweight*[1] prevalence increased significantly for all children between 2 and 19 years of age (Ogden et al., 2006). Similarly, a two-decade examination of children between birth and 6 years showed comparable trends in all age groups, including infants under 6 months of age (Kim et al., 2006). Because of the notable tracking of overweight across childhood and into the adult years (Magarey, Daniels, Boulton, & Cockington, 2003; BMI > 85th percentile; Nader et al., 2006), understanding the developmental course of individuals who become overweight early in life is crucial for reversing these trends.

Overweight is detrimentally associated with children's development. Research shows links between childhood overweight and health problems (e.g., Must & Strauss, 1999), academic difficulties (e.g., Falkner et al., 2001), poor psychosocial functioning (e.g., Hesketh, Wake, & Waters, 2004), behavior problems (e.g., Lumeng, Gannon, Cabral, Frank, & Zuckerman, 2003), and social isolation within peer networks (e.g., Strauss & Pollack, 2003). For the purpose of this chapter, we focus on overweight and a single area of development—children's academic achievement.

The school context is especially salient because it brings together children, peers, and important adults. School has been mentioned as the most common setting for weight-based stigmatization, such as peer teasing, and over half of junior and senior high school teachers, nurses, and social workers view overweight as a condition that is under a child's control (Neumark-Sztainer et al., 2002; Neumark-Sztainer, Story, & Harris, 1999). Schools play a significant role in overweight children's development and day-to-day well-being.

Our chapter begins with a framework that helps to organize the different sources of influence in overweight children's lives. Next, research on overweight and children's school performance is reviewed and evaluated. We then address, by age group, the psychosocial processes that may put overweight children at risk for less-than-optimal academic performance. Not all overweight children have problems at school and identifying the factors that link weight problems and academic challenges may improve our ability to identify those overweight children most at risk. The chapter concludes with ideas for future research.

A BIO-ECOLOGICAL FRAMEWORK
TO UNDERSTAND THE IMPLICATIONS
OF OVERWEIGHT

Bronfenbrenner's bio-ecological theory is useful for organizing the various levels of influence in individual development (Bronfenbrenner & Morris, 1998). His theory uses four components—process, person, context, and time—to explain variations in human development. What makes this framework helpful is that it considers how overweight at different ages may interfere with normative development and subsequently compromise children's scholastic potential. Moreover, it permits examination of factors that are in close proximity to overweight children (e.g., television habits, peer relationships) and those that are at a distance (e.g., societal beliefs) and that, in combination or on their own, may lead to academic problems.

In its simplest portrayal, overweight reflects an imbalance between calories consumed and calories burned. As straightforward as this sounds, overweight is a complex problem with roots in the genetic makeup of individuals and the social and physical environment. To date, research shows that risk for overweight and overweight itself are associated with various aspects of eating (e.g., parent restriction of access to foods; Birch, Fisher, & Davison, 2003) and sedentary activity (e.g., time spent watching television; Gable, Chang, & Krull, 2007). Overweight thus results from processes that occur within the individual and during interactions with the social and physical world.

Comparable processes may also put overweight children at risk for academic problems. For instance, overweight children may have qualitatively different relationships with peers and teachers than their non-overweight counterparts. Similarly, children with weight problems may spend their out-of-school time engaged in different kinds of activities than their peers without weight problems. Moreover, these processes may vary by children's age and gender. Gender plays a noteworthy role in the messages children receive about their physical appearance (McCabe & Ricciardelli, 2005). Thus, while the clinical fact of overweight may be the same over time, its meaning and consequences for boys' and girls' scholastic performance may change with age and experience.

The larger social context must also be acknowledged. Overweight is widely viewed as a stigmatizing condition and society holds many derogatory stereotypes against overweight people of all ages (Brownell, Puhl, Schwartz, & Rudd, 2005). Overweight individuals are seen as responsible for their weight problems and this belief in the controllability of weight is the foundation from which prejudice grows (Crandall & Reser, 2005). A recent study of school-aged children's perceptions of various physical disabilities shows that children are not immune to such biases. In their replication of a study done by Richardson, Goodman, Hastrof, and Dornbusch (1961), Latner and Stunkard (2003) asked 5th and 6th graders to rank a set of six drawings on the basis of "how well you like" each child and 70 percent of the children rated the overweight child as second to last or last.

Living under the cloud of stigma can be very stressful. Among adults, stigma-based expectations and stress can manifest in women as heightened self-awareness (Fredrickson & Roberts, 1997) and, in men and women alike, as poor intellectual performance (Fredrickson, Roberts, Noll, Quinn, & Twenge, 1998; Steele & Aronson, 1995). For children, the school setting provides countless opportunities for the stress of stigma to manifest. As mentioned earlier, most weight-based teasing takes place in schools (Neumark-Sztainer et al., 2002), and a number of school personnel endorse negative attributions to children with weight problems (Neumark-Sztainer, Story, & Harris, 1999). Indeed, some believe that the impact of stigma appears in overweight children's scholastic performance (Latner & Schwartz, 2005). Consequently, with a multivariate approach, we can examine the person, process, and contextual factors that underlie the relationship between overweight and academic difficulties at different periods of development. First, however, a review of the research on overweight and children's school performance will be provided.

CHILDHOOD OVERWEIGHT AND ACADEMIC ACHIEVEMENT

The academic achievement of overweight children is not as well researched as other developmental correlates and consequences of overweight (e.g., physical health, psychosocial well-being). Nonetheless, the research suggests that overweight is associated with academic difficulties in children of all ages, both concurrently and, in some cases, across time. For instance, a study of 106 clinic-referred overweight children between ages 5 and 18 years found that overweight children and their parents both reported lower school functioning than parents and children in a healthy group and a group of children receiving chemotherapy (Schwimmer, Burwinkle, & Varni, 2003). A prospective study using a large national sample examined overweight at ages 16 to 24 and educational attainment and economic well-being seven years later (Gortmaker, Must, Perrin, Sobol, & Dietz, 1993). The results indicated that the young women who were overweight at the start of the study had later completed fewer years of education, had lower household incomes, and evidenced more poverty than their female peers who were not overweight when the study began.

Cross-Sectional Studies

Some research has been conducted with age-limited samples of children from disadvantaged backgrounds. Specifically, Tershakovec, Weller, and Gallagher (1994) examined child obesity, school performance, and behavior problems in a sample of 104, 3rd and 4th grade students from a predominantly black, urban, economically-disadvantaged area. Triceps skinfold thickness measures were used to identify children who were overweight (> 85th percentile on these measures). Parents reported on child behavior and information about children's absences, and placement in special education classes was taken from school records. Data analyses controlled for childbirth weight, age, gender, family income, and school absences. Findings indicated that overweight children were more often placed in special education classrooms than their non-overweight peers.

Another cross-sectional study utilized a much larger and more diverse sample of older students and examined, among other factors, the educational correlates of adolescents' weight status (Falkner et al., 2001). Close to 10,000 females and males in 7th, 9th, and 11th grade completed a 225-item questionnaire that included self-reports of height and weight, and questions about academic performance and future educational goals. Data analyses controlled for grade level, race, and parental socio-economic status and were conducted separately by gender. In comparison to average weight peers, the results indicated, that overweight girls were more likely to view themselves as poor students, to report being held back a grade, and to expect not to finish college. Overweight boys similarly viewed themselves as poor students and were more likely to expect to drop out of school.

In summary, the cross-sectional research indicates a negative relationship between children's weight status and measures of school performance and future educational goals. From these studies, it appears that children who are overweight have different school experiences than their peers who are not overweight.

Prospective and Longitudinal Studies

A handful of studies have examined prospective and longitudinal relations between overweight and academic achievement. For instance, Crosnoe and Muller (2004) utilized the Adolescent Health data (n = 11,658, 7th through 12th graders from 126 schools) to study weight status and academic achievement at two time points separated by one year. The teens self-reported their height and weight, and risk-for-overweight was defined as more than 85th percentile of the body mass index. Academic achievement was represented by student reports of the letter grade earned in math, science, English, and social studies. Data analyses controlled for gender, age, race, parent education and family structure, prior academic achievement, athletic status, educational aspirations, attendance, effort, frequency of non-athletic school activities, and several school-level factors. The findings revealed a concurrent, negative relationship between risk-for-overweight and 7th through 12th graders' grade point average (i.e., lower GPA's than teens not-at-risk for overweight). No significant associations emerged between early weight status and later academic achievement.

In another prospective study, Datar, Sturm, and Magnabosco (2004) investigated overweight status at kindergarten entry and children's academic abilities, both concurrently and at the end of first grade, in a large, nationally representative sample (n = 11,192; the Early Childhood Longitudinal Study—Kindergarten Cohort [ECLS-K]). Child height and weight were measured by trained staff and reading and math skills were directly assessed. A wide range of child and family covariates were controlled in data analyses (e.g., child television time and birth weight, parent-child interactions, maternal education, household income). The results indicated that overweight boys had lower concurrent math scores than their non-overweight male peers at kindergarten entry and that overweight girls were not different from their non-overweight female peers. No prospective relationships emerged between baseline overweight status, and math and reading abilities at the end of first grade.

A more recent longitudinal study used additional data points of the ECLS-K and examined the academic trajectories of children with varying histories of overweight onset and persistence at four times between kindergarten entry and third grade spring (Gable, Krull, & Chang, 2006). Eight thousand children participated and four mutually exclusive overweight groups were identified: (1) children who were overweight from kindergarten through third grade; (2) children who were not overweight during kindergarten and who were overweight at first and third grade; (3) children who were not overweight during kindergarten and first grade and who were overweight for the first time at third grade; and (4) children who were never overweight between kindergarten entry and third grade. Growth models estimated trajectories of children's directly assessed reading and math abilities. Analyses controlled for race and a composite measure of family socioeconomic status and tested the effects of time, overweight group, and gender, and the interactions among these variables. The results showed an overweight effect on direct assessments of children's academic abilities, with several of the effects moderated by time.

Specifically, for children who were overweight persistently from kindergarten through third grade, their reading and math skills were similar to their never-overweight peers at kindergarten entry and lower than their never-overweight peers at first and third grade spring. For children who were overweight at first grade spring and remained so at third grade spring, their reading scores were similar to their never-overweight peers at kindergarten entry and first grade spring and lower than their never-overweight peers at third grade spring. Their math scores were similar to their never-overweight peers at kindergarten entry and lower than their never-overweight peers at first and third grade spring. Being overweight for the first time at third grade spring showed no effects on children's reading and math abilities at kindergarten entry, first grade spring, or third grade spring. Overall, the effects of overweight were not moderated by child gender when predicting academic performance. Results were similar for boys and girls. This study highlights the temporal nature of the relationship between overweight and academic achievement, with overweight status preceding the onset of scholastic difficulties in most cases. Furthermore, as future ECLS-K data points become available (5th grade data were released in 2006, and plans are in place to gather additional data in grades 8, 10, and 12), it will be possible to determine if the age at overweight onset contributes uniquely to the relationship between overweight and academic problems. For example, are children whose overweight persists from kindergarten entry through the school years at greater risk for poor school performance than children whose overweight appears later?

In general, the prospective and longitudinal studies concur somewhat with the findings from the cross-sectional research: overweight and academic achievement are negatively related. However, the findings reveal very little about the complexity of the relationship between childhood overweight and academic achievement, particularly from an ecological perspective. Consequently, a critical review of the research follows.

LIMITATIONS OF RESEARCH BASE

At present, the research on overweight and children's school performance is beset by two broad limitations. The first concerns the varying research methods employed. For example, overweight is measured and defined differently across studies. In some instances, children are directly weighed and measured and in others, participants self-report their height and weight. Moreover, overweight is defined on the basis of different cut-points of the body mass index. Current best practices define overweight as a body mass index at or above the 95th percentile for age and gender (Committee on Prevention of Obesity in Children and Youth, 2005). Some studies follow these guidelines and others do not. Another methodological concern is how academic achievement is measured and defined. In the studies reviewed, academic achievement is variously represented by self-reports of school-functioning, academic performance, future goals, children's experience with remedial learning, and direct assessments of children's academic abilities. To have a more accurate estimate of the effect of overweight on children's academic achievement, more research is needed that utilizes agreed-upon measures and definitions of overweight and academic achievement.

The second broad limitation reflects the limited developmental orientation present in the research. For example, although most studies illustrate a detrimental relationship between overweight and children's scholastic performance, weight status is considered as a static condition that has the same meaning and impact regardless of age at onset and duration. This may not be the case; the strength of the relationship may be dependent on the age at which overweight emerged and how long it has persisted.

Similarly, child gender has not been uniformly considered as a potential moderator of overweight effects. Boys and girls experience different pressures associated with physical appearance, and controlling for gender does not permit the examination of how these different pressures may emerge in overweight children's academic achievement.

Another pressing challenge to this area of research is establishing the temporal sequence of associations between overweight and poor outcomes. With the exception of Gable et al. (2006), no other studies addressed if overweight precedes problems or if particular problems bring about overweight. Furthermore, there is the question of a tipping point; must overweight (i.e., a BMI > 95th percentile for age and gender) be in place before academic problems appear or can they surface before children reach overweight status? Moreover, does the tipping point vary by age and gender? And finally, none of the studies addressed the underlying processes that link overweight with poor academic achievement. It seems unlikely that the relationship between overweight and academic achievement is a straight line. Not all overweight children have problems at school and for those who do, we have little knowledge of the intra- and interpersonal factors that may compromise their academic performance.

One direction we could take would be to argue that some of the same factors that are associated with overweight onset—in this case, diet and television time—explain the relationship between overweight and academic achievement. For instance, research indicates that children who eat breakfast tend to have better diets and that breakfast eating may improve memory, test grades, and attendance (for an extensive review, see Rampersaud, Pereira, Girard, Adams, & Metzl, 2005). Similarly, children who live in food-insufficient households have academic difficulties, among other challenges (Alaimo, Olson, & Frongillo, 2001). Unfortunately, the links between childhood overweight and these particular measures of child diet (i.e., breakfast eating, food insufficiency) are not well understood, thus limiting our ability to argue that overweight and academic problems can be explained by dietary factors.

Similar to measures of child diet, time spent watching television is associated with children's academic abilities. Moreover, time spent watching television is a reliable correlate of risk for and actual overweight status (e.g., Gable et al., 2007). For children ages 6 through 18 years, time spent watching television is detrimentally associated with standardized test scores and class grades (Cooper, Valentine, Nye, & Lindsay, 1999), and less time on homework, studying, and leisure reading (Shin, 2004). Borzekowski and Robinson (2005) found that having a television in the bedroom was associated with lower scores on standardized tests of math, reading, and language arts. Having a television in the bedroom is also associated with greater risk for overweight in preschoolers from low-income families (Dennison, Erb, & Jenkins, 2002). For today's children, screen media are ubiquitous and complex aspects of daily life and when the content of what children view is considered, the complexity grows.

For instance, with detailed television viewing data gathered in the early 1980s, Anderson and colleagues (2001) reported a significant and positive relationship between watching Sesame Street as a preschooler and adolescent boys' English grades and adolescent boys' and girls' science grades (both self-reports and transcripts). When children's time spent watching television is placed in the context of societal standards of physical appearance, the potential risks grow far beyond sedentary activity and time away from academically oriented pursuits. Television is a prime vehicle for transmitting the social stigma of overweight (Greenberg & Worrell, 2005). Content analyses of popular situation comedies indicate that television depicts misrepresentations of the distribution of weight status among females, with a high percent of underweight characters and few overweight ones. Moreover, overweight female characters are more often the target of disparaging comments that are typically followed by audience laughter (Fouts & Burggraf, 2000). When compared to thin characters, those male and female characters who are overweight tend to be less involved in romantic relationships and participate in fewer positive interactions (Greenberg, Eastin, Hofschire, Lachlan, & Brownell, 2003). Viewing such distorted realities and hurtful messages may place overweight children at risk for adopting society's stereotypes as true representations of themselves, which may then compromise their sense of self as a thinking person with dreams of scholastic success.

Despite the simplicity and attractiveness of this argument (i.e., that the same factors that bring about overweight underlie its poor outcomes), it is a limited approach that does not fully consider person, process, context, and time. For instance, child age at overweight onset and gender are important considerations and the quality of an overweight child's peer relationships and social standing may also link weight status with school performance. Consequently, to identify the intra- and interpersonal factors that may clarify the relationship between overweight and academic achievement, we examine how overweight may disrupt aspects of normative development that are associated with concurrent or future school success. The discussion is organized by developmental periods and framed by society's focus on physical appearance and stigmatization of overweight individuals.

INFANCY AND EARLY CHILDHOOD

We begin with infancy and early childhood. Although children have not yet entered formal school settings, the developmental changes that occur during the first five years create a foundation that accompanies children into school. Moreover, the increased prevalence of overweight among children under the age of six (Kim et al., 2006) and its notable tracking across childhood (BMI > 85th percentile; Nader et al., 2006) suggests that attention to this period of development is warranted. The study of overweight during the early years is limited, especially in terms of how it may influence children's scholastic potential. However, in keeping with our goals, we address overweight and young children's motor development (an important facilitator of early cognitive development), time spent with screen media, and early experiences of weight-based stigma.

Motor Development

The field of motor development is guided by two overarching theoretical perspectives (for an extensive review, see Adolph & Berger, 2006). One views motor development as the outcome of processes that occur within the organism (e.g., brain development and changes in perception) and compel an infant to use her body. The other considers motor development as proceeding because of the reorganization in the components of motor functioning itself. Rather than following changes of a higher order, motor development sets the stage for later perceptual and cognitive development. For instance, when infants engage in self-produced locomotion (e.g., crawling, walking), they actively create opportunities to acquire new skills and thoughts about the physical and social world.

For our discussion, we adopt the second perspective and ask, what happens if the onset of self-produced locomotion is delayed and potentially constrained by an excess of body weight? Are other areas of development affected and, if so, how? While there is limited research on infant overweight and motor development, several studies show associations between measures of body composition and large motor delays (Jaffe & Kosakov, 1982), later onset of crawling (Adolph, Vereijken, & Denny, 1998), and less experience with walking (Adolph, Vereijken, & Shrout, 2003). Do overweight infants have fewer opportunities to actively explore the social and object world? Are they at risk for developing less proficient large motor skills? If early overweight is associated with less optimal early cognitive development, infants could be embarking on an unfavorable trajectory for future academic achievement. Moreover, if large motor activity brings little pleasure, infants may be at risk for developing a preference to be sedentary.

When these ideas are placed in the context of infants' access to screen media, the potential emerges for overweight to interfere with the processes that lay the foundation for later scholastic performance. Zelazo's (1972) observation of the changes that accompany learning to walk and, in turn, serve as the built-in rewards of the activity leads one to wonder what happens if the rewards of sedentary activity prevail. It is easy to imagine that television viewing can become an inherently reinforcing and preferred activity. The relationships between motor development, screen media, and early cognitive development are not well-understood and may contribute to the study of overweight and school achievement.

Screen Media

Television and media use in children under age six is receiving considerable attention. A new report from the Kaiser Family Foundation (Rideout & Hamel, 2006) indicates that in a typical day, 6- to 12-month-olds spend 49 minutes with screen media (i.e., television, videos, and computers), 2- to 3-year-olds spend 1 hour and 51 minutes, and 4-to 6-year-olds spend 1 hour and 50 minutes, compared with 33, 42, and 42 minutes reading or being read to, respectively, in a typical day. The percent of children who spend more than two hours per day with screen media is 14 percent (6- to 12-month-olds), 41 percent, (2- to 3-year-olds) and 43 percent (4- to 6-year-old) and the percent of children with a television in their bedroom is 19, 29, and 43, respectively. Screen media occupies a noteworthy place in young children's lives and displaces time that could be spent in other, more school-oriented or physical, activities.

A review by Anderson and Pempek (2005) suggests that television exposure may have detrimental consequences for young children's development. Such effects are evident in children who live in "heavy television exposure" households (Vandewater et al., 2005). The authors identified household where the television is "always on" or "on most of the time" and determined that 38 percent of 6-month to 2-year-olds, 37 percent of 3- to 4-year-olds, and 27 percent of 5- to 6-year olds lived in such homes. Compared with children in non-heavy television households, children who lived in heavy television homes spent more time using electronic media and less time reading or being read to. After controlling for parent education, income, and family structure, 3- to 4-year-olds who were unable to read were 2.38 times more likely to be from television-heavy households than 3- to 4-year-olds who were reading; 5- to 6-year olds who were unable to read were 2.86 times more likely to be from heavy television households than 5- to 6-year-olds who were reading. The review above indicates that television time is a reliable correlate of childhood over-weight (e.g., Gable et al., 2007) and is negatively associated with school performance (Cooper et al., 1999). These cross-sectional findings suggest that early and heavy exposure to television may also have a detrimental impact on young children's early preparation for school.

Early Experiences of Weight-Based Stigma

Although young children do not necessarily understand stigma, research shows that children as young as three years of age use physical appearance as the basis for making attributions (Cramer & Steinwert, 1998). Four stories were presented to 30, 3- to 5-year olds, two stories about a pair of boys and two about a pair of girls. In each story, one character was thin and one was chubby and one was explicitly mean (e.g., knocked over the other child's sand castle) and one was explicitly nice (e.g., complimented the other child's sand castle). After hearing the stories, children were asked to identify which child was mean and which was nice. The results showed that the chubby target child was more often labeled as the mean child. Furthermore, in a replication and extension with a larger sample, the effects were moderated by child age, with older children more strongly endorsing negative descriptors and less strongly endorsing positive descriptors about the target chubby children. If experi-mentally produced findings such as these are evident in preschool or child care settings, preschoolers with weight problems are likely encountering weight-based prejudice that could negatively impact their immediate and later social and academic experiences.

How are young children learning these negative stereotypes? Research on parenting practices offers one answer. A study of middle-income 5-year-old girls and their families found that, independent of daughters' weight status, mothers who reported higher concern about their daugh-ters' weight had daughters who reported lower self-perceptions of their cognitive and physical abilities (Davison & Birch, 2001). Furthermore, when actual weight status was examined, more maternal restriction of access to foods was associated with girls' self-reports of lower cognitive and physical ability only for those girls with a higher weight status (i.e., > 85th percentile of BMI) and not for girls with a lower weight status. These findings suggest that regardless of girls' weight status, the negative stigma associated with bigness was conveyed through mothers' worry and actions, and appeared in disparaging self-perceptions of one's cognitive and physical abilities.

A follow-up with the same sample at age seven indicated that weight-related parent criticism and peer teasing mediated the relationship between girls' body mass index and self-reports of perceived cognitive ability (Davison & Birch, 2002). Thus, peers have joined mothers as transmitters of derogatory stereotypes about weight status, which brings the discussion to middle childhood .

MIDDLE CHILDHOOD

Middle childhood presents a unique opportunity to study childhood overweight. The social and cognitive changes that children experience, combined with entry to formal school, marks this as a period for social-ization into the larger society. Children become more attuned to others' perspectives and feelings, especially others' thoughts about them, and as the self develops, others' evaluations become increasingly critical "self-guides" (Harter, 1999). Children also become more sophisticated in recognizing what thoughts or beliefs may motivate one's interpersonal behavior. Between the ages of 6 and 10, children's awareness of others' endorsement of stereotypes unfolds (McKown & Weinstein, 2003). It begins with virtually no awareness, proceeds to recognition of individu-als' stereotypes (e.g., person A is behaving that way to person B because person B is __), then culminates with a generalized understanding of societal stereotypes (e.g., many people behave that way to people who are __). Thus, prior to school entry, children with weight problems are likely unaware that their physical appearance may elicit prescribed reac-tions from others. However, after some time in the school setting, children begin to understand that their physical appearance may influence others' thoughts about and actions toward them.

Social Stigma and Stereotype Threat

The social-cognitive advances of middle childhood likely contribute to the relationship between overweight and academic achievement. Specifically, overweight children may be responding to what Steele and Aronson (1995) refer to as *stereotype threat*. That is, because of the negative stigma attached to overweight and children's burgeoning understanding of how stereotypes manifest themselves (McKown & Weinstein, 2003), overweight children may be caught in a harmful cycle of striving to fulfill societal beliefs and expectations. Children of this age are ever-attuned to others' thoughts about them. If overweight children are directly or indirectly experiencing weight-based prejudice at school (i.e., the stereotype that big is bad), they may respond by performing more poorly in the classroom because they believe it is expected.

These are not new ideas. In *Pygmalion in the Classroom,* Rosenthal and Jacobson (1968) described such processes in teachers with students from different racial backgrounds and characterized them as "interpersonal self-fulfilling prophecies." For overweight children who live in a society where weight problems are widely viewed as under the control of the individual (Crandall & Reser, 2005), fulfilling such no-win expectations may come at the cost of academic success. The means by which children come to learn about society's weight-based stereotypes is an important link between overweight and children's academic achievement.

The Transmission and Consequences of Appearance-Based Stigma

For school-age children and adolescents, the stigma associated with weight status is transmitted primarily through the media and peer culture (Latner & Schwartz, 2005). Two recent studies examined how societal standards of physical appearance are communicated and later associated with children's developing self-esteem. McCabe and Ricciardelli (2005) examined external sources of pressure on school-age boys' and girls' feelings about their physical appearance. They followed 443 children, ages 8 to 12, over a 16-month period and measured parent, peer, and media influences on children's body satisfaction. For boys, body dissatisfaction was predicted by messages from mothers to increase muscles and messages from the media to lose weight. For girls, body dissatisfaction was predicted by messages from mothers and from best friends to lose weight.

Dohnt and Tiggeman (2006) similarly investigated the contribution of peer and media influences to girls' body satisfaction and self-esteem. Ninety-seven, Caucasian, 5- to 8-year old females participated and were extensively interviewed at two time points separated by one year. Their results indicated that girls who reported socializing with peers who wanted to be thin later reported their own desire to be thin, were less satisfied with their bodies, and reported lower self-esteem. Moreover, exposure to appearance-oriented television programs at baseline predicted decreases over time in girls' satisfaction with how they looked. In sum, these studies document the power of peer and media endorsement of ideal body standards on school-age children's developing sense of self and body satisfaction. For children who experience such pressures, the costs emerge in a shaky sense of self-worth that is based, in part, on others' ideals of physical appearance.

These findings also reveal how children can learn from peers, parents, and the media that bigness is undesirable. However, what is less clear is the impact of such appearance-oriented, external pressures on overweight children's developing sense of self. Overweight children have already violated U.S. society's ideals for how boys and girls/men and women are to look. Consequently, how do overweight children respond to similar external messages about being big? How are their responses subsequently internalized as part of the developing self? And lastly, how do these internalized messages from the outside world manifest as poor academic achievement?

Earlier we posited that overweight children perform poorly in school because they believe it is expected of them. Over time the cumulative stress of such felt stigma and stereotype threat can interfere with intellectual performance (Steele & Aronson, 1995). Objectification theory similarly posits that cognitive functioning may be negatively affected, especially for girls, by the stresses associated with meeting society's standards of feminine physical appearance (Fredrickson & Roberts, 1997). However, research on these topics has, for the most part, been conducted with older, post-pubertal participants. Mapping these findings onto pre-adolescent children who have not achieved the cognitive developments that permit adolescent thought would be careless. Thus, investigating the transmission and manifestation of weight-based stigma in overweight children during middle childhood—a time when children are especially apt to consider external perspectives in their construction of self—will illuminate the links between overweight and academic achievement.

ADOLESCENCE

During adolescence, typical development includes the search for one's identity and the onset of puberty and sexual maturity. Both of these changes play an important role in understanding how overweight might influence teens' academic performance. Because physical appearance and interpersonal relationships play a central role in adolescent identity formation, teens with weight problems may be particularly vulnerable to the consequences of societal stigmatization (Neumark-Sztainer, Story, & Harris, 1999). Perhaps at no other time during development is the following statement quite so salient: *"What others believe about fat people is the same as what fat people believe about themselves"* (Crandall & Reser,

2005, p. 91). During middle childhood, overweight children are learning of society's stigmatization of overweight individuals and possibly internalizing those beliefs as part of their self-perception. Once internalized, these beliefs can become the foundation for what overweight teens think about themselves as they form their identity. An overweight teen's burgeoning identity has the potential to be indelibly linked with societal stereotypes about overweight people.

Moreover, for virtually all adolescents, these years are accompanied by increases in weight and changes in physical appearance. Such normative changes can actually make teens more likely to feel overweight and these perceptions are associated with lower self-esteem and more depressed mood, particularly among 7th and 8th grade Caucasian males and females and Hispanic females (Ge, Elder, Regenerus, & Cox, 2001). Due to society's tendency to judge females in part on the basis of their physical appearance (Fredrickson & Roberts, 1997), and a growing tendency to view males in a similar fashion (McCabe & Ricciardelli, 2004), the stresses that accompany typical physical growth and development are not surprising. For adolescents who are overweight, there is reason to believe that these stresses are magnified.

The Transmission and Consequences of Appearance-Based Stigma

Similar to middle childhood, societal standards about physical appearance and weight-based stigma are conveyed to adolescents through peer culture and visual media (Neumark-Sztainer & Eisenberg, 2005). A study of 13- to 18-year-olds' social networks indicated that overweight teens were less likely to be selected by others as a friend and were more frequently on the periphery of peer networks (i.e., connected to fewer others) than normal-weight teens (Strauss & Pollack, 2003). Although these findings do not reveal the explicit transmission of stigma, they show that overweight teens are less connected with their peers via intermediate-level relationships, leaving them with a marginalized social standing.

Overweight teens are also at risk for stigma-based teasing from peers. In a sample of 4,746 adolescents, 45 percent of overweight girls and 50 percent of overweight boys reported weight-related teasing more than a few times a year (Neumark-Sztainer et al., 2002). In fact, all teens who were not of average weight (average weight = BMI > 15th percentile and < 85th percentile) were significantly more likely to report ever being teased. Lieberman, Gauvin, Bukowski, and White (2001) similarly examined the role of peers in the transmission of societal ideals about body size and how girls felt about themselves in a sample of 876 females from grades 7 to 10. Their findings indicated that as body mass index increased, girls were more likely to be teased about their weight and to take the perspective of their peers when describing themselves. Additionally, bigger girls were more likely to have internalized the societal message that being thin and physically attractive will bring about greater popularity and interest from the opposite sex. During adolescence, teens are engulfed in a culture that actively endorses bias against those who do not conform to social ideals of physical appearance. These biases manifest in weight-related teasing, social marginalization, and teens' internalization of society's standards (and presumed rewards) of an acceptable physical appearance.

The media similarly transmits social standards of physical appearance that may impact what adolescents think about their bodies and how they treat them. With a sample of 366 males and females from grades 6, 9, and 12, Harrison (2001) examined the potential mediating role of body-specific self-discrepancies in the relationship between exposure to thin-ideal media and symptoms of disordered eating. Harrison utilized Higgins' Self-Discrepancy Theory (1987) which proposes that when individuals hold discordant views of how they would like to look and how they actually describe themselves, they experience emotional discomfort when reminded of the appearance-oriented discrepancies. The emotional discomfort, in turn, elicits self-regulatory behaviors believed to lessen the bad feelings and reduce the discrepancies. The study's findings supported this hypothesis. In analyses that controlled for body mass index, the relationship between adolescents' "thin-ideal" television viewing and reading habits (the "reminding" variable) and self-reports of disordered eating thoughts and habits (the "self-regulatory" variable) was mediated by the degree of discrepancy in how participants described their bodies and what they wanted their bodies to look like.

Harrison's (2001) study is important because it illustrates that intrapersonal conflicts over one's physical appearance can increase the potency of visual representations of idealized bodies on one's self-directed and, in this case, potentially harmful regulatory behaviors. How do teens who are overweight see themselves and what would they like to look like? Moreover, what are the upper limits for the impact of media representations of ideal male and female bodies on overweight adolescents' self-regulatory behaviors? The affective and cognitive energy required to cope with such visual reminders yields insight into why overweight youth may have a hard time at school.

The pervasive emphasis on physical appearance in U.S. culture can divert energy and attention away from other cognitive pursuits, particularly for adolescents who have the added burden of overweight status. With the pressures associated with maintaining an idealized physical appearance, teens may be engaging in near-constant monitoring of their observable selves. For women, such self-monitoring can produce feelings of anxiety and shame, interfere with optimal cognitive functioning and reduce awareness of the functioning of one's body (Fredrickson et al., 1998; Fredrickson & Roberts, 1997). Moreover, although objectification theory is intended to explain the female experience, there is sufficient cause to believe that young men in contemporary society are increasingly subject to a male version of objectification (McCabe & Ricciardelli, 2004). Thus, for some overweight adolescents, the school setting is likely a stressful environment where one's appearance-oriented limitations are on constant display and available for comparison with society's idealized vision of how males and females should look. At such an important time in human development, it is disheartening to imagine that for some young people, their emerging identity becomes entwined with physical appearance and not with personal qualities.

FUTURE RESEARCH

Throughout the chapter, we identified several areas in need of additional research, such as the direction of causality between overweight and academic difficulties, the possible existence of a tipping point between weight status and problems of development, and the developmental consequences of overweight that appears early in life. To further our understanding of the links between overweight and academic achievement, we propose three additional areas.

First, because rates of overweight are increasing for both genders, all ages, and all racial and ethnic groups, studies on the psychosocial processes that link societal standards of physical appearance with developmental outcomes need to include males and females from diverse cultural and economic backgrounds. Second, explicit model-testing is needed for some of the ideas proposed in the current chapter, specifically, those purporting links between overweight status, exposure to appearance-oriented media and peer influences, intrapersonal distress, and academic achievement. And finally, strategic efforts must be made to disseminate developmentally oriented research findings to professionals who are engaged in overweight prevention and treatment. Children in today's society are caught between the stresses of everyday life and society's standards of physical appearance. On the one hand, children are spending more time with screen media, experiencing less physical education, and establishing more sedentary lifestyles. On the other, children are bombarded with visual media depicting unrealistic portrayals of ideal bodies and disparaging messages about overweight individuals. If overweight trends are to reverse, action is needed in all areas of children's lives.

ACKNOWLEDGMENT

Preparation of this chapter was made possible in part by a grant from the United States Department of Agriculture, Economic Research Service, Food Assistance, and Nutrition Research Programs (43–3AEM-1–80077) to Sara Gable, Jo Britt-Rankin, and Jennifer L. Krull.

NOTE

1. Throughout this chapter, unless otherwise noted, childhood overweight and obesity is defined as a body mass index (BMI; child weight in kilograms divided by height in meters squared) at or above the 95th percentile for age and gender (Committee on Prevention of Obesity in Children and Youth, 2005).

REFERENCES

Adolph, K. E. & Berger, S. A. (2006). Motor development. In W. Damon & R. Lerner (Series Eds.), & D. Kuhn & R. S. Siegler (Vol. Eds.), *Handbook of child psychology: Vol 2: Cognition, perception, and language* (6th ed., pp. 161–213). New York: Wiley.

Adolph, K. E., Vereijken, B., & Denny, M. A. (1998). Learning to crawl. *Child Development, 69*(5), 1299–1312.

Adolph, K. E., Vereijken, B., & Shrout, P. E. (2003). What changes in infant walking and why. *Child Development, 74*(2), 475–497.

Alaimo, K., Olson, C. M., & Frongillo, E. A. (2001). Food insufficiency and American school-aged children's cognitive, academic, and psychosocial development. *Pediatrics, 108,* 44–53.

Anderson, D. R., Huston, A. C., Schmitt, K. L., Linebarger, D. L. & Wright J. C. (2001). Early childhood television viewing and adolescent behavior. *Monographs of the Society for Research in Child Development. 66*(1, Serial No. 264).

Anderson, D. R., & Pempek, T. A. (2005). Television and very young children. *American Behavioral Scientist, 48*(5), 505–522.

Birch, L. L., Fisher, J. O., & Davison, K. K. (2003). Learning to overeat: Maternal use of restrictive feeding practices promotes girls' eating in the absence of hunger. *American Journal of Clinical Nutrition, 78,* 215–220.

Borzekowski, D. L. G., & Robinson, T. N. (2005). The remote, the mouse, and the No.2 pencil: The household media environment and academic achievement among third grade students. *Archives of Pediatric Adolescent Medicine, 159,* 607–613.

Bronfenbrenner, U., & Morris, P. A. (1998). The ecology of developmental processes. In R. M. Lerner (Ed.), *Handbook of child psychology* (Vol. 1, 5th ed., pp. 993–1028). New York: Wiley.

Brownell, K. D., Puhl, R. M., Schwartz, M. B., & Rudd, L. (2005). *Weight bias: Nature, consequences, and remedies.* New York: Guilford Press.

Committee on Prevention of Obesity in Children and Youth. (2005). *Preventing childhood obesity: Health in the balance.* Washington, DC: National Academy Press.

Cooper, H., Valentine, J. C., Nye, B., & Lindsay, J. L. (1999). Relationships between five after-school activities and academic achievement. *Journal of Educational Psychology, 91,* 369–378.

Cramer, P., & Steinwert, T. (1998). Thin is good, fat is bad: How early does it begin? *Journal of Applied Developmental Psychology, 19,* 429–451.

Crandall, C. S., & Reser, A. H. (2005). Attributions and weight-based prejudice. In Brownell, K. D., Puhl, R. M., Schwartz, M. B., & Rudd, L. (Eds.) *Weight Bias: Nature, consequences, and remedies* (pp. 54–67). New York: Guilford Press.

Crosnoe, R., & Muller, C. (2004). Body mass index, academic achievement, and school context: Examining the educational experiences of adolescents at risk of obesity. *Journal of Health and Social Behavior, 45,* 393–407.

Datar, A., Sturm, R., & Magnabosco, J. L. (2004). Childhood overweight and academic performance: National study of kindergartners and first-graders. *Obesity Research, 12*(1), 58–68.

Davison, K. K., & Birch, L. L. (2001). Weight status, parent reaction, and self-concept in five-year-old girls. *Pediatrics, 107*(1), 46–53.

Davison, K. K., & Birch, L. L. (2002). Processes linking weight status and self-concept among girls from ages 5 to 7 years. *Developmental Psychology, 38*(5), 735–748.

Dennison, B. A., Erb, T. A., & Jenkins, P. L. (2002). Television viewing and television in bedroom associated with overweight risk among low-income preschool children. *Pediatrics, 109*(6), 1028–1035.

Dohnt, H., & Tiggeman, M. (2006). The contribution of peer and media influences to the development of body satisfaction and self-esteem in young girls: A prospective study. *Developmental Psychology, 42*(5), 929–936.

Falkner, N. H., Neumark-Sztainer, D., Story, M., Jeffrey, R. W., Beuhring, T., & Resnick, M. D. (2001). Social, educational, and psychological correlates of weight status in adolescents. *Obesity Research, 9*(1), 32–42.

Fouts, G., & Burggraf, K. (2000). Television situation comedies: Female weight, male negative comments, and audience reactions. *Sex Roles, 42*(9/10), 925–932.

Fredrickson, B. L., & Roberts, T. (1997). Objectification theory: Towards understanding women's lived experiences and mental health risks. *Psychology of Women Quarterly, 21,* 173–206.

Fredrickson, B. L., Roberts, T., Noll, S. M., Quinn, D. M., & Twenge, J. M. (1998). That swimsuit becomes you: Sex differences in self-objectification, restrained eating, and math performance. *Journal of Personality and Social Psychology, 75*(1), 269–284.

Gable, S., Chang, Y., & Krull, J. L. (2007). Television watching and frequency of family meals are predictive of overweight onset and persistence in a national sample of school-age children. *Journal of the American Dietetic Association, 107*(1), 53–61.

Gable, S., Krull, J. L., & Chang, Y. (2006). *The developmental implications of overweight from kindergarten through third grade.* Unpublished manuscript. The University of Missouri, Columbia.

Ge, X., Elder, G. H., Regenerus, M. K., & Cox, C. (2001). Pubertal transitions, perceptions of being overweight, and adolescents' psychological maladjustment: Gender and ethnic differences. *Social Psychology Quarterly, 64*(4), 363–375.

Gortmaker, S. L., Must, A., Perrin, J., Sobol, A. M., & Dietz, W. H. (1993). Social and economic consequences of overweight in adolescence and young adulthood. *New England Journal of Medicine, 329,* 1008–1012.

Greenberg, B. S., Eastin, M., Hofschire, L., Lachlan, K., & Brownell, K. D. (2003). Portrayals of overweight and obese individuals on commercial television. *American Journal of Public Health, 93*(8), 1342–1348.

Greenberg, B. S., & Worrell, T. R. (2005). The portrayal of weight in the media and its social impact. In Brownell, K. D., Puhl, R. M., Schwartz, M. B., & Rudd, L. (Eds.) *Weight bias: Nature, consequences, and remedies* (pp. 42–53). New York: Guilford Press.

Harrison, K. (2001). Ourselves, our bodies: Thin-ideal media, self-discrepancies, and eating disorder symptomatology in adolescents. *Journal of Social and Clinical Psychology, 20*(3), 289–323.

Harter, S. (1999). *The construction of the self.* New York: Guilford Press.

Hesketh, K., Wake, M., & Waters, E. (2004). Body mass index and parent-reported self-esteem in elementary school children: Evidence for a causal relationship. *International Journal of Obesity, 28,* 1233–1237.

Higgins, E. T. (1987). Self-discrepancy: A theory relating self and affect. *Psychological Review, 94,* 319–340.

Jaffe, M., & Kosakov, C. (1982). The motor development of fat babies. *Clinical Pediatrics, 21*(10), 619–621.

Kim, J., Peterson, K. E., Scanlon, K. S., Fitzmaurice, G. M., Must, A., Oken, E., et al. (2006). Trends in overweight from 1980 through 2001 among preschool-aged children enrolled in a health maintenance organization. *Obesity, 14*(7), 1107–1112.

Latner, J. D., & Schwartz, M. B. (2005). Weight bias in a child's world. In Brownell, K. D., Puhl, R. M., Schwartz, M. B., & Rudd, L. (Eds.) *Weight bias: Nature, consequences, and remedies* (pp. 54–67). New York: Guilford Press.

Latner, J. D., & Stunkard, A. L. (2003). Getting worse: The stigmatization of obese children. *Obesity Research, 11*(3), 452–456.

Lieberman, M. Gauvin, L., Bukowski, W. M., & White, D. R. (2001). Interpersonal influence and disordered eating behaviors in adolescent girls: The role of peer modeling, social reinforcement, and body-related teasing. *Eating Behaviors, 2,* 215–236.

Lumeng, J., Gannon, K., Cabral, H., Frank, D. A., & Zuckerman, B. (2003). Association between clinically meaningful behavior problems and overweight in children. *Pediatrics, 112*(5), 1138–1145.

Magarey, A. M., Daniels, L. A., Boulton, T. J., & Cockington, R. A. (2003). Predicting obesity in early adulthood from childhood and parental obesity. *International Journal of Obesity, 27,* 505–513.

McCabe, M. P., & Ricciardelli, L. A. (2004).Weight and shape concerns of boys and men. In J. K. Thompson (Ed.), *Handbook of eating disorders and obesity* (pp. 606–634). Hoboken, NJ: John Wiley and Sons, Inc.

McCabe, M. P., & Ricciardelli, L. A. (2005). A longitudinal study of body image and strategies to lose weight and increase muscles among children. *Applied Developmental Psychology, 26,* 559–577.

McKown, C., & Weinstein, R. S. (2003). The development and consequences of stereotype consciousness in middle childhood. *Child development, 74*(2), 498–515.

Must, A., & Strauss, R. S. (1999). Risk and consequences of childhood and adolescent obesity. *International Journal of Obesity, 23*(Suppl 2), S2–S11.

Nader, P. R., O'Brien, M., Houts, R., Bradley, R., Belsky, J., Crosnoe, R., et al. (2006). Identifying risk for obesity in early childhood. *Pediatrics, 118,* 594–601.

Neumark-Sztainer, D., & Eisenberg, M. (2005). Weight bias in a teen's world. In Brownell, K. D., Puhl, R. M., Schwartz, M. B., & Rudd, L. (Eds.) *Weight Bias: Nature, consequences, and remedies* (pp. 68–79). New York: Guilford Press.

Neumark-Sztainer, D., Falkner, N., Story, M., Perry, C., Hannan, P. J., & Mulert, S. (2002). Weight-teasing among adolescents: Correlations with weight status and disordered eating behaviors. *International Journal of Obesity, 26,* 123–131.

Neumark-Sztainer, D., Story, M., & Harris, T. (1999). Beliefs and attitudes about obesity among teachers and school health care providers working with adolescents. *Journal for Nutrition Education, 31,* 3–9.

Ogden, C. L., Carroll, M. D., Curtin, L. R., McDowell, M. A., Tabak, C. J., & Flegal, K. M. (2006). Prevalence of overweight and obesity in the United States, 1999–2004. *Journal of the American Medical Association, 295*(13), 1549–1555.

Rampersaud, G. C., Pereira, M. A., Girard, B. L., Adams, J., & Metzl, J. D. (2005). Breakfast habits, nutritional status, body weight, and academic performance in children and adolescents. *Journal of the American Dietetic Association, 105,* 743–760.

Richardson, S. A., Goodman, N., Hastrof, A. H., & Dornbusch, S. M. (1961). Cultural uniformity in reaction to physical disabilities. *American Sociological Review, 26*(2), 241–247.

Rideout, V., & Hamel, E. (2006). *The media family: Electronic media in the lives of infants, toddlers, preschoolers and their parents.* Menlo Park, CA: Kaiser Family Foundation.

Rosenthal, R., & Jacobson, L. (1968). *Pygmalion in the classroom: Teacher expectation and pupils' intellectual development.* New York: Holt, Rinehart, & Winston, Inc.

Schwimmer, J. B., Burwinkle, T. M., & Varni, J. W. (2003). Health related quality of life of severely obese children and adolescents. *Journal of the American Medical Association, 289,* 1813–1819.

Shin, N. (2004). Exploring pathways from television viewing to academic achievement in school age children. *The Journal of Genetic Psychology, 165*(4), 367–381.

Steele, C. M., & Aronson, J. (1995). Stereotype threat and intellectual test performance of African Americans. *Journal of Personality and Social Psychology, 69*(5), 797–811.

Strauss, R. S., & Pollack, H. A. (2003). Social marginalization of overweight children. *Archives of Pediatric and Adolescent Medicine, 157,* 746–752.

Tershakovec, A., Weller, S., & Gallagher, P. (1994). Obesity, school performance and behavior of black, urban, elementary school children. *International Journal of Obesity, 18,* 323–327.

Vandewater, E. A., Bickham, D. S., Lee, J. H., Cummings, H. M., Wartella, E. A., & Rideout, V. J. (2005). When the television is always on: Heavy television exposure and young children's development. *American Behavioral Scientist, 48*(5), 562–577.

Zelazo, P. R. (1972). "Walking" in the newborn. *Science, 176,* 314–315.

Chapter 4

ADIPOSITY AND INTERNALIZING PROBLEMS: INFANCY TO MIDDLE CHILDHOOD

Robert H. Bradley, Renate Houts, Phillip R. Nader, Marion O'Brien, Jay Belsky, and Robert Crosnoe

The rapid rise in childhood obesity has induced health and social scientists to search for biological and psychosocial factors that may be implicated in the rise (Agras, Hammer, McNicholas, & Kraemer, 2004). Because of the social stigma attached to being overweight, obesity has consequences that go well beyond such physical problems as metabolic disorder and cardio-vascular disease. There is evidence that links obesity to low self-esteem, mood disorders, and depression in children (Braet, Mervielde, & Vandereycken, 1997; French, Story, & Perry, 1995; Goodman & Whitaker, 2002; Manus & Killeen, 1995; McElroy, et al., 2004; Strauss, 2000; Young-Hyman, Schlundt, Herman-Wenderoth, & Bozylinski, 2003; Zametkin, Zoon, Klein, & Munson, 2004). However, the relation appears neither consistent nor simple, with variations noted by gender, age, family context, and duration of obesity (Goodman & Whitaker, 2002; Krahnstoever Davison & Lipps Birch, 2002; McElroy, et al., 2004; Mustillo, et al., 2003; Zametkin, et al., 2004). The limited literature on young children provides scant evidence of a relation between obesity and internalizing problems prior to age seven. However, granting the considerable methodological limitations of most studies, it appears that the association becomes somewhat more consistent, albeit modest, for adolescents and young adults (French et al., 1995; Friedman & Brownell, 1995; Goodman & Whitaker, 2002; Zametkin et al., 2004).

The purpose of this study is to further delineate the complex interplay of internalizing problems and adiposity in a diverse sample of children followed prospectively from birth to determine (a) when the relation emerges, and (b) the primary causal direction of influence. The National Institute of Child Health and Human Development (NICHD) Study of Early Child Care and Youth Development sample is a particularly useful one in that data on height and weight and on internalizing behavior were gathered periodically beginning in infancy (Nader, et al., 2006). The study is also useful because of its large sample size ($n = 1364$) and the diversity of the participants, in terms of ethnicity, socioeconomic status, and geography. A secondary purpose of the study is to determine whether the pattern of relations observed may be different for children who show high levels of negative emotionality early in life and for children who live in highly unstable life circumstances.

The prevailing belief is that overweight children suffer from social stigmatization associated with their obesity and that they gradually become dissatisfied with their body image (Friedman & Brownell, 1995; Harrison, 2001). As a consequence, they are prone to loss of self-esteem and depression (Goodman & Whitaker, 2002). Although logical, the evidence in favor of such an argument is far from compelling. Most of the studies are cross-sectional and a significant number utilize clinical populations, making attributions to causal connections in the general population of obese children suspect. The available evidence suggests that most obese children do not suffer from depression or mood disorders (McElroy et al., 2004; Sheslow, Wallace, & DeLancey, 1993) and that the strength of the relation is considerably stronger for children who are chronically obese than for those who did not become obese until adolescence or who lost weight during adolescence (Mustillo et al., 2003). As well, there are studies indicating that depression may precede rather than result from obesity (Goodman & Whitaker, 2002; Pine, Goldstein, Wolk, & Weissman, 2001). However, Tanofsky-Kraff, and colleagues (2006) found no evidence that depression was related to body fat gain in children at high risk for obesity.

In sum, there is considerable inconsistency in findings of studies that have examined relations between obesity and depression. Part of the inconsistency lies in differences in study design and sampling methodology. Part also derives from differences in how obesity is defined and the failure to have adequate controls in statistical analyses. A major difficulty with the current literature is that so little is known about the emergence of the association between obesity and depression, owing to the fact that there are very few studies of children under the age of seven and to the fact that most studies are cross-sectional or do not have measures of both BMI and depression at all data points. There is little to suggest a significant association between obesity and depression prior to middle childhood as the presumed mechanisms linking the two would not likely be operative in young children. Making comparisons between one's own body and either idealized images or the bodies of others is the presumed connection between obesity and low self-esteem; and there are studies showing that once body image is accounted for the relation between obesity and depression is non-significant (Goodman & Whitaker, 2002). Harter (2006) argues that the ability to make such social comparisons for the purpose of self-evaluation does not seriously emerge until middle childhood.

There is little to suggest the internalizing problems would contribute to adiposity in children prior to adolescence. The only three studies suggestive of a causal effect in that direction had significant technical flaws. The Goodman and Whitaker (2002) study did not control for earlier BMI, and the Pine et al. (2001) and Christoffel and Forsyth (1989) studies involved clinical samples that were extreme either for internalizing problems or weight. In a fourth study of the impact of depression on obesity, there was no consistent relation between adolescent depression and adult obesity (Pine, Cohen, Brook, & Coplan, 1997) and in a fifth there was no relation at all (Tanofsky-Kraff et al., 2006).

In sum, there is little to suggest that internalizing problems and obesity will be consistently related prior to middle childhood. The evidence indicative of direction of causality is somewhat equivocal, but with theory and some evidence suggesting that being obese is more likely to lead to internalizing problems than the reverse except perhaps when children are chronically and extremely obese. For example, depression and mood disorders are relatively common in patients who seek treatment for obesity (McElroy et al., 2004). The likely impact of early anxiety and stressful life events on these patterns is difficult to predict. Both may directly contribute to weight gain (Haas, et al., 2003; Mustillo et al., 2003); but it's not clear whether the relation between internalizing problems and adiposity would change as a function of either.

The current study was designed to advance inquiry into the interrelation of adiposity and internalizing problems using data from the NICHD Study of Early Child Care and Youth Development (Nader, et al., 2006). The first goal of this study was to determine whether lagged relations exist between BMI and internalizing problems, either in the form of earlier BMI predicting to later internalizing problems or in the form of earlier internalizing problems predicting to later BMI, after taking into consideration the stability in both BMI and internalizing problems. In addition, we sought to determine whether such lagged relations might be moderated by child gender, infant negative emotionality, or life instability. The question of whether relations between body mass index and adaptive functioning are different for males and females is one of long standing (French et al., 1995). Although research on the question provides mixed evidence, it seemed important to examine the possibility that the lagged relations were different for boys and girls. Somewhat by contrast, there is both empirical and theoretical support for the proposition that overweight children who score high in negative emotionality might be more strongly affected by adverse social feedback that often occurs as a consequence of being heavy (Belsky, 2005; Boyce & Ellis, 2005). The case for the moderating role of life instability is a little less clear, but appears worth pursuing. There is evidence that family instability is associated with internalizing problems in children and that negative life events induce depressive cognitions (Adam & Chase-Lansdale, 2002; Bruce, et al., 2006; Milan & Pinderhughes, 2006). Unstable family circumstances both increase felt insecurity about the family and reduce the likelihood of maintaining important supportive relationships (Forman & Davies, 2003). The loss of a sense of predictability, control, and social support may well make it more difficult to contain physiological stress responses that derive from poor body image and negative social feedback (Adam, 2004). In such circumstances, overweight children might be at advanced risk of succumbing to internalizing problems. For purposes of this study, life instability was indexed in terms of changes in household composition, changes in residence, changes in childcare arrangements, changes in school, and changes in parental employment status.

FAMILIES PARTICIPATING IN THE NICHD STUDY

Participants were a subset of the families in the NICHD Study of Early Child Care and Youth Development. Families in the study were recruited during the first 11 months of 1991 from 24 hospitals in the vicinity of 10 data collection sites (Charlottesville, VA; Irvine, CA; Lawrence, KS; Little Rock, AR; Madison, WI; Morganton, NC; Philadelphia, PA; Pittsburgh, PA; Seattle, WA; and Wellesley, MA). A total of 8,986 women who gave birth during selected 24-hour periods and their infants were screened in the hospital for participation in the study.

Mother-newborn dyads were excluded from the study if: the mother was under 18 years old, did not speak English, had known or acknowledged substance abuse, was too ill to participate, was placing her infant for adoption, or refused the hospital screening interview or a follow-up telephone call two weeks later; if the infant had serious medical complications or was a multiple birth; or if the family lived more than an hour's drive from the lab site, planned to move from the area within one year, lived in a neighborhood deemed by police too unsafe for visitation, or was enrolled in another study. A total of 5,416 families met the eligibility criteria. Study participants were selected from among eligible families based on conditionally random sampling to insure that the sample would include at least 10 percent single-parent households, 10 percent mothers with less than a high school education, and 10 percent ethnic minority mothers. Recruitment and selection procedures are described in detail in previous study publications (e.g., NICHD Early Child Care Research Network [ECCRN], 1997) and on the study Web site (http://secc.rti.org).

A total of 1,364 families with healthy newborns were ultimately enrolled in the study, with approximately equal numbers of families at each site. The study sample was demographically similar to the population of families with young infants in the communities from which it was recruited.

Analysis Sample

The analysis sample for the current study consisted of 1254 children ($n = 608$ girls; $n= 646$ boys). Children were included in these analyses if they participated any of the study's repeated assessments of body mass index (BMI) or internalizing problems (see below). In the analysis sample, mothers had completed an average of 14.33 years of education and were living with a spouse or partner an average of 82.5 percent of measurement occasions from the time the child was six months of age until the child was in sixth grade. Their average family income, assessed in terms of income-to-needs averaged from the period six months to sixth grade, was higher than the U.S. government-determined poverty line by a factor of 3.91. The participants differed in several ways from the 110 children who were recruited at birth but not included in this analysis due to a total absence of data on BMI and Internalizing Problems. Children were more likely to be white than minority (77.5% vs. 63.6%, $p < 0.001$); mothers of participants had more education (M = 14.33 vs. 13.08, $p < 0.0001$), higher income-to-needs (M = 3.91 vs. 2.34, $p < 0.0001$) and lived with a husband or partner a greater proportion of the time (M = 83.5% vs. 65.9%, $p < 0.0001$).

PROCEDURES FOR THE LONGITUDINAL STUDY

The children in the study were followed from birth through age 14 ½. Families were visited at home when the children were 1, 6, 15, 24, 36, and

54 months of age, and when they were in firstthirdfifth, sixth grades. At each home visit, mothers responded to a demographic interview and completed questionnaires about themselves, the child, and their family, and children were observed in interaction with one or both parents. Mothers and children also came to university laboratories when the children were 15, 24, 36, and 54 months old, and again during first, third, fourth, fifth, and sixth grades. At these visits the children completed various standardized assessments and developmental tasks and were observed during play and interaction with their mothers. Beginning when they were approximately 9 ½ years old, children received an annual health and physical development assessment from a nurse practitioner or physician. Between visits, data were obtained using periodic telephone interviews and questionnaires (see below for schedule).

Measures Drawn from the NICHD Longitudinal Study

This section describes the specific measures used in this study. Additional details about all data collection procedures and measures are documented in the study's Manuals of Operation, which are available on the study Web site, http://secc.rti.org.

Body Mass Index (BMI): Height and Weight

Standardized procedures were used to measure height and weight at 24, 36, and 54 months, and at 7, 9, 11 and 12 years. Height was measured with children standing with shoes off, feet together, and their backs to a calibrated 7-foot measuring stick fastened to a wall. Children were asked to stand straight and tall, while a research assistant lowered a level T-square to rest on the top of the child's head to read the height value. Height was measured to the nearest eighth of an inch (0.32 cm) and recorded two times. If the first two height measures differed by more than a quarter of an inch (0.64 cm), two more height measurements were taken. Weight was measured using a physician's 2-beam scale. Scales were calibrated monthly using certified calibration weights. Weight was measured with children in minimal clothing (i.e., no shoes, no outer layers of clothing and other items that could add weight such as belts, keys, or watches). As with height, weight was measured twice, each time to the nearest quarter pound (0.1 kg). If the two weight measurements differed by more than four ounces, two more measurements were taken. BMI was calculated by converting height from inches to meters and weight from pounds to kilograms, and then dividing weight by height squared.

Internalizing Behavior Problems

Mothers completed the Child Behavior Checklist (CBCL) at 24, 36, and 54 months and again at first, third, fifth, and sixth grades. The CBCL-2/3 (Achenbach, 1992), used at 24 and 36 months, lists 99 problem behaviors, which the mother rated as not true (0), somewhat true (1), or very true (2) of her child over the previous two months. The CBCL-4/18 (Achenbach, 1991), completed by mothers at 54 months and first, third, fifth, and sixth grades, lists 113 problem behaviors rated on the same three-point scale. Scores on the Internalizing Problems subscale (e.g., "Too fearful and anxious") were converted to T-scores, based on normative data for children of the same age. Correlations across adjacent time points ranged from 0.54 to 0.64.

Gender

During home interviews at one month, mothers reported the study children's sex.

Negative Emotionality

Negative emotionality was operationalized as the mean level of observed infant distress during the three separation episodes of the Strange Situation administered at 15 months of age (Ainsworth, Blehar, Waters & Wall, 1978; NICHD ECCRN, 1997). Distress during each episode was rated on a 5-point scale, with a rating of 1 reflecting no overt distress (and no attenuation of the child's exploration) and a rating of 5 reflecting immediate, high distress resulting in termination of the separation. Cronbach's alpha for the composite score was 0.83.

Life Instability

Children's life instability was calculated as the number of changes in life circumstances a child experienced between 3 months and sixth grade (across the entire BMI/Internalizing data collection range). Areas included in the instability index included (1) changes in maternal and paternal employment status, (2) changes in residence, (3) changes in household composition, (4) changes in the type of child care a child experienced between 3 and 54 months, (5) changes in the amount of child care a child experience between 3 and 54 months, and (6) changes in schools within a school year (from Kindergarten through sixth grade). Each of these is explained in more detail below.

Changes in Maternal and Paternal Employment Status

At 3, 6, 9, 12, 15, 24, 36, 42, 46, 50, 54 months, fall kindergarten, spring first grade, fall and spring second grade, and in third, fourth, fifth, and sixth grades, mothers reported whether they and their husband or partner were employed outside of the home. Each change in maternal or paternal employment status from one time period to the next (i.e., from either employed to not employed or vice versa) resulted in one point added to the instability index. If a time period was missing, the comparison was made to the next time point with available data.

Changes in Residence

Each time a family in the study changed residences, information regarding when the move happened was recoded into a separate database. The number of moves a family experienced prior to the child's sixth grade assessment (age 11.5 for Wave 1 children, age 12 for Wave 2 children) was included in the instability index.

Changes in Household Composition

Data on changes in household composition were gathered via maternal interview at 3 month intervals between 3 and 36 months, at 4-month intervals between 42 and 54 months and at 6-month intervals between kindergarten and second grade and at yearly intervals between third and sixth grade. A child received one point on the instability index for each time someone moved into or out of the household.

Changes in the Type and Amount of Child Care

Data on type and hours of child care were gathered via maternal report at 3-month intervals between 3 and 36 months and at 4-month intervals between 42 and 54 months of age. If a child changed type of care (i.e., exclusive maternal, father care, grandparent care, in-home care, family day home, center care) from one reporting period to the next (either into or out of a particular type), the child received one point on the instability index. Additionally, if the total hours of non-maternal care changed by more than 10 hours per week (either up or down) the child received one point on the instability index. As with changes in maternal and paternal employment status, if a time period was missing data, the comparison was made to the next time point with available data.

Changes in Schools within a School Year

For each school year (kindergarten through sixth grade) mothers reported the number of schools a child attended. For each school greater than one, a child received one point on the instability index.

Statistical Methods Used to Analyze the Data

Descriptive Statistics

Sample description was completed by calculating means, standard deviations, and frequencies as appropriate. Independent sample t-tests and chi-square tests were conducted to determine how those included in the analysis sample differed from those who were lost to attrition.

Primary Analysis

The primary analysis model involved a cross-lagged structural equation model tested using AMOS 4.01 (Arbuckle & Wothke, 1995–1999). AMOS uses full information maximum likelihood (FIML) of missing data and utilizes the maximum sample size for each pathway to be estimated without deletion or imputation (Arbuckle & Wothke, 1995–1999).

The original model included stability coefficients between the various measurements of BMI and the various measurements for Internalizing; additionally, cross-lagged paths were included from one measurement of BMI to the next measurement of Internalizing and vice versa (see figure 4.1).

We tested a series of nested models in an attempt to discern the most parsimonious model that adequately fit the data. In each case, chi-square difference tests were completed to determine whether the imposed model constraints significantly influenced model fit. In trimming the initial model, we examined the following: (1) whether the model required cross-lags from BMI to Internalizing; (2) whether the model required cross-lags from Internalizing to BMI; and (3) whether required cross-lags could be constrained to particular time periods (i.e., preschool and/or elementary).

Once the baseline model was finalized, we tested three moderators (gender, negative emotionality, and life instability) one at a time via a series of multi-group models. Chi-square difference tests were completed to determine how close the models for the two groups could be made without incurring a significant detriment to model fit. For negative emotionality, two groups were formed via a median split (low emotionality,

Figure 4.1
Original Cross-Lagged Model Relating BMI and Internalizing

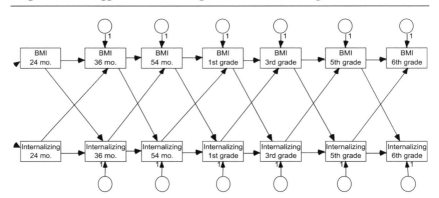

$n = 560$; high emotionality, $n = 612$); for life instability, the sample was split into tertiles and comparisons were made between those in the upper ($n = 451$) and lower tertile ($n = 365$).

What did We Find?

Sample descriptives are presented in table 4.1; correlations between BMI and internalizing behavior at the various ages are presented in table 4.2. The sample was predominantly white. Mothers had, on average, more than a high school education and were partnered an average of 83% of the time when children were between the ages of 6 months and sixth grade. Families had income-to-needs ratios that were almost four times above the U.S. government-determined poverty line.

Families varied considerably on the number of instability incidents they experienced with an average 18.5 occurring between the time children were 3 months old and their sixth grade assessment. Children's average BMI declined between 24 and 54 months, before rising steadily between 54 months and sixth grade. Average internalizing scores reached a high of 51.2 when children were 36 months old and a low of 47.3 when children were 54 months old.

As the correlations in table 4.2 show, BMI was highly stable beginning at age two. Correlations between adjacent assessments were typically in the 0.8 to 0.9 range; and the correlation between BMI at 24 months and BMI in sixth grade was moderate ($r = .42$). Internalizing behavior was relatively stable as well. Correlations between scores at adjacent time periods were typically in the 0.5 to 0.6 range; and even the correlation

Table 4.1
Sample characteristics and descriptive statistics for primary analysis variables

Description of Sample	N	Mean	SD
Mother's Education	1254	14.33	2.50
% Partner in Home (6mo – G6)	1254	0.83	0.29
Income-to-Needs (6mo – G6)	1251	3.91	3.03
Ethnicity (% white)	1254	77.51	NA
Gender (% male)	1254	51.52	NA
Family Instability (3mo – G6)	1254	18.54	11.13
Body Mass Index			
24mo	991	16.77	1.37
36mo	1087	16.16	1.31
54mo	1031	16.05	1.56
Grade 1	990	16.82	2.55
Grade 3	931	18.39	3.70
Grade 5	913	20.00	4.64
Grade 6	899	20.80	4.86
Internalizing Problems (T-score)			
24mo	1189	50.27	9.26
36mo	1175	51.21	9.50
54mo	1061	47.29	8.88
Grade 1	1028	48.27	8.94
Grade 3	1026	48.43	9.90
Grade 5	1017	48.74	9.78
Grade 6	1022	47.72	9.99

between internalizing reported at age 2 and sixth grade was significant ($r = .25$). By contrast, correlations between BMI and internalizing were non-significant from age 24 months through first grade. Correlations between BMI and internalizing behavior during middle childhood (grades 3 to 6) were significant but low (never higher than $r = .14$). There were also some instances of significant low correlations between BMI in early childhood and internalizing in middle childhood (all $< .10$). The correlations between internalizing at first grade and BMI at fifth and sixth grades was also significant ($r = 0.10$ and 0.09 respectively).

Table 4.2
Correlations between BMI and internalizing problems.

Stability of BMI

	BMI					
	36mo	54mo	G1	G3	G5	G6
BMI (24mo)	0.82	0.66	0.52	0.43	0.40	0.42
BMI (36mo)	--	0.79	0.64	0.55	0.51	0.51
BMI (54mo)	--	--	0.83	0.75	0.71	0.70
BMI (Grade 1)	--	--	--	0.92	0.87	0.85
BMI (Grade 3)	--	--	--	--	0.94	0.93
BMI (Grade 5)	--	--	--	--	--	0.97

Stability of Internalizing Problems

	Internalizing Problems					
	36mo	54mo	G1	G3	G5	G6
Int (24mo)	0.65	0.46	0.35	0.32	0.30	0.25
Int (36mo)	--	0.54	0.44	0.39	0.35	0.32
Int (54mo)	--	--	0.57	0.51	0.48	0.41
Int (Grade 1)	--	--	--	0.63	0.63	0.57
Int (Grade 3)	--	--	--	--	0.67	0.63
Int (Grade 5)	--	--	--	--	--	0.73

BMI & Internalizing Problems

	BMI						
	24mo	36mo	54mo	G1	G3	G5	G6
Int (24mo)	.02	.05	.03	.02	.02	.04	.03
Int (36mo)	.04	.06	.01	.03	.04	.08	.08
Int (54mo)	.05	.05	.04	.03	.02	.06	.09
Int (G1)		.02	.03	.05	.05	.05	.06	.11
Int (G3)		.03	.00	.05	.05	.07	.07	.13
Int (G5)		.07	.02	.06	.10	.08	.10	.14
Int (G6)		.05	.03	.06	.09	.09	.12	.16

Refining the Baseline Model

The baseline model was tested to determine which cross-paths were needed for adequate model fit. When constraining the cross-paths from internalizing to BMI to be zero, no detriment to model fit was noted,

χ^2 (6, n = 1254) = 7.65, p = 0.27. However, when constraining the cross-paths from BMI to internalizing to be zero, model fit declined significantly, χ^2 (6, n = 1254) = 18.11, p = 0.01, indicating that, as a set, the paths from BMI to internalizing could not be omitted from the model (see figure 4.2).

Next, we tested whether we could restrict the BMI to internalizing cross-lags to only the preschool period (i.e., 24 to 36 months; 36 to 54 months, 54 months to first grade) or to only the elementary period (i.e., first to third grade; third to fifth grade, and fifth to sixth grade). Constraining the BMI to internalizing cross-paths to just the preschool period led to a significant decline in model fit, χ^2 (3, 1254) = 14.13, p = 0.003, but constraining the cross-paths to just the elementary period did not lead to a decline in model fit χ^2 (3, 1254) = 4.16, p = 0.24. Thus, the model needed cross-paths from BMI to internalizing, but not from internalizing to BMI. Furthermore, we could restrict the BMI-to-internalizing paths to only the elementary period without any detriment to overall model fit. In the final model, standardized stability coefficients for BMI ranged from 0.81 to 0.97 (p < 0.001), standardized stability coefficients for internalizing ranged from 0.55 to 0.72 (p < 0.001), paths from BMI to internalizing were significant between third and fifth grade (0.05, p < 0.05) and between fifth and sixth grade (0.07, p < 0.01), but not between first and third grade (0.02, p = 0.40).

In overview, having more internalizing problems at any point during early and middle childhood did not increase the likelihood of subsequent internalizing problems. However, being heavier was associated with later increases in internalizing problems, even accounting for the stability of internalizing problems.

Figure 4.2
Final Cross-Lagged Model Relating BMI and Internalizing

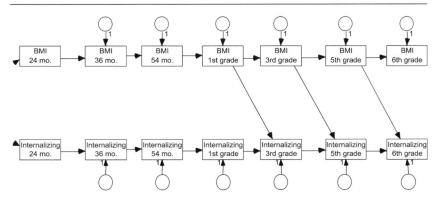

Testing Moderators

Once the baseline model was pared down to a more parsimonious model we began testing whether our three moderators influenced the remaining cross-paths of the model. We initially allowed other parameters to vary as a function of the moderator (e.g., means and intercepts, stability paths, error variances) when testing whether the cross-paths could be constrained to be equal. In all cases, adding constraints requiring the cross paths to be equal in the two groups under study did not significantly effect model fit [Gender: χ^2 (3, n = 1254) = 0.61, p = 0.90); negative emotionality: χ^2(3, n = 1172) = 1.35, p = 0.72; life instability, 3 months—sixth grade: χ^2 (3, n = 816) = 3.57, p = 0.31]. When additional constraints for various portions of the model were added (e.g., constraining means to be the same in the two groups), results regarding the cross-paths did not change.

MEANING OF THESE ANALYSES

Like a number of other prospective studies of children's growth, we found BMI to be highly stable during early and middle childhood (Harter, 2006; Wardle, Brodersen, Cole, Jarvis, & Boniface, 2006). Mother-reported internalizing behavior was also quite stable within and across these two periods. Although we found evidence that BMI and internalizing were related, the findings suggest minimal association prior to age seven. This finding is not surprising in that the social-cognitive processes that are presumed to forge the connection (feelings of stigmatization, social comparisons, dissatisfaction with body image) remain undeveloped in most children prior to school entry (Harter, 2006). Nonetheless, those children who are extremely obese may begin the process slightly earlier as a function of experiencing lots of negative feedback, but the majority of children who are overweight are less likely to. However, once children reach middle childhood, the alliance between BMI and internalizing behavior appears to strengthen, as would be expected on account of the fact that children's capacities for self-evaluation and making social comparisons increase. That said, the findings do not indicate a strong connection between BMI and internalizing. As has been shown in other studies, the majority of overweight children do not suffer from depression and serious mood disorders (McElroy et al., 2004; Mustillo et al., 2003; Sheslow et al., 1993).

Somewhat contrary to expectations, some of the simple bivariate correlations between early BMI and later internalizing were significant; likewise, the correlations between first grade internalizing and later BMI (fifth and sixth grades) were significant. What might account for these apparent lagged relations? The most likely explanation is the high stabilities in both variables. Because BMI at 36 and 54 months is highly correlated with BMI at fifth and sixth grades and the latter is correlated with internalizing at fifth and sixth grades, these latter correlations effectively carried the former. Had we looked for a relation between early BMI and later internalizing, the partials would have almost certainly been non-significant. The same situation applies to the observed lagged association between first grade internalizing and BMI at fifth and sixth grades. The absence of significant correlations with the intervening assessments is telling in this regard. There is no theory that supports such lagged associations; that is, no reasonable arguments for the kinds of mechanisms that would need to be operative. These findings point to what may well be a quite significant problem with much of the existing literature; namely, most studies do not control for account for contemporaneous relations between BMI and internalizing when trying to estimate prediction from early time points to later time points. Potentially, this is a quite significant limitation given the high stability of both.

Although the association between BMI and internalizing appears relatively weak in middle childhood, findings from this study are consistent with research suggesting that being obese can lead to depression and other forms of internalizing behavior (Braet et al, 1997; French et al., 1995; Friedman & Brownell, 1995; Mustillo et al., 2003; Strauss, 2000; Zametkin et al., 2004). The SEM analyses showed significant lagged associations between BMI at third grade and internalizing at fifth grade and between BMI at fifth grade and internalizing at sixth grade.

By contrast, there was no support for the hypothesis that internalizing behavior contributes to being overweight. To date, there is no convincing support that being somewhat depressed increases the likelihood of becoming overweight. There is a small amount of evidence suggesting that serious depression might increase such a tendency, but no general population studies have provided evidence for such an effect. The only study that showed a link between earlier depression and later obesity in children who did present for clinical treatment failed to control for earlier BMI, so the findings remain suspect (Goodman & Whitaker, 2002).

Because the relation between BMI and internalizing is quite modest, it was not surprising that neither negative emotionality nor life instability served to moderate the relation. Neither was there any evidence for a gender effect. The multiple group comparisons done for each of these moderators showed no evidence that they played a significant role in the relation. In sum, there appears to be a small, but meaningful, relation between BMI and internalizing behavior that begins in middle childhood, a time when self-evaluations and social comparisons begin to have a meaningful impact on children's moods and self-attributions. Being overweight appears to increase the likelihood of having negative self-attributions and, thus, internalizing problems. In the United States, the process appears to operate more or less the same for all children, irrespective of whether they are male or female, manifested high or low levels of negative emotionality as infants, or experienced many or few life changes during early and middle childhood. However, there were too few children from most socio-cultural groups in the NICHD SECCYD to conduct subgroup analyses, so it would be worthwhile to perform analyses similar to those done in this study on minority populations within the United States as well as samples drawn from other countries.

Thus, we find that BMI and internalizing are very stable between 24 months and sixth grade; BMI leads to internalizing, starting at the third to fifth grade lag and that the magnitude of the connections between BMI and internalizing are not moderated by gender, early negative emotionality or life instability.

ACKNOWLEDGMENTS

The NICHD Study of Early Child Care and Youth Development was funded under cooperative agreement with the National Institute of Child Health and Human Development (U.S. Department of Health & Human Services).

Members of the steering committee for the study include (in alphabetic order): Jay Belsky (Birbeck College, University of London), Cathryn Booth-LaForce (University of Washington), Robert Bradley (University of Arkansas at Little Rock), Celia Brownell (University of Pittsburgh), Peg Burchinal (University of North Carolina, Chapel Hill), Elizabeth Cauffman (University of California, Irvine), Martha Cox (University of North Carolina, Chapel Hill), Robert Crosnoe (University of Texas at Austin), Sarah Friedman (NICHD project scientist), Bonnie Halpern-Fisher (University of California, San Francisco), Willard Hartup (University of Minnesota), Kathryn Hirsh-Pasek (Temple University), Aletha Huston (University of Texas at Austin), Daniel Keating (University of Michigan), Bonnie Knoke (RTI International), Tama Levanthal (Johns Hopkins University), Kathleen McCartney (Harvard University), Vonnie McLoyd (University of North Carolina, Chapel Hill), Fred Morrison (University of Michigan), Philip Nader (University of California, San Diego), Marion O'Brien (University of North Carolina, Greensboro), Margaret Tresh Owen (University of Texas at Dallas), Ross Parke (University of California, Riverside), Robert Pianta (University of Virginia), Kim Pierce (University of Wisconsin), Vijaya Rao (RTI International), Glenn Roisman (University of Illinois at Champaign-Urbana), Susan Spieker (University of Washington), Laurence Steinberg (Temple University), Elizabeth Susman (Pennsylvania State University), Deborah Vandell (University of California, Irvine), and Marsha Weinraub (Temple University).

REFERENCES

Achenbach, T. M. (1991). *Manual for the Child Behavior Checklist/ 4–18 and 1991 Profile.* Burlington: University of Vermont Department of Psychiatry.

Achenbach, T. M. (1992). *Manual for the Child Behavior Checklist/ 2–3 and 1992 Profile.* Burlington: University of Vermont Department of Psychiatry.

Adam, E. K. (2004). Beyond quality: Parental and residential stability and children's adjustment. *Current Directions in Psychological Sciences, 13,* 210–213.

Adam, E. K., & Chase-Lansdale, L. (2002). Home sweet home(s): Parental separations, residential moves, and adjustment problems in low-income adolescent girls. *Developmental Psychology, 38,* 792–805.

Agras, W., Hammer, L., McNicholas, R., & Kraemer, H. (2004). Risk factors for childhood overweight: A prospective study from birth to 9.5 years. *Journal of Pediatrics, 145,* 20–25.

Ainsworth, M. D., Blehar, M. , Waters, E., & Wall, S. (1978). *Patterns of attachment: A psychological study of the strange situation.* Hillsdale, NJ: Erlbaum.

Arbuckle, J. L., & Wothke, W. (1995–1999). *Amos 4.0 User's Guide.* Chicago: SmallWaters Corporation.

Belsky, J. (2005). Differential susceptibility to rearing influence. In B. J. Ellis & D. F. Bjorklund (Eds.), *Origins of the social mind: Evolutionary psychology and child development* (pp. 139–163). New York: Guilford Press.

Boyce, W. T., & Ellis, B. J. (2005). Biological sensitivity to context. *Development and Psychopathology, 17,* 271–301

Braet, C., Mervielde, I., & Vandereycken, W. (1997). Psychological aspects of childhood obesity: A controlled study in a clinical and nonclinical sample. *Journal of Pediatric Psychology, 22,* 59–71.

Bruce, A. E., Cole, D. A., Dallaire, D. H., Jacquez, F. M., Pineda, A. Q., & La-Grange, B. (2006). Relations of parenting and negative life events to cognitive diatheses for depression in children. *Journal of Abnormal Child Psychology, 34,* 321–333.

Christoffel, K. K., & Forsyth, B. W. (1989). Mirror image of environmental deprivation: Severe childhood obesity of psychosocial origin. *Child Abuse and Neglect, 13,* 246–256.

Davison, K. K., & Birch, L. L. (2002). Processes linking weight status and self-concept among girls from age 5 to 7 years. *Developmental Psychology, 38,* 735–748.

Forman, E. M., & Davies, P. T. (2003). Family instability and young adolescent maladjustment: The mediating effects of parenting quality and adolescent appraisals of family security. *Journal of Clinical Child and Adolescent Psychology, 32,* 94–105.

French, S. A., Story, M., & Perry, C. L. (1995). Self-esteem in children and adolescents: A literature review. *Obesity Research, 3,* 479–490.

Friedman, M. A., & Brownell, K. D. (1995). Psychological correlates of obesity: Moving to the next research generation. *Psychological Bulletin, 117,* 3–20.

Goodman, E., & Whitaker, R. C. (2002). A prospective study of the role of depression in the development and persistence of adolescent obesity. *Pediatrics, 109,* 497–504.

Haas, J. S., Lee, L. B., Kaplan, C. P., Sonneborn, D., Phillips, K. A., & Liang, S. (2003). The association of race, socioeconomic status, and health insurance status with the prevalence of overweight among children and adolescents. *American Journal of Public Health, 93,* 2105–2110.

Harrison, K. (2001). Ourselves, our bodies: Thin-ideal media, self-discrepancies, and eating disorder symptomatology in adolescents. *Journal of Social and Clinical Psychology, 20,* 289–323.

Harter, S. (2006). Developmental and individual difference perspectives on self-esteem. In D. K. Mroczek & T. D. Little (Eds.), *Handbook of personality development* (pp. 311–334). Mahwah, NJ: Erlbaum.

Manus, H. E., & Killeen, M. R. (1995). Maintenance of self-esteem by obese children. *Journal of Child & Adolescent Psychiatric Nursing, 8,* 117–27.

McElroy, S. L., Kotwal, R., Malhotra, S., Nelson, E. B., Keck, P. E., & Nermeroff, C. B. (2004). Are mood disorders and obesity related? A review for the mental health professional. *Journal of Clinical Psychiatry, 65,* 634–651.

Milan, S., & Pinderhughes, E. E. (2006). Family instability and child maladjustment trajectories during elementary school. *Journal of Abnormal Child Psychology, 34,* 43–56.

Mustillo, S., Wortham, C., Erkanli, A., Keeler, G., Angoold, A., & Costello, E. J. (2003). Obesity and psychiatric disorder: Developmental trajectories. *Pediatrics, 11,* 851–859.

Nader, P. R., O'Brien, M., Houts, R., Bradley, R., Belsky, J., Crosnoe, R., et al. (2006). Identifying risk for obesity in early childhood. *Pediatrics, 118*(3), e1–e8.

NICHD Early Child Care Research Network. (1997). The effects of infant child care on infant-mother attachment security: Results of the NICHD Study of Early Child Care. *Child Development, 68,* 860–879.

Pine, D. S., Cohen, P., Brook, J., & Coplan, J. (1997). Psychiatric symptoms in adolescence as predictors of obesity in early adulthood: A longitudinal study. *American Journal of Public Health, 56,* 573–579.

Pine, D. S., Goldstein, R. B., Wolk, S., & Weissman, M. M. (2001). The association between childhood depression and adult body mass index. *Pediatrics, 107,* 1049–1056.

Sheslow, D., Wallace, W., & DeLancey, E. (1993). The relationship between self-esteem and depression in obese children. *Annals of the New York Academy of Sciences, 699,* 289–291.

Strauss, R. (2000). Childhood obesity and self-esteem. *Pediatrics, 105,* e15.

Tanofsky-Kraff, M., Cohen, M. L., Yavonvski, S. Z., Cox, C., Theim, K. R., Keil, M., et al. (2006). A prospective study of psychological predictors of body fat gain among children at high risk for adult obesity. *Pediatrics, 117,* 1203–1209.

Wardle, J., Brodersen, N., Cole, T., Jarvis, M. & Boniface, D. (2006). Development of adiposity in adolescence: Five year longitudinal study of an ethnically and socioeconomically diverse sample in Britain. *BMJ, 332*(7550).

Young-Hyman, D., Schlundt, D. Herman-Wenderoth, L., & Bozylinski, K. (2003). Obesity, appearance, and psychosocial adaptation in young African American children. *Journal of Pediatric Psychology, 28,* 463–472.

Zametkin, A. J., Zoon, C., Klein, H., & Munson, S. (2004). Psychiatric aspects of child and adolescent obesity: A review of the past 10 years. *Journal of the American Academy of Child and Adolescent Psychiatry, 43,* 134–150.

Chapter 5

FOOD MARKETING GOES ONLINE: A CONTENT ANALYSIS OF WEB SITES FOR CHILDREN

Elizabeth S. Moore

Childhood obesity is a serious public health problem. Among preschool children (ages 2–5) in the United States, obesity rates have more than doubled over the last three decades, and they have more than tripled among children ages 6–11 (Ogden et al., 2006; Ogden, Flegal, Carroll, & Johnson, 2002). This problem has attracted the attention of policymakers, consumer interest groups, health professionals, and industry leaders. Particular questions are being raised about the impacts of food marketing. Two comprehensive studies have been published, one by the Institute of Medicine (IOM) in the United States, and another by the Food Standards Agency (FSA) in the United Kingdom that try to assess marketing's contribution to obesity (Hastings et al., 2003; IOM, 2005). In its analysis, the IOM concluded that exposure to advertising influences key dietary precursors including children's (ages 2–11) food-related beliefs, preferences, purchase requests, and choices. Correlational evidence also links advertising exposure and children's adiposity although a causal relationship has not been established.

Both the IOM and FSA reviews focus on the impacts of television advertising because this has been the research emphasis over time. Advergaming or advertising embedded in commercial computer games and on Web sites for children is becoming more prevalent, and is cause for concern among some consumer advocates and government officials.

The author thanks Victoria J. Rideout for her many thoughtful contributions to this project.

Calls for an assessment of online marketing to children have come from groups representing diverse interests including Congressional leaders, the Center for Science in the Public Interest (CSPI), the National Advertising Review Council (NARC), and the IOM (see e.g., Harkin in FTC, 2005; IOM, 2006; NARC, 2005). To this point these groups have had to rely primarily on anecdotal evidence. The study reported in this chapter was designed to inform decision makers about the nature and scope of online food marketing that targets children.

BACKGROUND

Articles appearing in the business press typically assume that advergames are a common feature of Web sites for children. These advertiser-sponsored video games embed selling messages, and are created by a firm for the explicit purpose of promoting one or more of its brands. Children appear to be willing consumers of these marketing communications. Approximately 64 percent of American children (ages 5–14) who access the Internet do so to play games (U.S. Dept. of Education, 2003). More than 13.1 million children ages 2 to 11 use the Internet, and their numbers are increasing rapidly (Larson, 2004). Nielsen/Net Ratings reported that usage among this age group increased 34 percent in October 2005 over the same time period the year before (Goetzl, 2006). Even very young children are participants. Sixty-six percent of 4-to 6-year-olds live in homes with Internet access, 56 percent can use the computer by themselves, and 30 percent have visited a Web site for children (Rideout, Vandewater, & Wartella, 2003). Recent studies also suggest that new media are supplementing rather than displacing TV viewing (Roberts, Foehr, & Rideout, 2005).

When a child is exposed to food advertising online, it is a different type of exposure than what he or she experiences via television or print media. Children's Web sites are designed to be playful and involving, with brand immersion as a key objective (Ferrazzi & Benezra, 2001). On the Internet, children have to actively seek out desired content rather than being passively exposed to it. Online marketing provides the opportunity for advertisers to interact with children for several minutes, rather than capturing their attention for only 30 seconds. Estimates suggest that visitors spend an average of 25 minutes on a gaming site (e.g., Bertrim, 2005; Fattah & Paul, 2002).[1]

The fact that marketing messages may be embedded in an advergame or other Web site activity also has the effect of blurring the lines between advertising and entertainment (Montgomery, 2001; Moore,

2004). Marketing practitioners have suggested that inserting ads in entertainment can be an effective way to reduce children's skepticism, and create more openness to a brand message (Lindstrom & Seybold, 2003). Thus online advertising can be more covert, with the intentions of the marketer less immediately apparent to a young audience.

Children's capacity to understand and to resist commercial messages may be particularly taxed on these Web sites (Moore, 2004; Moses & Baldwin, 2005). Even in traditional media, young children are readily persuaded because they do not yet possess the cognitive skills needed to fully evaluate advertising messages (see John, 1999 for a review). Although policy makers have raised questions about advergaming Web sites, until recently there has been very little empirical evidence to inform their decision making. With more and more children gravitating to the Internet, greater insight into the nature and impacts of these Web sites is needed.

In this chapter, key results from the first systematic study of the content of online food marketing to children are presented. Topics such as advergaming, viral marketing, nutritional information, media tie-ins, sales promotions, and direct purchase inducements are addressed (a more detailed report of study findings can be found in Moore, 2006).

RESEARCH METHOD

A content analysis of major food advertisers' Web sites (e.g., Master Foods' skittles.com; Wrigley's juicyfruit.com) was conducted in the summer and fall of 2005. This observational research method is used to scientifically analyze message content, and has been applied to a range of social science topics, including advertising (e.g., Alexander, Benjamin, Hoerrner, & Roe, 1998; Maher & Childs, 2003). This observational method also produces an analysis that is objective and quantifiable (Kassarjian, 1977; Kolbe & Burnett, 1991). A number of systematic steps were taken to identify study brands, and to locate relevant Web sites.

Selection of Brands and Web Sites

Researchers identified the top food brands advertised to children on TV, and then searched for corporate or brand Web sites for those products.[2] The food brands with the largest TV advertising expenditures targeted at children were identified through Competitive Media Reports (CMR) data. Any child-oriented brand that was in the top 80 percent of advertising spending in its product category was included: a total of 96 brands were identified.[3] Web sites for these brands were included in the study if they had content for children ages 12 and under. In most cases, these were sites whose primary audience was children; in some cases, the primary audience appeared to be either teens or all ages, with content or separate sections likely to appeal to children. Only Web sites sponsored by a food manufacturer were included in the study; food ads appearing on sites such as Nick.com or Neopets.com were excluded. A total of 77 unique Web sites were identified through this procedure (list available from the author). Because some sites contained multiple study brands, and some brands appeared on multiple sites, the final sample included a total of 107 brand and site pairs.

Data Analysis

Study Web sites were independently coded by two judges. Each of five judges received approximately 20 hours of training to code Web sites that were similar to, but outside the research sample. Coders were given detailed written instructions as part of the training process. After a preliminary site was coded, judges were brought together to review question definitions, and resolve disagreements. Through this process, a satisfactory level of preliminary agreement was achieved among each pair of coders. Once the training process was complete, two coders were randomly assigned to each site. All pages of the Web sites were coded, totaling over 4,000 unique pages including games.[4] Screenshots (i.e., pictures) were also captured. Any disagreements that arose were resolved through discussion after coding was completed by both judges. The average interjudge agreement across all items was 96 percent.

FINDINGS?

Overview

Of the brands originally identified for study, 85 percent had a Web site with content for children. Among these, more than three-quarters of the brands (77%) had Web sites specifically created for children or teens, 12 percent had child-oriented sections embedded within Web sites designed for a more general audience, and 11 percent had content that would likely appeal to each of these age groups. This indicates that the majority of food brands that are heavily advertised to children on television are also promoted to them through food marketers' Web sites. Based on an analysis of proprietary Nielsen/Net Ratings data, study Web sites receive an estimated 49 million total visits by children ages 2–11 annually. Yet, there are sizeable differences in the number of young visitors individual Web sites attract. Children spend anywhere from a few seconds on these Web sites to well over an hour per visit.

Seventy-three percent of study Web sites advertised only a single brand. Among the remaining 27 percent, as many as 41 food brands were promoted (some more prominently displayed than others). Brand marks including logos, brand characters, product packages, pictures of food items, and corporate logos were prominently placed throughout these Web sites. For example, on every page within a Web site a child was exposed to an average of two different *types* of brand reminders.[5] Seventy-five percent of the Web sites also included a brand or corporate logo on almost all pages in the site. Thus, for visitors to these Web sites it was rare to encounter content that did not provide some brand reinforcement.

Some Web sites in the study sample were quite simple, and others were much more elaborate incorporating not only games but sales promotions, viral marketing, membership offers, and media tie-ins. Figure 5.1 lists 10 specific features of the Web sites. Findings relevant to each of these are discussed in the following sections.

Brand Reinforcement via Advergames

One of the advantages of a advergame from a marketer's perspective is the ability to draw attention to a brand in a playful way, and for an extended period of time. Online games can provide a more involving brand experience than is possible with conventional media. At least one commentator has characterized gaming sites as "virtual amusement parks" (Goetzl, 2006). On the kids.icecream.com site, for example, children are invited to imagine that "Nestle Push-up Frozen Treats are popping up all over the place, and it's your job to bop 'em back down." For every pop that you bop points are awarded, and as your skills develop through repeated play you can progress from an easy to a medium or hard level of play. The package is the visual centerpiece of the game (it pops up repeatedly), making the brand easier to recall later.

Food marketers make abundant use of advergames in marketing to children. Almost three of four (73%) study wWeb sites included advergames, ranging from 1 to over 65 games per site (mean = 7). In total, 546 games containing one or more food brands were counted on the sites (431 games involving study brands and the remainder containing related brands). Almost all games were animated and most incorporated lively music or sound effects (90%). Arcade, sports, and adventure games were the most

Figure 5.1
Ten Key Features of Food Marketers' Web Sites for Children

I	*Brand Reinforcement via 'Advergames'*
II.	*Exposure to Specific Advertising Claims*
III.	*Availability of Nutritional Information*
IV.	*Viral Marketing Efforts*
V.	*Marketing Partnerships: Promotions and Sponsorships*
VI.	*Use of Television and Movie Characters to Promote Food Brands*
VII.	*Offers of Website Membership*
VIII.	*Extending the Online Experience Offline*
IX.	*Incentives for Product Purchase and Consumption*
X.	*Website Protections for Children*

common (together accounting for 57% of the total). The focus across all game types was brand reinforcement through play.

How much children actually learn about a brand is a function of the volume of product exposure gained during game play. One way to measure exposure is to assess how prevalent brand marks (i.e., food item, product package, brand character, brand logo) are within advergames. Because these marks are pictorial in nature, they may aid brand recall particularly among younger children who are not as verbally proficient. Ninety-seven percent of the games included at least one *type* of brand mark, and 80 percent contained two or more. One or more brand marks was prominent in almost two-thirds (64%) of the games in which they appeared (e.g., object of the game is to catch as many Froot Loops as possible in a bowl as they fall from the sky), thus providing substantial reinforcement of the brand imagery during game play.

Brand exposure levels are also a function of the time spent playing a game. Game designers have incorporated features into games to sustain a child's interest and encourage return Web site visits. One way to increase player engagement is to enable some customization of the game experience (e.g., let a child to choose his player, select an opponent, or design the game space): 39 percent of games offered this option. Another mechanism to help maintain high interest is to structure a game so that players can measure their personal progress. For example, games with multiple levels (e.g., easy vs. hard), those that set time limits, or tally scores may each motivate players to try to improve their performance and play again. Forty-five percent of games offered multiple levels of play, 40 percent had time limits, and 69 percent awarded game points. Designers also use more overt mechanisms to encourage extended play. Explicitly asking a player if they would like to "play again" at the end of a game is one example (71% of games included this option). Recommendations of other games also extend time spent on site, and expand the range of activities worth returning for (22% of games offered suggestions). And, 39 percent of the games invited players to post their high scores to a leader board. This public display of scores invites competition, encourages gamers to return to the site to see how well they are faring, and may motivate them to try to improve their position in the overall standings.

Gaming was the primary activity on some study Web sites (e.g., candystand.com, nabiscoworld.com, postopia.com). Such sites contained a large number of games and they attract more children (ages 2–11). To illustrate, Web sites that were more popular with this age group averaged 22.4 games per site, while those that were less popular averaged 4.5 games (F = 25.44, p < .0001).[6] Gaming sites also had more food brands associated with them, and thus many additional opportunities for brand exposures (16.4 games per multi-brand site vs. 3.6 on single brand sites, F = 19.13, p < .0001).

Exposure to Specific Advertising Claims

In addition to advergames, children are exposed throughout the Web sites to food companies' products, characters, and logos—and to specific claims promoting brand benefits. Some advertising claims are embedded in television commercials that are available online.

Television Commercials Online

The increasing popularity of the Internet has prompted children's advertisers to reassess how they are allocating their marketing budgets (Steinberg & Flint, 2006). Planning challenges have surfaced, in part, because technological developments have eliminated traditional boundaries between one ad medium and another. For example, television commercials now frequently appear on Web sites, enabled by faster connection speeds, and increased broadband access (Larson, 2004).

Among study Web sites, just over half (53%) had television commercials available for viewing. These appeared more often on child-oriented sites (60%) than on sites targeted at a more general audience (32%) ($\chi = 4.76$, p < .03).[7] Some marketers use this as an opportunity to solicit feedback from visitors about their TV ads (e.g., on Campbell's mysoup.com, children were asked to rate commercials posted on the site). Television ads may be embedded among other site features. For example, on Kellogg's FunKtown site children can go to a town theater to watch cereal commercials, meet brand characters, or see trailers for movies the firm sponsors. If children are registered Web site members they can earn stamps for viewing the ads (registration possible only with parental permission). Stamps are then redeemed to gain access to special games. In so doing, Web site activities reinforce the television ad, and vice versa.

Explicit Brand Benefit Claims

In addition to online television ads, children may be exposed to specific brand claims in other sectors of food marketers'wWeb sites. Almost eighty percent (79%) of study brands included one or more benefit claims on their Web sites (e.g., statements touting a brand's taste, convenience, popularity, variety or fun). There were 1,500 of these claims, accounting for 80 percent of all claims made on the Web sites. For example, "see the candy magically change color in your mouth" appeared on wonka. com. Similarly, the claim that "you can find new yummy smelling Rub 'n' Sniff Froot Loops cereal boxes in stores with the new Cherry Cherry loops, here for a limited time" was listed on one of Kellogg's sites. Benefit claims were more numerous on Web sites appealing to a general audience (mean = 24.7) than on those focused exclusively on children and teens (mean = 10.8; $F = 7.15$, $p < .009$). Taste claims were most common (27%). Claims focused on suggested uses were also prevalent (13%), as were appeals to fun and feelings (10%). Comparative appeals (1%) and price claims (1%) were used much less often. This is consistent with early studies of children's TV advertising that revealed price and informational appeals to be a rarity during children's programming (e.g., Barcus, 1980). Exposures to other types of informational claims are possible however, such as those related to a brand's nutrition.

Availability of Nutritional Information

One of the options that food marketers have in creating a Web site is to use this space, at least in part, to educate site visitors about the nutritional qualities of their brands and how they may fit into a healthy lifestyle. In fact, it could be argued that the Internet has unique capabilities which make it particularly well-suited for this purpose. The capacity for sight, sound, and animation enables creative and exciting content (like television), and at the same time, more detailed information can be provided to both inform and persuade (like print media). As part of this study, Web sites were analyzed to see the extent to which food marketers use their Web sites to provide nutrition and health-related information.

Just over half of the sites (51%) presented basic nutritional information about their brands. Nutrition facts (as displayed on a package) were most frequently communicated (39%), followed by ingredient lists (24%), allergens (17%), and information about how a brand fit within a balanced diet (13%). This information appeared more often on Web sites with a general audience (88%) than on those targeting children and teens exclusively (38%), (F = 19.31 p < .0001), suggesting that adults are more often the target of these communications. One potential explanation for this result is that younger children may not be able to read and readily interpret this information, and more child-friendly approaches are needed.

Specific nutrition claims were also recorded, using a categorization scheme derived from a Federal Trade Commission study of advertising and nutrition (Ippolito & Pappalardo, 2002). One or more nutrition claims were listed for 44 percent of the brands studied. Most prevalent were vitamin and mineral claims (e.g., 100% daily value of Vitamin C) and general nutrient claims (e.g., "perfect kid food for growing bones") (each representing 14% of all nutrition claims). Specific nutrient, fat, calcium, and sugar content claims were also common. It should be noted that nutrition claims typically referred to only a subset of the flavors or types offered (e.g., low sugar content in Diet 7-Up). Fewer nutrition claims were made on gaming Web sites containing multiple brands than on single brand Web sites, thus providing further support for the supposition that this information is primarily intended for adults (multi brand mean = 1.0; single brand mean = 5.8; F = 5.18, p < .03). There is also directional evidence suggesting that fewer nutrition claims are made when children and teens are the primary audience (mean = 2.4), than when a more general audience is targeted (mean = 7.3), (F = 3.68, p < .058).

Overall, our results indicate that children are much more likely to encounter brand benefit claims than nutrition claims (at almost a 4 to 1 ratio) on the Web sites they visit. This suggests that there may be something of an informational imbalance, with nutrition coming up short. Child-oriented sites are less focused on making explicit brand claims (either benefit or nutrition-related) than on providing other forms of entertainment for this audience. However, it is also the case that some marketers are making efforts to inform site visitors about nutrition. Online efforts to help children learn about the foods they eat and to help them make better choices is a realistic goal in the context of corporate Web sites. However, this information has to be provided in a format that young children can readily understand.

Viral Marketing Efforts

Recognizing the power of personal information sources, managers have developed approaches such as buzz and viral marketing to encourage consumers to talk to one another about their firm's brands (e.g., Dye, 2000). Peers are a key source of influence on children's preferences (see e.g., Moschis, 1987), so this is likely to be an effective marketing tool to reach them. One type of viral marketing encourages site visitors to send email to friends containing brand-related greetings (e-cards) or invitations to a Web site: this occurred on 64 percent of study Web sites. This technique turns email into advocacy or a word of mouth endorsement because news, activities, and entertainment that are favorable to a brand are embedded in the email. These efforts were more prevalent on sites focused on children and teens (74%) than those that include adult content as well (32%) ($\chi = 11.20$, p<.0008). On all of the Web sites that were more heavily visited by children, there was an attempt to enlist peers.

The most frequent activities targeted at friends were e-greetings, site invitations, and personal challenges or links to specific games. These messages were highly brand focused, containing the brand name, logo, and often a brand character. To participate, a sender was asked to provide a friend's first name and email address as well as their own (this data was discarded once a message is sent.) In some cases, the sender was given the opportunity to design the message by choosing the layout, colors, or text. For example, on Keebler's Hollow Tree Web site, children were invited to send a friend some "Elfin Magic" or a birthday or seasonal greeting. The friend receives a personalized brand message from someone they know and like, which may enhance both its appeal and credibility.

Marketing Partnerships: Promotions and Sponsorships

Marketing partnerships, whether through promotions or sponsorships are a common practice in today's marketplace. Almost two-thirds (65%) of study Web sites offered at least one promotion in which children could participate. Forty-three percent had a sweepstakes or contest, and 31 percent made a premium offer. Some 90 brand partners were incorporated in promotional activities on the Web sites. Approximately 70 were non-food brands (e.g., Six Flags, Play Doh, Little League Baseball); the others were food brands outside the study sample (e.g., Taco Bell, Dole, Quiznos).

Sweepstakes are a popular promotional tool. Seventy-five percent of packaged goods marketers use them, and one-third of U.S. households participate each year (Shimp, 2007). The offered prizes can be an exciting inducement for children. For example, on pfgoldfish.com site, children could win a trip to Nickelodeon Studios. Campbell's mysoup.com offered a continuing series of "Souperstar" sweepstakes (e.g., "Souperstar" Island—win a trip to a Caribbean island) that overtly encouraged visitors to frequently return to the site to learn about upcoming events. Web site promotions were generally structured to involve parents, either to enter or to claim a prize. This may help to reduce the possibility that young children will develop unrealistic expectations about their chances of winning. Because this potential is known to exist, the Children's Advertising Review Unit [CARU] (2006) specifies how advertisers should communicate promotional offers to children in their self-regulatory guidelines.

Other online promotions offered premiums or free brand-related merchandise. Some premiums required purchases however. For example, on Hershey's kidztown.com, visitors were able to obtain free movie tickets for the re-release of *E. T.*, but multiple purchases of Reese's candy were needed to do so. On chefboy.com a free Chef Boyardee Superball offer was made to children. However, to obtain the ball they had to register in the Chef Club (requires parent permission), and play a game on the site which was then emailed to a friend. This example illustrates how premiums can be used to stimulate specific consumption-related behaviors, in this case, word-of-mouth among children.

Use of Television and Movie Characters to Promote Food Brands

In the current debate about marketing to children, critics have questioned whether it is appropriate to link television shows or movies to food brands (see, e.g., CSPI, 2003). Underpinning these concerns is the assumption that a food brand will be more appealing to children when associated with a well-liked TV or movie character. Forty-seven percent of study Web sites incorporated a television or movie tie-in. Thirty-one percent had a movie tie-in; 25 percent had a link to one or more television shows, and 9 percent incorporated both.

Brands were generally partnered with large blockbuster films, and it was not uncommon for a film to be promoted by multiple brands. For example, *Star Wars: Revenge of the Sith* was involved in marketing events on seven study Web sites. So, a child can encounter several promotions involving a popular movie and various food brands as they visit different sites. A movie tie-in is typically part of a larger integrated marketing communications effort that extends beyond the Internet. For example, in the summer of 2005 Mars partnered with the producers of Star Wars to create a multi-faceted campaign. To highlight the movie tie-in, Mars created the "Chocolate Mpire" within its M&Ms Web site. There were Star Wars screen savers, wallpapers and e-cards incorporating the M&M brand. Television commercials and video linked to the movie were also available for viewing and special themed packaging was highlighted. Children could play a Light Saber Training game and download a paper light saber. Each of these elements reinforces the association between the brand and the film.

Television tie-ins were also evident on 25 percent of study Web sites. More than half of these incorporated multiple children's programs: one included as many as nine shows. Some television tie-ins simply announced special packaging (e.g., Nestle Pop-Ups with Scooby Doo boxes). Others were tied in with promotions or offered as a reward to members (e.g., special MTV previews on the Starburst site). Tie-ins were also used to educate young consumers. For example, on gotmilk.com SpongeBob and the Powerpuff Girls helped to communicate the benefits of milk.

Evidence shows that children do pay substantial attention to advertisements containing a movie or television tie-in. They exhibit high levels of recognition of cartoon characters and their product associations, as well as liking for the characters and advertised brands (e.g., Henke, 1995; Mizerski, 1995). However, the impacts on children's product choices are not as clear. Some studies suggest that children's choices shift when linked to a cartoon character (Kotler 2005) and others indicate that they remain unchanged (Neeley & Schumann, 2004). Additional research is needed to isolate those circumstances in which children's food choices are affected (and not).

Offers of Web Site Membership

Getting visitors to spend time on a Web site and then return later is a key challenge Internet marketers face. Memberships that offer access to special promotions or games are a way to encourage repeat visits. Children (age 12 and younger) had the option to become a member on 25 percent of study Web sites. On a subset of these (12% of total sample), they could become members without providing much identifying information (e.g., screen name, password) and parental permission was not required. Other Web sites (13%) requested personal data: on these sites corporate sponsors did attempt to obtain parental permission before collecting any information, in accordance with the Children's Online Privacy Protection Act (see FTC, 2006). Consent was obtained via an email to parents, written parental permission or a parent's input of a credit card number (to verify adult status).

Membership provides children with access to special Web site features. Some sites offer gaming enhancements such as bonus power, access to special games, or the opportunity to post scores to a leader board (see e.g., nabiscoworld.com). Members may also be informed about new brand developments, such as line extensions, exclusive promotional offers, or new TV ads. Other sites allow members to customize space on the Web site. For example, on General Mill's millsberry.com a child creates a character (including gender, clothing, hairstyle), and then chooses a neighborhood and house in which to live. The character can shop (e.g., at the grocery store, bookstore, toy store), check out library books, visit the post office, make a charitable contribution, go to a museum, or an arcade. Millbucks are the currency: these are earned by playing games and are spent on the site. The grocery store stocks many foods from produce to branded items. General Mills' cereals are available, but there are many sectors on the site where there is no visible brand presence. Other sites (e.g., nesquik.com, lunchables.com) had some similar features but were much less elaborate. The primary significance of Web site memberships is that by individualizing the experience, brand exposures may be more memorable and more likely to lead to a continuing relationship with a young consumer.

Extending the Online Experience Offline

One way that marketers may try to extend children's interactions with a product is to provide brand-related items that visitors can keep once they leave the Web site. These are items that can be downloaded, or printed and saved. Among study brands, 76 percent offered at least one extra item and 52 percent offered two or more.

Extras are of many forms (approx. 70 in this study), and are typically very brand-centered. The most common (39%) were desktop items such as a brand wallpaper or screensaver for a child's computer, or a brand logo or character that can live on a desktop (e.g., Mountain Dew's "Do the Dew" screensavers). Reminders including pictures of brand characters or logos were also common, as were brand-related art activities, games and toys. For example, on the Lunchables site there was a branded calendar that children could print and save. Such extras have the capacity to reinforce and augment a brand message over an extended period of time.

Incentives for Product Purchase and Consumption

Beyond providing brand information or entertainment, some marketers also use the Internet to directly encourage children to consume their products. Almost 4 out of 10 study Web sites (39%) had programs to encourage consumers to collect brand points, codes, stamps, or unit pricing labels (UPCs) that they could then exchange for rewards (e.g., access to new games, brand-related toys, or clothing). For example, children were encouraged to purchase specially marked packages of Bubble Tape gum and then enter codes online to get free Nintendo game tips. As another example, children were encouraged to collect postokens from the inside flap of Post cereal boxes, which they could then enter on postopia.com to either unlock secret game levels or to see exclusive TV bloopers from Nickelodeon's *Fairly Odd Parents*. For almost all brands, points, or codes were only available on the product package. So, in virtually all cases where a points program was offered, a brand purchase was required to reap the reward. Although parents may act as gatekeepers, young children can exert substantial influence on family purchase decisions (e.g., Isler, Popper, & Ward 1987).

Through these incentives, a marketer has the opportunity to establish a direct connection between the entertainment on a Web site and consumption of a specific brand. When multiple points are required, repeat brand usage and return visits to the site are encouraged. From a child's perspective a link is created between the brand he or she chooses, and the fun experienced on a Web site. This may have potentially powerful reinforcing effects, even among older, more cognitively sophisticated children. Evidence suggests that older children (11- to 12-year-olds) are more attentive to the entertainment in an ad than younger children (7- to 8-year-olds), and more likely to allow it to shape their perceptions of product use (Moore & Lutz, 2000).

Web Site Protections for Children

Because children are a vulnerable audience, advertising needs to be conducted in a way that takes into account their level of maturity, cognitive capacity, and domain-relevant knowledge. The Internet has enabled new ways of communicating with children, and the need for unique forms of protections may arise. Major emphasis to date has been on protecting children's online privacy via COPPA regulations. CARU (2006) has also recently instituted a set of general guidelines (in addition to privacy) to advise advertisers on how to communicate with children in an age appropriate way on the Internet. One of the goals of this study was to examine the protective mechanisms already in place.

Information for Parents

Almost all Web sites (97%) provided information explicitly labeled for parents. Among these, 96 percent specified what data was (or was not) to be collected from children. Legal information and disclaimers were also present on most of these sites (91%), as were statements about the use (or not) of cookies (84%). Explicit statements about compliance with COPPA regulations were found on 76 percent of the Web sites and 47 percent specified adherence to CARU's guidelines. Less common were tips on children's Internet safety (35%). Many sites (87%) also provided a mechanism to contact the firm (via a contact us link, mailing address or phone number). So, there is information available for parents if they choose to access it.

Privacy Protections and Age Blocks

The marketers in our sample were careful to screen children under the age of 13 when necessary. Some did not request any information from site visitors (adults or children) so no age screening device was needed. Others collected only basic identifying data, such as a screen name to recognize site visitors, or a first name, and email address (used on one occasion to send an e-card or greeting). Still others excluded children under 13 from participating in site activities that involved registration, a promotional entry, or online purchase. On all Web sites where personal data was requested (and children were permitted to participate), mechanisms were in place to ensure that they did not submit information without parent permission. For example, to register on Kellogg's FunKtown site a parent had to input a credit card number, thus making it quite difficult for a child to subvert the age block.

Ad-Break Reminders

One of the long standing concerns about children's processing of television advertising centers on their capacity to distinguish between editorial and ad content. To help children make this distinction, the Federal Communications Commission prohibits "program length commercials" and "host selling" (FCC, 2006). These policies are intended to avoid misleading children who may be confused when commercial characters are embedded in programs. The FCC has also requested that advertisers insert commercial bumpers, short segments before and after commercial breaks, in children's programs (Kunkel, 2001). These bumpers (approx. 5 seconds) remind children they are watching ads and encourage them to be vigilant.

The boundaries between advertising and other content may be harder for children to distinguish on the Internet, because there are not the natural breaks that typify television. As discussed earlier, online activities such as advergames and viral marketing provide a kind of camouflage for selling intent that may make it difficult for young children to discern. Yet, only a small number of advertisers in our sample provided ad-break reminders (18% of study Web sites). On those that did, most defined it, and presented it on multiple locations in the site (e.g., reminder was repeated on every page on postopia.com). However, ad break disclosures on the Web sites were small, and visually static, as compared to the animated and appealing nature of other Web site content. No published research yet exists indicating how effective these ad-break reminders are: questions related to the format(s), size, and placement of reminders should be pursued.

FUTURE DIRECTIONS AND CHALLENGES

The disturbing trend of a steady and alarming increase in obesity among the nation's youth has captured the attention of a broad set of citizens and institutions, with calls for action becoming increasingly powerful. Particular questions are being raised about the impacts of food marketing. As children have gravitated to the Internet in large numbers, online marketing activities are coming under increasing scrutiny. The study reported in this chapter is the first to systematically examine online food marketing to children. Our results show that the majority of food brands advertised to children on television are also promoted to them through food marketers' Web sites. On the Internet, children are exposed to an array of advergames, promotions, media tie-ins, viral marketing, membership offers, and explicit purchase incentives. When a marketing message is embedded in Web site games and activities, it may be more difficult for children to understand and resist (Montgomery, 2001; Moore, 2004; Moses & Baldwin, 2005). Children that are the target of these online efforts (ages 2–11) are still in the process of developing the information processing skills needed to evaluate advertising effectively.

In response to public pressures, some initial steps have been taken by industry leaders. Recent announcements of the formation of the Children's Food and Beverage Advertising Initiative (NARC, 2006) and revision of the Children's Advertising Review Unit self-regulatory guidelines (CARU 2006) are two primary examples. As part of the Initiative, participating firms have pledged to dedicate at least half of their children's advertising to communications that promote healthier dietary choices and/or messages that encourage good nutrition or healthy lifestyles (both in traditional media and on the Internet). They also made the commitment to either limit the brands shown in advergames to healthier options, or to incorporate healthy lifestyle messages into their games. In its revised guidelines, CARU has incorporated new provisions specifying the depiction of serving size, balanced nutrition, and healthy lifestyles. Given the recentness of these developments, it remains to be seen how these industry efforts will be implemented and what impacts they will ultimately have on children's food preferences and choices (see Moore & Rideout, in press, for an extended analysis of the public policy issues).

Although young children are rapidly adopting new media, research efforts have not kept pace. Little is known about what children understand, believe, or do as a consequence of their exposure to brand messages on marketers' Web sites. This study is intended to be a first step towards understanding the online commercial environment in which many children are spending time. Now the challenge is to learn more about how this young audience responds within it, and what impacts it may have on their diet and health.

APPENDIX: LIST OF STUDY WEB SITES

3musketeers.com

7up.com

airheads.com

applejacks.com

bk.com (kids' section)

bubblegum.com

bubbletape.com

butterfinger.com

candystand.com

capncrunch.com

caprisun.com

cheetos.com

chefboy.com

chuckecheese.com

cuatmcdonalds.com

danimalsxl.com

dannon.com

dewbajablast.com

doritos.com

drpepper.com

frootloops.com

funkyfaces.com

gotmilk.com

got-milk.com

gushers.com

hersheys.com

honbatz.com

jello.com

juicyjuice.com (just for kids' section)

juicyfruit.com

keebler.com/brand/onthegosnacks

kelloggsfunktown.com

kelloggs.com/products/treats/index.html

kfc.com (kids' section)

kids.icecream.com

kidztown.com

kool-aid.com

lifecereal.com

littledebbie.com

luckycharmsfun.com

lunchables.com

millsberry.com

mountaindew.com

mycoke.com

mypasta.com

mysoup.com

nabiscoworld.com

nestlecrunch.com

nesquik.com

nutritioncamp.com

pepsi.com

pfgoldfish.com

popsicle.com

poptarts.com

postopia.com

pringles.com

quakeraday.com (family fun section)

ronald.com

sillyrabbit.millsberry.com

skittles.com

smuckers.com

snickers.com

sprite.com

starburst.com

subway-kids.com

sunnyd.com

thecheesiest.com

thehollowtree.com

tonguetracks.com

tonythetiger.com

topps.com

twinkies.com

us.mms.com

wendys.com (kids section)

whymilk.com

wonderball.com

wonka.com

NOTES

1. These estimates are typically based on visitors of all ages.

2. Analysis proceeded for all product categories in which advertising for *any* child-oriented brands appeared. These included: (1) breads and pastries, (2) candy and gum, (3) breakfast cereals, (4) cookies and crackers, (5) fruit juices and other

non-carbonated drinks, (6) ice cream and frozen novelties, (7) peanut butter and jelly, (8) prepared foods and meals, (9) restaurants, (10) salty snacks, (11) carbonated soft drinks, and (12) other snacks (e.g., yogurt, fruit snacks, granola bars).

3. As noted above, the study sample includes brands that have been heavily advertised to children on TV, and so mirrors the nutritional profile of foods advertised in that medium. With this caveat in mind, the Director of Nutrition Policy at the Center for Science in the Public Interest (CSPI) examined the brands promoted on the Web sites in this study and concluded that 90 percent of them were of poor nutritional quality (Wootan, 2006).

4. There was one exception. On sites with a distinct children's section, only the pages designated as within that section were coded in detail (e.g., juicyjuice. com). So, information such as data for stockholders and career opportunities with the company were not coded. If material of specific interest in this study such as information for parents or privacy policies appeared within the larger site, these were coded and are included in our reported results.

5. This measure actually underrepresents the level of brand exposure because it captures the *types* of visible brand marks on each page *not the total number of appearances* (that is, when a brand character was depicted on a page it was counted as one whether it was pictured one time or five times). Even with the more conservative measure, it is clear that it is rare to encounter site content that does not contain some brand reinforcement.

6. To explore whether differences existed between the more and less popular sites with children, Nielsen data was used to divide the sample into two groups based on audience size among 2–11 year olds. Natural clustering in the data suggested a split such that the so-called more popular group represents 27 percent of study Web sites, and the so-called less popular group includes the remaining 73 percent. Although this may appear to be a somewhat arbitrary split, it reflects the distribution reasonably well. To be certain of this, other possible grouping methods were tried. Each of these revealed the same pattern in terms of statistical relationships to other site descriptors, thus lending confidence in the validity of the split. Given the unequal cell sizes, Type III sum of squares were used to ensure the validity of the statistical tests (Iacobucci, 1995). Type III sum of squares were used in all comparisons of variables where cell sizes are unequal (e.g., single vs. multi-brand sites, popular vs. less popular sites), not only in the specific comparison referenced here.

7. Web sites emphasizing children and teen-oriented content (77% of the sample) were compared to those that also include information for adults (23% of the sample) in this analysis.

REFERENCES

Alexander, A., Benjamin, L. M., Hoerrner, K., & Roe, D. (1998). We'll be back in a moment: A content analysis of advertisements in children's television in the 1950s, *Journal of Advertising, 27*(Fall), 1–9.

Barcus, F. E. (1980). The nature of television advertising to children. In E. L. Palmer & A. Dorr (Eds.), *Children and the Faces of Television,* New York: Academic Press, 287–305.

Bertrim, B. (2005). It's how you play the games, *Marketing Magazine, 110(16),* 18.

Center for Science in the Public Interest (2003). *Pestering parents: How food companies market obesity to children.* Washington, DC.: Author.

Children's Advertising Review Unit (2006). *Self-regulatory program for children's advertising,* 8th ed., New York: Council of Better Business Bureaus. Retrieved November 21, 2006, from http://www.caru.org/guidelines/index.asp

Dye, R. (2000, November/December). The buzz on buzz, *Harvard Business Review,* 139–146.

Fattah, H., & Paul, P. (2002, May). Gaming gets serious, *American Demographics,* 39–43.

Federal Communications Commission (2006). Children's Educational Television, FCC Consumer Facts. Retrieved June 30, 2006, from http://www.fcc.gov/cgb/consumerfacts/childtv.html

Federal Trade Commission (2006, March 15). *Children's online privacy protection rule, retention of rule without modification,* 16 CFR Part 312, Washington, DC.

Ferrazzi, K., & Benezra, K. (2001, April 16). Journey to the top, *Brandweek,* 28–36.

Goetzl, D. (2006, February 20). Television has competition in pursuit of kids, *Television Week,* 8, 10, 10.

Harkin, T. (2005). *Marketing, self-regulation, and childhood obesity.* Comments at a Joint Workshop of the Federal Trade Commission and the Department of Health and Human Services. Transcript retrieved on April 4, 2006, from http://www.ftc.gov/bcp/workshops/foodmarketingtokids/index.htm

Hastings, G., et al. (2003). *Review of research on the effects of food promotion to children,* Report to the Food Standards Agency, Glasgow, UK: Center for Social Marketing, University of Strathclyde.

Henke, L. L. (1995). Young children's perceptions of cigarette brand advertising symbols: Awareness, affect and target market identification, *Journal of Advertising,24*(Winter), 13–28.

Iacobucci, D. (1995). Analysis of variance for unbalanced data. In D. W. Stewart & N. J. Vilcassim (Eds.), *Marketing theory and practice: AMA Winter Educators' conference proceedings* (pp. 337–343), Chicago: American Marketing Association.

Institute of Medicine (2006). *Food marketing to children and youth: Threat or opportunity?* Washington, DC: National Academies Press.

Ippolito, P. M., & Pappalardo, J. K. (2002). *Advertising, nutrition & health – Evidence from food advertising 1977–1997,* Bureau of Economics Staff Report, Federal Trade Commission.

Isler, L., Popper, E. T., & Ward, S. (1987, October/November). Children's purchase requests and parental responses: Results from a diary study, *Journal of Advertising Research, 27,* 28–39.

John, D. R. (1999, December). Consumer socialization of children: A retrospective look at twenty-five years of research. *Journal of Consumer Research, 26,* 183–213.

Kassarjian, H. H. (1977, June). Content analysis in consumer research, *Journal of Consumer Research, 4,* 8–18.

Kolbe, R. H., & Burnett, M. S. (1991, September). Content-analysis research: An examination of applications with directives for improving research reliability and objectivity, *Journal of Consumer Research, 18,* 243–250.

Kotler, J. (2005, July 5). *The healthy habits for life initiative at sesame workshop.* Presented at the Marketing, Self-Regulation, and Childhood Obesity workshop of the Federal Trade Commission and the Department of Health and Human Services. Retrieved April 26. 2006, from http://www.ftc.gov/bcp/workshops/foodmarketingtokids/index.htm, accessed

Kunkel, D. (2001). Children and television advertising. In D. G. Singer & J. L. Singer (Eds.), *Handbook of Children and the Media* (pp. 375–394). Thousand Oaks, CA: Sage.

Larson, M. (2004, February 9). Nick swims upstream. *Media Week,* 14.

Lindstrom, M., & Seybold, P. B. (2003). *Brand Child.* London: Kogan Page.

Maher, J. K., & Childs, N. M. (2003). A longitudinal content analysis of gender roles in children's television advertisements: A 27 year review. *Journal of Current Issues and Research in Advertising, 25*(1), 71–81.

Mizerski, R. (1995, October). The relationship between trade cartoon character recognition and attitude toward product category in young children. *Journal of Marketing, 59,* 58–70.

Montgomery, K. C. (2001). Digital kids—The new on-line children's consumer culture. In D. G. Singer & J. L. Singer (Eds.), *Handbook of Children and the Media* (pp. 635–650). Thousand Oaks, CA: Sage.

Moore, E. S. (2004, June). Children and the changing world of advertising. *Journal of Business Ethics, 52,* 161–167.

Moore, E. S. (2006). *It's child's play: Advergaming and the online marketing of food to children.* Menlo, Park, CA: Kaiser Family Foundation Report.

Moore, E. S., & Lutz, R. J. (2000, June). Children, advertising, and product experiences: A multimethod inquiry. *Journal of Consumer Research, 27,* 31–48.

Moore, E. S., & Rideout, V. J. (in press). The online marketing of food to children: Is it just fun and games?, *Journal of Public Policy & Marketing.*

Moschis, G. P., (1987). *Consumer socialization.* Lexington, MA: Lexington Books.

Moses, L. J., & Baldwin, D. A. (2005). What can the study of cognitive development reveal about children's ability to appreciate and cope with advertising. *Journal of Public Policy & Marketing, 24,* 186–201.

National Advertising Review Council (2005, September 15). *NARC announces key initiatives to strengthen self-regulation of advertising to children* (NARC news, press release).

Neeley, S. M., & Schumann, D. W. (2004). Using animated spokes-characters in advertising to young children. *Journal of Advertising, 33*(Fall), 7–23.

Ogden, C. L., Carroll, M. D., Curtin, L. R., McDowell, M. A., Tabak, C. J., & Flagel, K. M. (2006). Prevalence of overweight and obesity in the United States 1994–2004, *Journal of the American Medical Association, 295*(13), 1549–1555.

Ogden, C. L., Flegal, K. M., Carroll, M. D., & Johnson, C. L. (2002). Prevalence and trends in overweight among U.S. children and adolescents 1999–2000. *Journal of the American Medical Association, 288*(14), 1728–1732.

Rideout, V. J., Vandewater, E. A., & Wartella, E. A. (2003). *Zero to six: Electronic media in the lives of infants, toddlers and preschoolers.* Menlo Park, CA: Kaiser Family Foundation.

Roberts, D. F., Foehr, U. G., & Rideout, V. J. (2005). *Generation M: Media in the lives of 8–18 year-olds.* Menlo Park, CA: Kaiser Family Foundation.

Shimp, T. A. (2007). *Advertising, promotion and other aspects of integrated marketing communications,*(7th ed.), Mason, OH: Thomson South-Western.

Steinberg, B., & Flint, J. (2006, March 13). Kids-TV "upfront" season kicks off under cloud. *The Wall Street Journal,* p. B2.

U.S. Department of Education (2003). Computer and internet use by children and adolescents in 2001, National Center for Education Statistics, NCES 2004–014.

Wootan, M. (2006, July 19). Comments at Kaiser Family Foundation Forum. Transcripts retrieved on October 1, 2006 from http://www.kff.org/entmedia/entmedia071906pkg.cfm

Chapter 6

FAMILIES AND OBESITY: A FAMILY PROCESS APPROACH TO OBESITY IN ADOLESCENTS

Matthew P. Thorpe and Randal D. Day

Obesity at all ages has risen sharply since, 1980 (figure 6.1). This steady and uncontrolled increase has alarmed the health community because once established, obesity is notoriously difficult to treat. Though concerns about obesity in youth have customarily been centered on a well-documented increased risk for adult disease, it is now clear that childhood and adolescent obesity promote multiple, often serious health conditions prior to adulthood. This problem is not confined to the United States or even to developed countries and has been called a global epidemic by the World Health Organization.

Family life is emerging as a key element in the development, prevention, and treatment of obesity. Early patterns of eating behavior and physical activity are established in a family setting. This chapter introduces the intersection of family life and the problem of childhood obesity. We will discuss the measurement and costs of obesity, and introduce a few key resources in the obesity literature. We will highlight the role of family processes and discuss their importance to obesity. Lastly we will provide an example of how family processes might be used as a tool in obesity research using data from the National Longitudinal Study of Adolescent Health (or Add Health for short).

Acknowledgements: This work was funded by the Brigham Young University Honors Program and Office of Research and Creative Activities. Matthew Thorpe is supported by a United States Department of Agriculture National Needs Fellowship. Thanks to Dr. Brent Webb, Elicia Hansen, Dr. Mark Rowe, Rudy Valentine, and April Thorpe for contributions and support.

Figure 6.1
Rates of Overweight and Obesity in the United States By Age Group 1960–2002

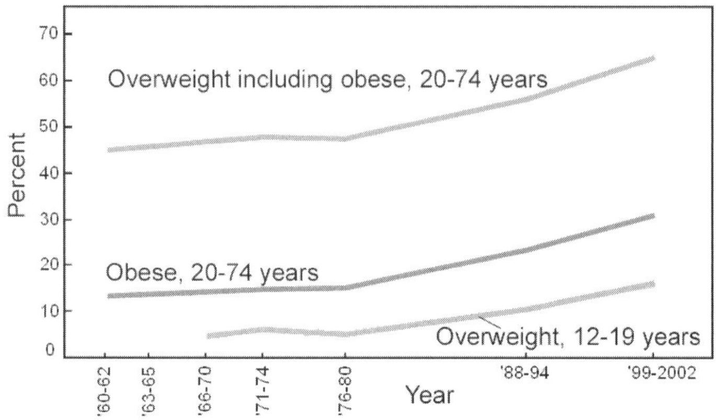

Adapted from: Centers for Disease Control and Prevention, National Center for Health Statistics, *Health, United States 2005*, figure 15.

DEFINING OBESITY

Obesity is defined simply as excess fat for age and sex. Obesity is most commonly measured in field research by calculating the body mass index, or weight in kilograms divided by height in meters squared (BMI = kilograms/meters^2). This index correlates well to more precise lab estimates of obesity among adults and children. The BMI is certainly not a perfect indicator of obesity, however, and is often misrepresentative among very tall, very short or very muscular individuals. Despite these limitations the BMI remains standard due to its simplicity and general accuracy.

In adult populations, absolute values of BMI are used to classify weight: a BMI more than 25 is considered overweight and a BMI more than 30 is considered obese. For children and adolescents BMI is determined using percentiles from a reference population of the same age and sex. The Centers for Disease Control and Prevention (CDC) published growth charts for children through age 20 (Kuczmarski, Ogden, Grummer-Strawn, et al., 2000). These charts provide growth percentile curves of a reference population that is unaffected by the recent obesity trends. BMI-for-age charts provide smoothed percentile curves (figure 6.2) for boys and girls. Expert recommendations regarding these growth charts prescribe cutoff values of the 85th percentile for the designation, at risk of overweight, and the 95th percentile for, overweight. Programming for SAS statistical software is available from the CDC

Figure 6.2
A 2000 BMI-for-age and Sex Growth Chart from the Centers for Disease Control and Prevention

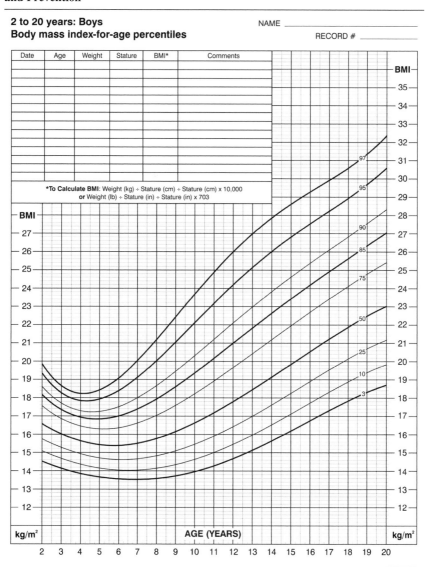

2 to 20 years: Boys
Body mass index-for-age percentiles

NAME _____

RECORD # _____

*To Calculate BMI: Weight (kg) ÷ Stature (cm) ÷ Stature (cm) x 10,000
or Weight (lb) ÷ Stature (in) ÷ Stature (in) x 703

Published May 30, 2000 (modified 10/16/00).

SAFER·HEALTHIER·PEOPLE™

(Continued)

Figure 6.2 (*Continued*)

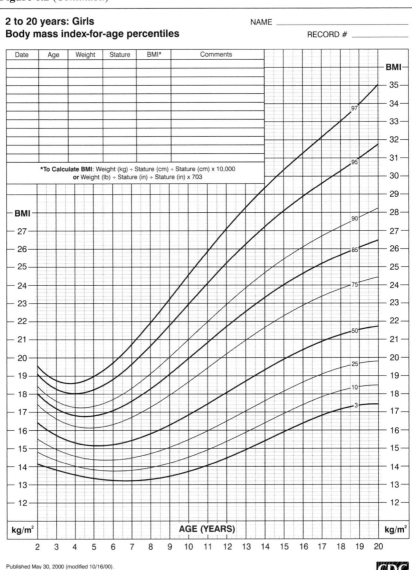

Source: Developed by the National Center for Health Statistics in collaboration with the National Center for Chronic Disease Prevention and Health Promotion (2000).

Web site (www.cdc.gov/growthcharts/) to calculate reference percentiles given height, weight, age, and gender.

Self-reports of height and weight have been validated for the calculation of BMI, but self- or parental report of weight status (e.g., "Are you overweight?") does *not* correlate well to measured BMI. Additionally, female adolescents tend to slightly under-report weight, while males tend to slightly over-report weight. Accordingly actual measurements are preferred wherever plausible. As general rules, digital scales are more precise than spring scales, and more expensive scales are more precise (let the buyer beware!). Height should be measured using a non-stretchable measuring tape or electronic stadiometer. Participants should be measured while standing with heels, back and head pressed against a wall or other even surface.

WHY WE CARE

Health Costs

Obesity in childhood and particularly during adolescence predicts adult obese status. Traditionally the concern over increasing childhood obesity is an increased risk of adult disease, mediated by continued obesity into adulthood. The National Institutes of Health (NIH) published a comprehensive evidence report, *Clinical Guidelines on the Identification, Evaluation and Treatment of Overweight and Obesity in Adults* (1998). This evidence report identifies strong epidemiological evidence that obesity increases all-cause mortality and risk for cardiovascular disease, type 2 diabetes, stroke, gallbladder disease, osteoarthritis, sleep apnea, respiratory problems, some cancers, and depression. Importantly the panel concludes there is extensive, strong, causal evidence that if obese, weight loss will improve blood pressure and cholesterol levels, two key risk factors for heart disease, and reduce hyperglycemia, a precursor to type 2 diabetes. Of 832.7 total age-adjusted deaths per 100,000 population in 2003, the CDC attributes 285.8 (34.3%) to cardiovascular disease (heart disease and stroke), and an additional 25.3 deaths to diabetes (National Center for Health Statistics, 2005, p. 170). Diabetes itself is a key risk factor for cardiovascular and kidney diseases.

As obesity continues to increase among children and adolescents, obesity-related diseases are appearing earlier. Type 2 diabetes, long considered an adult disease, is now seen in obese children. So is insulin resistance, sometimes referred to as, pre-diabetes. Studies have also noted an early onset of cardiovascular risk factors in obese youth. Such early onset of these diseases is likely to shorten the lifespan of these youth.

Psychosocial Costs

Psychosocial illness related to obesity is more controversial. While some studies link obesity to increased depression, poorer self-esteem ,and suicidal ideation, other studies find no such associations (see Faith, Matz, & Allison, 2003 for a detailed review). On the other hand poor body image is consistently related to obesity. Part of this ambiguity may relate to variation in the way obesity is perceived. For example one study found an increased risk of depression among overweight females, but a decreased risk of depression among overweight men (Carpenter, Hasin, Allison, & Faith, 2000). Clear gender discrepancies exist in the meaning attributed to body weight, highlighting the need for gender-controlled study of obesity. Uncertainty about the psychosocial influence of obesity could also come from indirect causes. Obese children are more often on the fringes of social interaction, having fewer friends than their non-obese peers (Strauss & Pollack, 2003). These social considerations may be the immediate cause of some psychosocial problems.

Weight-based teasing is unambiguously linked to poor self-esteem and body image. Such teasing may be even more important than actual obesity in the child's formation of a body image and self-esteem (Eisenberg, Neumark-Sztainer, & Story, 2003). It seems that children who are teased by peers or family members about weight suffer measurable declines in self-esteem and body image, even in cases where children are not actually overweight. This suggests a causative role of teasing. Such social troubles accompanying obesity probably mediate other, less clear associations between obesity and psychosocial distress.

Economic Costs

Estimates of national expenditures attributable to obesity range from 46 to 75 billion U.S. dollars, and between 5.5 to 9.1 percent of recent U.S. medical expenditures (e.g., Thompson and Wolf, 2001). Approximately one half of this cost was directed to Medicare and Medicaid. A 1990 study estimated indirect costs of obesity due to work days or lifetime earnings lost to morbidity and mortality at 23.0 billion (Wolf & Colditz, 1994). Although actual costs are impossible to estimate precisely, these studies demonstrate a staggering economic cost imposed on society.

INDIVIDUAL FACTORS IN THE DEVELOPMENT OF OBESITY

Behavior

The physiological role of body fat is to store energy. The amount of energy expended in physical activity and biological housekeeping (the work of keeping the body running properly) subtracted from energy intake from food (measured in calories) determines our *energy balance.* A positive energy balance results in weight gain, while a negative energy balance results in weight loss.

Social changes over the past few decades have converted employment activities from primarily labor-intensive to sedentary work, as well as active leisure to more sedentary media use. Concurrent changes in the food industry have made, in many cases, energy dense snack and junk foods less expensive than more healthful food choices. The Institute of Medicine (IOM) has published multiple key reports on childhood obesity, which may be browsed at www.iom.edu (search for the term "obesity"). One such report, *Preventing Child Obesity: Health in the Balance,* concludes that at least 30 percent of the calories in the average American's diet come from sweet or salty snacks, soft drinks or fruit beverages (Koplan, Liverman, & Kraak, 2005). This trend is also reflected in youth. The report notes that children and adolescents are spending less time in active play and more time watching TV, using computers, or playing video games. The net effect of these changes is a more positive energy balance, promoting weight gain.

Genetic Predisposition

Genetic *heritability* measures how much of a population's variation in a particular trait (called a *phenotype* by geneticists) can be explained by variation in genes. Heritability estimates of BMI vary widely; the most common figures range from 50 to 70 percent. Estimates depend on the study method, the population of interest, and the specific sample. Among U.S. adolescents in the Add Health study, heritability is highest among black females, 85 percent, and lowest among white females, 45 percent, (Jacobsen & Rowe, 1998). Discrepancies notwithstanding, a considerable portion of variation in obese status can be explained by genetic factors, but another substantial part must be explained by environmental or behavioral factors. Furthermore the current upward trend in obesity rates is too rapid to be explained by changes in genetic programming. Obesity's causes are clearly not exclusive to nature or nurture.

Current theory in the role of genetics proposes a lipostat mechanism (from the Greek *lipos,* or fat). Like an internal thermostat, the lipostat is set through evolutionary and biological processes to maintain an appropriate energy balance. For most of human history, increased work was required to increase food intake. As noted previously, technological and social advances in the recent past have produced, for the first time, an abundance of high energy food that may be obtained with no practical increase in physical exertion. One explanation for the recent spike in obesity rates is that these rapid social changes may have overwhelmed biological compensatory machinery that has been fine tuned over thousands of years to conserve energy.

Genetic regulation of body weight occurs through several different mechanisms. For example, variation in one gene changes the way different individuals perceive feeling full, another regulates the amount of energy spent in background biological processes, and another changes the way fat is stored. Due to these and other biological processes, two people with the same food intake and the same amount of physical activity may differ in body fat. The term *thrifty genotype* describes an individual whose body uses or stores energy more efficiently. Such an individual can still reduce body fat with extra physical activity or reduced energy intake, but may have to work much harder than others to do so. Accordingly the behavioral causes of obesity are moderated by genetic factors.

FAMILY PROCESSES

Family processes are the strategies families use to achieve their goals. While much of the research in family life considers the content, or *what* of family life, a family processes perspective asks the question, *"how?"* (Sauber, L'Abate, Weeks, & Buchanan, 1993). Regarding eating behavior, "the family may exert powerful influence on family members' eating habits, though there is very little conclusive literature regarding the specific mechanisms" (Bourcier, Bowen, Meischke, & Moinpour, 2003, p. 265). This conspicuous gap in the literature falls into the realm of family process. Families matter, and the question of *how* families matter in the development of child and adolescent obesity is our present concern.

The process approach assumes families are made up of members whose individual character defines and drives a part of the larger family. It also assumes that families are goal-seeking entities (Broderick, 1993, p. 41). These goals and the strategies families employ to achieve them are the *how* of family life, the essence of family process. Day, Miller, and Cox (2006) assert that family processes occur in context of broader-than-the-family social forces, and upon bedrock composed of family *structure,* family *rules and ideologies,* and family *resources.* With one eye on these contextual considerations, they describe six domains encompassing the range of family processes: *inclusion, protection, nurturing, providing, regulation,* and *teaching.*

Domains of Family Process

Inclusion

Inclusion processes in families define membership and member roles. Families define themselves through various processes, including family- or even member-specific notions of what it means to be a member, value assigned to membership and what is expected of members. Membership may be ambiguous all together, or change during family rituals. As family structures and relationships are formed or dissolved existing rules concerning membership are challenged and may be redefined. Regarding obesity, inclusion processes become important in the ownership of obesity in the family. That is, does obese status make a child more different or more similar to the family? Who does responsibility for obesity belong to? (e.g., Kinston, Loader, & Miller, 1988).

Protection

Though protection processes are not frequently considered in process literature, the responsibility of members to protect each other is a dominating societal theme. Motivation and tactics employed by family members to keep one another healthy and free from chronic disease would intuitively fall under this domain.

Nurturing

Families seek to nourish members in every sense through the application of resources (including social capital) to meet member needs. This includes warmth and encouragement in addition to physical sustenance. The latter has obvious relevance to obesity, but the former has been implicated in eating disorders, suggesting that even nurturing unrelated to eating is relevant to eating behavior.

Providing

Providing is a universal family process that is most commonly conceptualized using household income. Unfortunately this concept is rarely studied in the sense of an interaction among members to generate, create, or transfer the necessities of living. This distinction is the difference between content and process. Income measures family access to resources and is relevant to inner family life, but does not tell us *how* resources are made, used, or shared to achieve families' goals. As a set of processes, providing in many families encompasses the types of foods available in the home and the amount of disposable income available to young children, who frequently spend their money on high calorie, low nutrient snacks.

Regulation

Regulation processes consist of making and enforcing rules. Much of the literature on familial roles in eating and physical activity taps into the regulation domain. *Monitoring* and *control* are two important regulating processes that have repeatedly appeared in explanations of the eating behavior of children.

Teaching

Teaching processes are synonymous with socialization. Again this process domain has enjoyed greater attention than most others in explaining child eating and activity. For example, parents influence a child's physical activity behavior through *modeling* and *encouragement.*

General Processes

Some specific processes intersect many or all of these domains, and are so prevalent in family literature they deserve particular mention. Communication is certainly important to the execution of all of the six domain areas. Communication is also relevant to obesity in families, and appears to play a role in disordered eating.

Routines and rituals represent additional family processes through which families include, protect, nurture, provide, regulate, and teach. Routines and rituals are not well differentiated, but each fall under the basic definition, "patterned interactions repeated over time" (Wolin & Bennett, 1984, p. 403). Three assumptions underpin routine and ritual in the family. First, interaction among members sets *family* routine apart from *individual* routine. Second, the beginning and ending of routines are plainly delineated. Members know when the routine has begun and when it is over. This idea is referred to as *bounded clarity.* Third, routines execute goal-seeking functions. These patterns exist to complete necessary tasks of family life in predictable, reliable, and efficient ways. This is not to say that routines and rituals are always efficient and beneficial to the family. To apply an example of routine gone awry, consider a family employing the rule, "dinner is not over until our plate is clean." In our current environment of abundant food and large portion sizes, this rule is likely to promote excessive food intake. The family confronted with burgeoning waistlines might reconsider the rule, or might dogmatically cling to it, promoting obesity.

FAMILY PROCESSES IN OBESITY LITERATURE

One early study to assess family process in obesity explored ideologies and communication strategies in families with obese children compared to families with children diagnosed with celiac disease, a food allergy that is treated by the complete exclusion of wheat and related grains from the diet (Kinston, Loader, & Miller, 1988). Both conditions are treated through modified nutritional behavior, but celiac disease (once diagnosed) is typically treated successfully, while obesity is not.

The study found that obesity is a persistent and moderately intense stressor to families and one that families have trouble coping with. While 100 percent of families with celiac children in this study were managing the disease, only 59 percent of families with obese children made any such attempts. The authors attributed this discrepancy to process. Families with celiac children held a belief that the condition was medical and only medical, and that adherence to the prescribed diet would prevent the disease's painful symptoms. Parents took leadership in regulation of the condition, read materials on the disorder and the diet, and communicated clearly with each other to tackle the situation as a unified team.

Families with obese children, however, had many conflicting beliefs about obesity's underlying causes—some medical, and some personal and negative such as "the child is lazy, greedy, and undisciplined." Different members of the family believed the condition should be managed in different ways, and the family communicated with less clarity, cooperation, and consensus. Families with obese girls also reported feeling that eating in the home was "out of control." The study demonstrated that family process, though not well utilized in obesity research, is a powerful framework for understanding the inner workings of families with obese members.

Family Influence of Energy Balance

Eating

Normally children are able to self-regulate food intake to their individual energy needs. Children whose parents are controlling of the child's eating behavior are less able to appropriately self-regulate, and are likelier to overeat (Johnson & Birch, 1994). In one study, obese children ate more quickly and took larger bites while the mother was present, but ate at normal pace in her absence. The mother's presence did not affect the rate of feeding in non-obese children (Laessle, Uhl, & Lindel, 2001). Appropriate regulation of meals and snacks such as providing healthy foods and limiting the amount of junk foods is thought to decrease the risk of obesity. Over-regulation and inappropriate rules regarding eating such as controlling the amount of food consumed represent processes gone awry. In this situation eating becomes out of control, and unhealthy eating attitudes develop, contrary to the intended effect of restricted or improved eating.

Family meals are a routine that provides monitoring of food choices and behavior, and may be a powerful process contributing to better adolescent nutrition. More frequent family meals are associated with more healthful diets (Videon & Manning, 2003). Routines such as family meals offer valuable opportunities for the family to regulate and teach health behaviors.

Activity

A review of 34 studies from 1985 to 2003 concludes that parenting consistently influences levels of child physical activity (Gustafson & Rhodes, 2006). Two mechanisms are proposed: *modeling* and *support* of active behavior. The term modeling, which has rich connotations in family literature, is applied theoretically to explain observed correlations between parent and child activity levels. None of the reviewed studies were designed to test modeling directly as a mechanism for increasing child activity. Additionally no study has investigated negative modeling, such as spending long periods of time watching television with or in the presence of the child, in contrast to positive modeling, such as exercising with or in the presence of the child. These gaps between content and mechanism represent an opportunity for the family process approach to make an important contribution.

Research on parental support of child activity has been more specific, and describes *encouragement,involvement,* and *facilitation* as forms of support. Encouragement connotes parental prompts or socialization for physical activity, and is somewhat ambiguously linked to child activity. Involvement includes coaching or coparticipation, which theoretically overlaps with modeling, and is positively correlated to child activity. Facilitation includes provision of necessary transportation, equipment, or access to opportunities for activity and is strongly correlated to child activity. Parental influence appears to have stronger associations among younger vs. older adolescents. A number of process domains are relevant here. Nurturing, providing, teaching, regulation, and inclusion are all represented in these processes and executed through the use of specific routines and communication tactics.

Structural moderators of the parent-child activity link are also apparent (Gustafson & Rhodes, 2006). Children from single vs. two parent homes exhibit differences in activity levels. Generally children in two-parent homes are described as more active, but not all studies agree. Reasons for these associations are not yet clear; they may be artifacts of socioeconomic status rather than actual family structure.

Sociodemographic Influences

Obesity rates vary according to family resources and structure as well. Specifically, low socioeconomic status and minority status are each risk factors for obesity. Furthermore, it appears that increased income and education are protective against obesity among whites, but not necessarily among minorities (Gordon-Larsen, Adair, & Popkin, 2003). Consensus has not emerged on the reasons for this differential effect of socioeconomic status by ethnicity.

The *nutrition transition* refers to the tendency for developing populations to shift from a low-fat diet grounded in staple foods to a diet high in fat and refined sugars (Popkin & Gordon-Larsen, 2004). In undeveloped countries, obesity is uncommon among the lower class and increases with income, as only the wealthy can afford rich foods and sedentary lifestyles. With development, however, such lifestyles become increasingly available to the lower class, and the incidence of obesity is redistributed. With further development it is thought that the upper class begins to spend a greater portion of copious resources seeking health and fitness. In the United States we see a reversal in the patterns of the developing world: obesity rates are greatest among the lower class and least educated and lowest among the upper class and most educated. While physical labor was once the currency to purchase the necessities of life, it seems progress has converted it to a commodity for purchase by those who can afford to exercise. Similarly the healthy foods that grew in the gardens of those who could not afford richer fare now are often costlier than dollar-menu burgers, fries, and soft drinks.

AN APPROACH TO FAMILIES AND OBESITY
USING ADD HEALTH

Our analysis includes 6,073 participants from wave I of the public-use version of the National Longitudinal Study of Adolescent Health (Add Health). These include 3,107 males and 2,966 females; 3,639 non-Hispanic whites, 1,429 non-Hispanic blacks, 690 Hispanics, 69 Native Americans, 219 Asians or Pacific Islanders, and 27 not identifying with any of the above groups. Adolescents reporting pregnancy (past or current) or disability are excluded due to confounding influence on body weight (431 subjects excluded). These data were collected over 1994 to 1995. Add Health includes a probability sample of 80 high schools stratified by region, urbanization, type of school, size, and ethnic mix. Students in each school were stratified by grade and sex, and about 17 students from each stratum participated in the in-home survey for each school. Additional details on Add Health surveys and sampling methods can be found in Udry (1998).

We screened Add Health for variables thought to tap into family structure, resources, and processes and to represent risk factors for obesity and calculated relative risks. Relative risks represent the probability of being overweight or at risk of overweight, defined by a BMI higher than the 85th percentile of the 2000 CDC Growth Charts for age and sex. Accordingly our data do not describe the risk of frank obesity, but of obesity as well as more modest levels of excess weight. We calculated BMI from self-report of height and weight because measured height and weight are not available for wave I of Add Health. Relative risks are presented for each variables, so cases with missing data were deleted in pairwise fashion. Significance was determined based on á = 0.05 using 95 percent confidence intervals (CI) of the relative risk. Missing responses for variables concerning fathers reflect 1740 cases (28.7%) with no residential father. Parental obesity and household income were reported by a responding parent; no responding parent was interviewed in 718 cases (11.8%). Of responding parents, 18.5 percent refused to report total household income. Missing data constituted less than 5 percent of cases across other variables. Among all included respondents, 23.8 percent had a BMI higher than the 85th percentile of the reference population. All data are reported as (relative risk, 95% confidence interval).

Structural Risk Factors

Structural risk factors include the number of parents in the home, the number of children in the household and the sex and ethnicity of the responding child. The structural component of family life modifies processes. Children with no or few siblings might expect to receive increased personal nurture and provision, compared to homes where resources are distributed among larger numbers. A greater number of children in the home creates complexity in all processes, as they must be executed across a greater number of people and a more intricate network of relationships. Responsibility over each of these processes in single parent homes is shifted to one parent, and often to a child who may not be developmentally prepared for these roles.

Adolescents from single parent homes were at increased risk of being overweight, but this effect was not significant (relative risk, 95% confidence interval: 1.10, 0.99–1.21). Significant reduction in obesity risk existed in homes with two children (0.89, 0.80–0.99) and three or more children (0.80, 0.71–0.89) compared to single child homes. Hispanics (1.23, 1.07–1.41) and non-Hispanic blacks (1.27, 1.14–1.41) were at increased risk relative to whites. Females were at lower risk than males (0.83, 0.76–0.91).

Risk associated with number of children in the home might reflect division of available food across more individuals. Additionally the task of feeding a larger family may be complex enough to force some level of structure and routine upon families who would otherwise leave eating unregulated. Conversely an only child may receive a greater share of not only family food, but also of monitoring; as we pointed out regarding eating, excessive monitoring of children's eating may promote unhealthy eating practices. These possible explanations are not testable with Add Health data. The increased risk among minorities demonstrated here is consistent with other research. In other research these effects persist after controlling for income and education. These differences could be caused by social inequalities not captured in conventional markers of socioeconomic status. Differences in risk between males and females may relate to the dominating social expectation that females conform to a particular body type.

Family Resource Risk Factors

Family resource risk factors include income-to-needs ratio, maternal education, and paternal education. Income-to needs-ratio is the ratio of household income to a family-size-adjusted poverty level. Ratios were calculated based on reported total income, household size, and membership, and poverty thresholds according to the 1995 U.S. Census report (ratio = total income / 1995 poverty threshold specific to the number of adults and children in the home). Resources most obviously influence the *providing* domain of family processes. High-calorie, low-nutrient foods are often less expensive to Americans today than healthier alternatives. Resources available to the family influence the kinds of food provided. In the context of obesity, increased education is drawn upon as families learn and decide what kinds of foods and activities are most beneficial to members. This kind of resource distills onto the way families choose to *nurture* and *provide*. We expect that the risk of being overweight will increase in lower income and less educated homes.

Compared to adolescents from the poorest third of households, those from the middle (0.86, 0.76–0.98) and the wealthiest thirds (0.77, 0.67–0.88) were at lower risk. Parental education also had a protective effect. Having a mother with a high school diploma reduced risk by about 15 percent (0.84, 0.75–0.95) and with a college, graduate or professional degree by about 30 percent (0.71, 0.62–0.81). For the father, a high school diploma reduced risk by about 12 percent (0.78, 0.68–0.90) and a college, graduate, or professional degree by more than 40 percent (0.57, 0.49–0.67).

Resources are important factors from which family process evolve. Income, for example, is not family life in its own right, but represents a

Figure 6.3
Income-to-needs Tertiles and Paternal Education on Adolescent Obesity Incidence

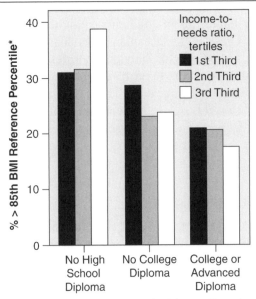

*Reference percentiles drawn from the Centers for Disease Control and Prevention 2000 Growth Charts.

key resource tapped into by family members in their efforts to achieve family goals (Day et al., 2006). Parental education is protective. This effect is attributed to improved diets and increased active recreation. This is an example of bedrock *resources* influencing family processes such as *providing*. Figure 6.3 reveals an interaction of paternal education and the income-to-needs ratio. Among children with the least educated fathers, increased income corresponds to an increase in obesity incidence. Among educated families increased income is protective.

This difference in trends with education is reminiscent of the nutrition transition discussed earlier. Recall that in undeveloped countries higher income is associated with increased obesity, while in developed countries income is protective. Education, like development, accompanies changes in the way income relates to obesity risk. Some attribute this effect to education's influence on behavior: more educated individuals may be more likely use resources in health-promoting pursuits. For a more detailed analysis of a race, income, and education interaction in incidence of adolescent obesity, refer to Gordon-Larsen, Adair, and Popkin (2003).

Family Processes

Eating

We anticipate that increased frequency of family meals will reduce the risk of being overweight, because family meals have been consistently shown to promote more healthful dietary choices. This effect represents *teaching* and *regulating* processes. Because parental control of eating interferes with normal self-regulation we anticipate decreased obesity risk among children reporting autonomy over diet. Finally we anticipate that increased servings of dairy, fruit, and vegetables will reduce risk of being overweight. These do not expressly measure family interactions involved in eating, but are intuitively connected to family decisions about foods *provided* and parental involvement or *nurturing* through feeding. Past literature has shown that skipping breakfast is associated with weight gain, apparently because breakfast suppresses appetite later in the day. Families may have rules or routines regarding breakfast, but direct assessment of such process is unavailable in Add Health.

An increased incidence of overweight was discovered in adolescents reporting seven family meals in the previous week relative to those reporting zero to three family meals (1.17, 1.05–1.30). No difference in risk was detected among those reporting four to six family meals. Adolescent report of autonomy over diet did not change risk. Consumption of dairy, fruits, and vegetables each had a protective effect. For dairy, two or more servings (0.85, 0.75–0.95) were not more protective than one serving (0.88, 0.77–0.99). This was also true of fruits: two or more servings (0.89, 0.79–0.99), one serving (0.88, 0.78–0.99). For vegetables, one serving was not protective but two or more servings conferred a significant risk reduction (0.88, 0.78–0.99). Skipping breakfast was associated with increased risk, as in other studies (1.24, 1.12–1.38).

Increased risk with seven family meals is counterintuitive given reports that family meals improve the diet (Videon & Manning, 2003). More specific measures of interactions surrounding family meals and eating behavior would tell us what is different about families eating dinner together nightly. Using Add Health variables we can only speculate, but perhaps food and eating are part of the family ideology. Where food takes a central position in the family, plates may be refilled as soon as they are empty and members may be encouraged through *teaching* and *providing* to consume excess food. These are merely guesses at the reasons for the unexpected result; in light of a substantial body of literature that family meals improve the overall quality of the diet and the observational nature of this analysis, it should *not* be interpreted from this result that family meals promote obesity. Risk was elevated only in adolescents reporting seven family meals weekly; no difference was detected in those reporting four to six weekly family meals.

Activity

Coparticipation in sport with parents represents *teaching* of a physically active lifestyle, and is expected to reduce risk of being overweight. We also expect that autonomy over television viewing will increase risk, as television viewing (unlike eating) is not biologically monitored and may be excessive without familial regulation. Increased use of media and decreased biking, sport, and exercise are expected to increase obesity risk. These last factors indirectly capture *rules* and *rituals* concerning recreational time.

Reports of playing an active sport with a parent in the last week were not significant, nor was reported autonomy over television viewing. Compared to the third of children viewing the least media, the middle third (1.12, 1.00–1.26) and the top third (1.43, 1.28–1.60) were at increased risk. Relative to the third practicing the lowest levels of physical activity, the middle third was not protected (1.04, 0.94–1.15) but the top third was (0.86, 0.76–0.97).

The ways family members spend recreational time are a function of family *goals* and *regulation* processes. Families may watch television together in the pursuit of greater cohesion, or allow children unlimited TV time seeking autonomy and freedom of members. Rules about TV viewing may be imposed in the pursuit of education, health or literacy, but if these rules are not enforced they do not matter. Alternatively a family may simply not consider it important to regulate child media use. Again, more detailed investigation into what rules families create—implicit or explicit—regarding recreational time, if and how these rules are enforced and the associated levels of active and sedentary behavior would allow for a clearer assessment of process. The current data support the role of active versus inactive recreation in obesity, but do not reveal insight into how families processes might be involved.

Inheritance

One additional family risk factor present in Add Health is difficult to classify due to problems with measurement. Responding parents were asked if the target child's biological mother and father were obese. The question was apparently directed at the genetic component of obesity, however 89.6 percent of public-use Add Health sample subjects live with the biological mother, and 67.3 percent with the biological father. In order to exert some measure of control over mutually confounding genetic and environmental influences, risk ratios for these two variables were calculated separately for adolescents living with and without the biological parent. Still, the question lacks precision, as the self-perception of obesity varies widely and is often not correct (Goodman, Hinden, & Khandelwal, 2000). These variables are included in the present analysis as inheritance of obesity is relevant to understanding obesity in the family context; they are expected to exhibit strong associations with obesity risk but should be interpreted with care.

Among adolescents living with the biological parent, identification of the mother as obese by the responding parent doubled risk of being overweight (2.10, 1.90–2.33). Identification of fathers as obese nearly doubled risk (1.84, 1.59–2.12). Among adolescents who did *not* live with the biological parent, obese status of the biological father conferred a similar risk (1.78, 1.40–2.16) but obese status of the biological mother was not a significant risk (1.33, 0.89–2.00). Though the confidence interval of this last risk estimate is wide, for all adolescents with reported obese mothers, the risk was greater in those living with the biological mother ($p<0.05$).

An adolescent living with an obese biological mother is expected to inherit generic risks, but also to learn obesity-promoting behaviors. Though the risk associated with an obese father was similar for children living with and without the biological father in question, it is possible that other sociodemographic risk factors mask true differences. Note that in most cases, the mother is the responding parent identifying obese status of parents. An obvious opportunity for reporting bias of own versus another's obese status complicates this analysis. Still these data provide some evidence that social inheritance of obese status occurs independently of genetic inheritance. Genetic inheritance of obesity represents a *structural* family element, whereas social inheritance represents a *teaching* process. This transmission of behavior relates to the *teaching* function of families, and ties into the idea that families cannot *not* teach. If parents fail to teach children healthy eating and activity behaviors, children learn that such behaviors are not important. Modeling of unhealthy practices by an obese parent is also likely to occur.

SUMMARY

Obesity among adolescents, as in the general population, is an increasingly pressing cause for concern. Obesity promotes several leading causes of death and illness, including heart attack, stroke, some cancers, and diabetes. Some traditionally adult illnesses such as diabetes and cardiovascular disease are beginning to appear in children. Obesity is also related to difficulties in body image and social development, depending somewhat on gender. These difficulties may promote poor self esteem, depression, and suicidal ideation, particularly if weight becomes an object of ridicule. Obesity is also expensive, incurring costs on the order of 50 to 100 billion U.S. dollars annually; as much as half of this may be paid by tax dollars through government programs.

The BMI or body mass index (weight in kilograms / height^2 in meters) is the most common measure of obese status. The BMI is not the best indicator of obesity, but it is the best that can be calculated without specialized training and equipment. In adolescents obesity is described using the CDC growth charts for age and sex. These provide percentiles from a reference population predating the current elevated obesity rates.

Obesity is caused most directly by the balance of energy expended in activity and background physiology with energy intake from food. Compared to past times, our modern work and play are more sedentary and our food is less expensive and more packed with energy. Excess eating combined with a sedentary lifestyle are the most immediate and obvious causes of obesity. These are influenced by biology, however, as in genetic programming for satiety (feeling full) or a thrifty metabolism. Downstream social factors also influence the risk of obesity: socioeconomic status, ethnicity, and education all factor into food and activity availability and preference.

Family processes refer to strategies families use to attain their goals. They are the how of family studies, and for our purposes here were divided into six domains: inclusion, protection, nurturing, providing, regulation, and teaching. Family processes also include routines and communication patterns, and depend partly on a broader family context of family structure, ideologies, and resources. Numerous studies have connected family processes to the causes of obesity. How a family copes with obesity depends on the meaning they attach to it. Parental over-regulation of a child's eating promotes poor eating habits. Also, patterns of eating and activity are established in the home through modeling, explicit teaching, and routines surrounding food and play. Most of our meals and recreational time happen in the family setting.

In Add Health, the risk of being overweight varies with family structure and family resources. Specifically children of single-child homes and of minority status were at increased risk, as were children with less educated parents and those from low income-to-needs homes. Males were more frequently overweight (defined for age and sex) than females. We speculate that gender and racial differences relate to social pressures and expectations, and that race, income, and education differences reflect disparity in access to health-promoting foods and recreation, but also in the way available resources are applied. Education in particular seems to be an important moderator of the relationship between income and obesity.

Family process measures such as reported autonomy over diet and TV viewing failed to predict differences in risk, as did parental participation in sports. Family meal frequency was predictive, as was actual time spent watching media. Reported consumption of dairy, fruit, and vegetables was protective, along with higher than average levels of physical activity. Obese status of the biological parents was the strongest predictor of being overweight, however this association is difficult to interpret due to the potential for reporting bias and mutually confounding influences of genetic inheritance and socialization, as the majority of Add Health respondents were also raised by the biological parent. Having an obese biological mother roughly doubled the risk of being overweight if the adolescent also lived with the obese mother, but not if the adolescent lived apart from that mother. Children with a reported obese biological father were approximately at 80 percent greater risk of being overweight compared to children without, regardless of whether the child lived with the biological father, however children living away from the biological father incur other sociodemographic risks. These results should be interpreted conservatively, but offer support for the idea that obesity can be inherited through socialization in addition to biology.

We assert that families matter in the development of obesity among adolescents. The why and the how of families' importance is a question of family process. Add Health variables provide a glimpse of differential risks of obesity across family structures, access to family resources, and some family processes. On the whole the large national data sets available to us measure a great deal of *content* but very little *process*. Though Add Health contains more process measures than most, there is a paucity of process measures specifically regarding family eating and activity patterns. Studies investigating routines, communication, and rules and their enforcement surrounding meals and recreation in the home are warranted.

REFERENCES

Bourcier, E., Bowen, D. J., Meischke, H., & Moinpour, C. (2003). Evaluation of strategies used by family food preparers to influence healthy eating. *Appetite, 41*(3), 265–272.

Broderick (1993). *Family processes.* Thousand Oaks, CA: Sage.

Carpenter, K. M., Hasin, D. S., Allison, D. B., & Faith, M. S. (2000). Relationships between obesity and DSM-IV Major Depressive Disorder, suicide ideation, and suicide attempts: Results from a general population study. *American Journal of Public Health, 90,* 251–257.

Day, R. D., Miller, R., & Cox, A. (2006). *Compelling family processes: Pilgrim's progress.* Family Process Symposium, Theory Construction and Research Methodology Workshop of the National Council on Family Relations..

Eisenberg, M. E., Neumark-Sztainer, D., & Story, M. (2003). Associations of weight based teasing and emotional well-being among adolescents. *Archives of Pediatric and Adolescent Medicine, 157,* 733–738.

Faith, M. S., Matz, P. E., & Allison, D. B. (2003). Psychosocial correlates and consequences of obesity. In R. E. Andersen (Ed.), *Obesity: Etiology assessment treatment and prevention* (pp. 17–31). Champaign, IL: Human Kinetics Publishers.

Goodman, E., Hinden, B. R., & Khandelwal, S. (2000). Accuracy of teen and parental reports of obesity and body mass index. *Pediatrics,106*(1), 52–58.

Gordon-Larsen, P., Adair, L. S., & Popkin, B. M. (2003). The relationship of ethnicity, socioeconomic factors, and overweight in U.S. adolescents. *Obesity Research 11*(1), 121–129.

Gustafson, S. L., & Rhodes, R. E. (2006). Parental correlates of physical activity in children and early adolescents. *Sports Medicine 36*(1), 79–97.

Jacobsen, K. C., & Rowe, D. C. (1998). Genetic and shared environmental influences on adolescent BMI: Interactions with race and sex. *Behavior Genetics, 4,* 265–278.

Johnson, S. L., & Birch, L. L. (1994). Parents' and children's adiposity and eating style. *Pediatrics, 94,* 653–661.

Kinston, W., Loader, P., & Miller, L. (1988). Talking to families about obesity: A controlled study. *International Journal of Eating Disorders, 7,* 261–275.

Koplan, J. P., Liverman, C. T., & Kraak, V. I. (Eds.) (2005). Committee on Prevention of Obesity in Children and Youth, Food and Nutrition Board, Board on Health Promotion and Disease Prevention. *Preventing childhood obesity: Health in the balance.* Washington, DC: The National Academies Press.

Kuczmarski, R. J., Ogden, C. L., Grummer-Strawn, L. M., et al. (2000). *Advance data from vital and health statistics.* Centers for Disease Control and Prevention growth charts: United States No. 314. Hyattsville, MD: National Center for Health Statistics.

Laessle, R. G., Uhl, H., & Lindel, B. (2001). Parental influences on eating behavior in obese and non-obese preadolescents. *International Journal of Eating Disorders, 30,* 447–453.

National Center for Health Statistics. (2005). *Health, United States, with trends in the health of Americans.* Hyattsville, MD: Author.

National Institutes of Health. (1998). *Clinical guidelines on the identification, evaluation, and treatment of overweight and obesity in adults* (U.S. Department of Health and Human Services: NIH Publication No. 98–4083). Bethesda, MD: NHLBI Obesity Education Initiative Expert Panel on the Identification, Evaluation, and Treatment of Overweight and Obesity in Adults.

Popkin, B. M., & Gordon-Larsen, P. (2004). The nutrition transition: Worldwide obesity dynamics and their determinants. *International Journal of Obesity, 28,* S2–9.

Sauber, S. R., L'Abate, L., Weeks, G. R., & Buchanan, W. L. (1993). *The dictionary of family psychology and family therapy.* Newbury Park, CA: Sage Publications.

Strauss, R. S., & Pollack, H. A. (2003). Social marginalization of overweight children. *Archives of Pediatrics & Adolescent Medicine, 157,* 746–752.

Thompson, D., & Wolf, A. M. (2001). The medical-care cost burden of obesity. *Obesity Review2*(3), 189–97.

Udry, J. R. (1998). *The National Longitudinal Study of Adolescent Health (Add Health), Waves I & II, 1994–1996* (Data sets 48–50, 98, A1-A3, Kelley, M. S. & Peterson, J. L.) [machine-readable data file and documentation]. Chapel Hill, NC: Carolina Population Center, University of North Carolina at Chapel Hill (Producer). Los Altos, CA: Sociometrics Corporation, American Family Data Archive (Producer & Distributor).

Videon, T. M., & Manning, C. K. (2003). Influences on adolescent eating patterns: The importance of family meals. *Journal of Adolescent Health, 32,* 365–373.

Wolf, A.M., & Colditz, G. A. (1994). The cost of obesity: the US perspective. *Pharmacoeconomics, 5*(1), 34–37.

Wolin, L., & Bennett, S. (1984). Family rituals. *Family Process, 23,* 401–411.

Part II

INDIVIDUAL DIFFERENCES AND ETHNIC VARIATION

Chapter 7

RESPONDING TO THE EPIDEMIC OF AMERICAN INDIAN AND ALASKA NATIVE CHILDHOOD OBESITY

Paul Spicer and Kelly Moore

In this chapter we review what is known about the prevalence and correlates of childhood overweight and obesity in American Indian and Alaska Native (AI/AN) communities. We then discuss some of the possible implications of this knowledge for policy change and program development in the areas of physical activity and nutrition. While much of what we see in AI/AN communities mirrors what we see in other U.S. racial and ethnic minority populations, the specific needs of AI/AN communities will require special attention as we move towards crafting culturally effective interventions. Our strategy is to position what we know or are starting to learn about obesity in AI/AN children and youth within the context of knowledge that is emerging more generally for U.S. children. We close by describing community-directed promising practices targeting AI/AN children and youth in specific communities and nationally, through the Special Diabetes Program for Indians grant programs.

THE CONSEQUENCES OF OBESITY

Obesity is a well-documented risk factor for several diseases at the center of efforts to address health disparities (Mokdad et al., 2003). Obesity is implicated in heart disease in both men and women (Carnethon et al., 2003; Hu et al., 2004; Lakka et al., 2002; Must, Jacques, Dallal, Bajema, & Dietz, 1992); a linear relation exists between body weight and blood pressure (Huang et al., 1998; Wing & Jeffrey, 1995; Witteman et al.,

1989); body mass index (BMI) and weight gain are directly correlated with risk for type 2 diabetes (Chan, Rimm, Colditz, Stampfer, & Willett, 1994; Weinstein et al., 2004; Weiss et al., 2004); and obesity is associated with several cancers (Calle & Kaaks, 2004; Calle, Rodriguez, Walker-Thurmond, & Thun, 2003; Hu et al., 2004; Huang et al., 1997). Given these multiple associations with severe and costly forms of disease, it is not surprising that obesity is associated with markedly decreased life expectancy (Fontaine, Redden, Wang, Westfall, & Allison, 2003) and dramatically higher medical costs in later life (Daviglus et al., 2004).

Among children, obesity increases the risk for type 2 diabetes, hypertension, dyslipidemia, gall bladder disease, orthopedic and osteoarticular problems, pseudotumor cerebri, and sleep apnea (de Sa Pinto, de Barros Holanda, Radu, Villares, & Lima, 2006; Friedlander, Larkin, Rosen, Palermo, & Redline, 2003; Must et al., 1999). Obesity also increases the risk of social and emotional morbidity in children and adolescents (Friedlander et al., 2003; Mustillo et al., 2003; Strauss, 2000). Furthermore, obese children are likely to remain obese into adulthood (Berkowitz & Stunkard, 2002; Serdula et al., 1993; Whitaker, Wright, Pepe, Kristy, & Dietz, 1997). Because the morbidity, mortality, and ensuing costs of the adult obesity epidemic are high (Allison, Fontaine, Manson, Stevens, & Vanitallie, 1999; Must et al., 1999; Wolf & Colditz, 1998), efforts to address obesity should begin at an early age. Recent data also have demonstrated the costs of childhood obesity are high. For instance, over a 20-year period, discharges related to diabetes doubled, discharges from gall bladder disease tripled, and those from sleep apnea increased five-fold. Not surprisingly, hospital costs increased almost fourfold overall (Wang & Dietz, 2002).

AI/AN communities are at a well-documented increased risk for health consequences that are highly correlated with obesity. Most notably, recent published data from the IHS confirm that, compared to overall U.S. population rates, AI/ANs experienced dramatically higher rates of death from type 2 diabetes mellitus (350%) and cardiovascular disease (13%) (Indian Health Service, 1999). Of equal concern, AI/ANs have not enjoyed the decreases that have been evident in the overall US death rates for cardiovascular disease in the past two decades. Although diabetes mellitus and heart disease are complex, multi-factorial disorders, obesity has clearly been shown to be an independent risk factor for both diseases (Knowler et al., 1991; Lee et al., 2002; Welty, 1991; Welty et al., 1995).

The most alarming health statistic in most AI communities is the rising prevalence of type 2 diabetes. Typically affecting adults, type 2 diabetes is increasingly being diagnosed at earlier ages in AI children and adolescents (Centers for Disease Control, 2003a); it has even been described in a three-year-old Pima child (Dabelea et al., 1998). Although the age of onset is more consistent with type 1 diabetes, most young AIs with diabetes lack islet cell and other autoantibodies characteristic of type 1 diabetes (Lee et al., 1995; SEARCH for Diabetes in Youth Study Group, 2006). Equally disturbing, Pima children 6–19 years of age have been shown to have higher fasting insulin levels than their white counterparts, even after controlling for age, glucose, and relative weight (Pettitt et al., 1993). Surveillance data reported from the Indian Health Service last year that the age-adjusted prevalence of diagnosed diabetes increased from 8.5 to 17.1 per 1,000 population among AI/ANs aged less than 35 years who use IHS health-care services (Centers for Disease Control, 2006). Also troubling is the increasing occurrence of gestational diabetes among AI women, which increases the risk of both mother and child for subsequent diabetes (Moum et al., 2004).

THE PREVALENCE OF OBESITY

Ongoing data collection from the National Health and Nutrition Examination Surveys (NHANES) continues to point to dramatic increases in the prevalence of overweight and obesity, at least for male adults and for all children. Between 1999–2000 and 2003–2004 the prevalence of obesity among men increased from 27.5 percent to 31.1 percent. During the same period the prevalence among women did not significantly change (generally around 33% in both years). For children, however, the prevalence of overweight for girls increased from 13.8 percent to 16.0 percent, and for boys from 14.0 percent to 18.2 percent (Ogden et al., 2006). Thus, although rates of obesity may have slowed or stabilized among women, they have continued to increase among men and children of both sexes, with racial and ethnic minorities continuing to be at increased risk for obesity. Significantly greater increases in childhood overweight in families living below the poverty line have also been reported (Miech et al., 2006).

Actual epidemiological data on the prevalence of AI/AN obesity are rare, in no small part because AI/AN populations have not been included in sufficient numbers in large national studies such as NHANES (Story et al., 1999). Data that do exist, however, paint a consistent portrait of AI populations with higher rates of obesity and overweight than the general U.S. population (Story et al., 1999). Data collected in the mid 1980s by the Indian Health Service (IHS) found that rates of overweight among AI adults were 10–15 percent higher than comparable U.S. rates (Broussard et al., 1991). The Strong Heart Study, a longitudinal study of risk factors for cardiovascular disease in 13 AI tribes, also documented rates of overweight among older AI men and women in Arizona, the Dakotas, and Oklahoma that were dramatically higher than U.S. averages for comparable age groups (Welty et al., 1995). Among adults, rates of obesity have ranged from 67 percent in the Dakotas (Welty et al., 1995) to 87 percent among Pima women (Knowler et al., 1991).

The few published rates of obesity and overweight in AI children indicate that high rates arise early in AI populations (Broussard et al., 1991; Zephier, Himes, & Story, 1999). One of the largest studies to assess childhood obesity among AI schoolchildren was conducted in 1990 in nine IHS service areas by the Centers for Disease Control and Prevention, IHS, and tribal nutrition programs. Overall, 39 percent of children ages 5–18 years were overweight or obese, defined as a BMI more than the 85th percentile (Jackson, 1993). Studies among the Navajo and among Northern Plains tribes of South Dakota, North Dakota, Iowa, and Nebraska have demonstrated similar rates (Eisenmann et al., 2002; Zephier et al., 1999). In the Northern Plains study, childhood overweight in tribal youth was more than twice as prevalent as in U.S. youth overall, and obesity was more than three times as prevalent (Zephier et al., 1999). In a recent follow-up on the Northern Plains research, rates of overweight and obesity among children again consistently exceeded those for all U.S. children and had increased by over 4 percent for each category from the mid-1990s (Zephier, Himes, Story, & Zhou, 2006). Excessive childhood obesity has also been reported in First Nation children and adolescents in Canada among the eastern James Bay Cree of Quebec (Bernard, Lavallee, Gray-Donald, & Delisle, 1995), the Mohawk community of Kahnawake (Trifonopoulos, 1995), and the Sandy Lake First Nation of central Canada (Hanley et al., 2000).

RISK AND PROTECTIVE FACTORS FOR OBESITY

Below we review the general and AI/AN-specific literature on factors associated with overweight and obesity. Although genetics clearly plays a role in obesity (Bell, Walley, & Froguel, 2005), and leading interventions may well work by altering the expression of genes, we focus here on efforts to change the patterns of physical activity and nutrition that appear to underlie the recent surge in childhood obesity, especially since interventions flowing from genetic knowledge have yet to be realized in childhood obesity (Stice, Shaw, & Marti, 2006; Whitlock, Williams, Gold, Smith, & Shipman, 2005).

Risk and Protective Factors in the General U.S. Population

Energy Gap

The most obvious risk factor for obesity is the energy gap, that is, the discrepancy between energy intake and energy expenditure (Hill, Wyatt, Reed, & Peters, 2003). Several social forces have converged to increase energy intake (e.g., availability of high-calorie foodstuffs, large portion sizes) and to decrease energy expenditure (e.g., increases in sedentary behaviors, decreases in activity). Although the actual energy gap may, in absolute terms, be small and amenable to small changes in behavior, its consequences for the prevalence of overweight and obesity are large (Hill et al., 2003). Underscoring these dynamics are recent results reported by the Nurses Health Study II, which documents strong associations between obesity, type 2 diabetes, sedentary behavior (Hu, Li, Colditz, Willett, & Manson, 2003), and soft drink consumption (Schulze et al., 2004).

Early Life Experiences and Parental Influences

Several sophisticated descriptive studies have provided valuable insight into the role of early experiences in shaping subsequent physical development. Among the early childhood risk factors identified are birth to a mother with diabetes (Plagemann, Harder, Kohlhoff, Rohde, & Dorner, 1997); conversely, breastfeeding may be a protective factor (Bergmann et al., 2003; Gillman et al., 2001; Owen, Martin, Whincup, Smith, & Cook, 2005), despite earlier equivocal results (Berkowitz & Stunkard, 2002) and recent findings demonstrating no association between breastfeeding and the likelihood of obesity during life course in participants in the Nurses Health Study (Michels et al., 2007),. Other factors predictive of weight gain include a child's weight gain in the first years of life (Dennison, Edmunds, Stratton, & Pruzek, 2006; Gunnarsdottir & Thorsdottir, 2003; Stettler, Zemel, Kumanyika, & Stallings, 2002; Toschke, Grote, Koletzko, & von Kries, 2004), maternal child-feeding patterns (Faith et al., 2003), dietary composition (Newby et al., 2003), duration of sleep (von Kries, Toschke, Wurmser, Sauerwald, & Koletzko, 2002), television viewing (Dennison, Erb, & Jenkins, 2002), participation in other sedentary activities (Vandewater, Shim, & Caplovitz, 2003), and participation in physical education (Datar & Sturm, 2004). In later childhood and adolescence, diet and sedentary behavior continue to be risk factors (Ebbeling et al., 2004; Giammattei, Blix, Marshak, Wollitzer, & Pettitt, 2003), with physical activity appearing to increase in importance (Aaron, Storti, Robertson, Kriska, & Laporte,

2002; Gordon-Larsen, Adair, & Popkin, 2002; Kvaavik, Tell, & Klepp, 2003; Patrick et al., 2004).

Food and activity choices of parents and children are also influenced by many factors, such as maternal depression and obesity (Burdette, Whitaker, Kahn, & Harvey-Berino, 2003), environmental barriers to physical activity (Centers for Disease Control, 2003b), cost and availability of healthier foods (Drewnowski, Darmon, & Briend, 2004; Horowitz, Colson, Hebert, & Lancaster, 2004), socioeconomic inequality (Zhang & Wang, 2004), and acculturation to the lifestyle of the U.S. majority culture (Goel, McCarthy, Phillips, & Wee, 2004; Gordon-Larsen, Harris, Ward, & Popkin, 2003). Interestingly, the BMI of mothers and their children have been shown to be highly associated in Hispanic families, but not in African American and European American families, although the reasons for this finding are not yet clear (Jago et al., 2004).

Parental Perceptions of Weight

Researchers have shown parents and caregivers may not initiate preventive changes unless they first perceive their child is overweight or at risk for some adverse outcome (Hazard & Lee, 1996; Uzark, Becvker, Dielman, Rocchini, & Kastch, 1988). The available evidence suggests that levels of awareness are low, especially among parents or caregivers with lower levels of income and education. A focus group study found low-income mothers believed that heavier infants were healthier, that their infants were not getting enough to eat and needed solid foods at ages earlier than recommended, and that food should be used to stimulate good behavior (Baughcum, Burklow, Powers, & Whitaker, 1998). In a subsequent study of primarily white mothers served by the Program for Women, Infants, and Children (WIC), most mothers of overweight children failed to recognize that their child had a weight problem (Baughcum, Chamberlin, Powers, & Whitaker, 2000). Likewise, parents of overweight children from a pediatric faculty practice invariably underestimated their children's weight (Etelson, Brand, Patrick, & Shirali, 2003). In NHANES III, which included 5,500 children 2–11 years of age, nearly one-third of mothers misclassified overweight children as weighing less than their actual measured weight (Maynard, Galuska, Blank, & Serdula, 2003). These findings contrast with earlier research suggesting that most parents accurately identify their child's weight status (Coates, Jeffrey, & Wing, 1978; Jackson, Strauss, Lee, & Hunter, 1990; Wing, Epstein, & Neff, 1980). Nevertheless, even this older literature documents that errors of weight underestimation are approximately five times as frequent as errors of overestimation (Jackson et al., 1990).

Parental Perceptions of Risks of Obesity

Another factor in preventing childhood obesity is recognizing the associated health risks. A study of caregiver perceptions of children's obesity-related health risk among African American families demonstrated that fewer than half of the caregivers perceived their child's weight to be a potential health problem, even though 57 percent of the children were obese and 12 percent were very obese (Young-Hyman, Herman, Scott, & Schlundt, 2000). Even when weight estimates appear to be correct, the level of parental concern may not reflect the actual risks of childhood obesity. For example, in a focus group of 18 young, low-income mothers participating in WIC, the majority correctly identified their child as overweight, but only two mothers worried about their child's present weight and only five were concerned about the child's weight in the future (Jain, 2001). Similarly, in Katz's research, some African American girls and their female caregivers were dissatisfied with the girls' body size, but body size was not viewed as a health risk (Katz et al., 2004) and, in a recent British study, parents were surprisingly unaware of overweight and obesity in themselves and their children and unconcerned about excess weight (Jeffery, Voss, Metcalf, Alba, & Wilkin, 2005).

Risk and Protective Factors in AI/AN Populations

Activity Levels

Research on risk and protective factors for obesity has rarely been conducted among AI populations, but a considerable body of work has consistently documented very low levels of activity in many communities. Among Strong Heart Study participants, for example, 38 percent of men and 48 percent of women reported no leisure-time physical activity during the past week (Welty et al., 1995). Other studies have generally substantiated this finding across many tribes: 25 percent of Navajo adults did not exercise during the past month (Mendlein et al., 1997); more than 50 percent of the members of two Montana tribes (Goldberg et al., 1991) and more than 90 percent of Yaqui adults aged 35 to 65 years had sedentary lifestyles (Molina & Campos-Outcalt, 1991); and 47 percent of Cree and Ojibwa tribes were physically inactive (Young, 1991). In the Intertribal Heart Project, the reported rate of inactivity was 28 percent, and was more common in women, older age groups, and persons with less formal education, lower income, and no employment (Centers for Disease Control and Prevention, 1996). Only 36 percent of participants aged 25 years and older were regularly active, compared to 42 percent of the U.S. population aged 18 and over. Regular activity did not differ by education or income, but was slightly higher among males and employed participants. Only in the Behavioral Risk Factor Surveillance Study was the prevalence of "no frequent exercise" much lower among AIs than non-Indians (Cheadle et al., 1994). Finally, the strong associations between television watching, physical activity, and obesity demonstrated in the majority culture have been replicated among Pima adults (Fitzgerald, Shannon, Kriska, Pereira, & De courten, 1997). While little is known, specifically, about AI/AN children, a recent investigation of very young Mohawk children has suggested that there is a gap between energy intake and expenditure that is measurable even in infancy and toddlerhood (Harvey-Berino, Wellman, Hood, Rourke, & Secker-Walker, 2000).

Early Life Experiences

The most recent national data on breastfeeding from the National Immunization Survey in 2005 indicate that AI/AN mothers are consistently low in all measures of breastfeeding, exceeded only by African Americans (Centers for Disease Control, 2007). What little AI/AN specific information we have suggests that, as in other populations, breastfeeding is a protective factor for childhood obesity (Thomas & Cook, 2005). Exclusive breastfeeding for the first two months of life has been associated with a large reduction in type 2 diabetes among Pima Indians (Pettitt, Forman, Hanson, Knowler, & Bennett, 1997). Furthermore, the Phoenix Indian Medical Center found that AI/AN children who were breastfed exclusively for the first six months of life experienced an overweight and obesity rate of 23 percent at the ages of three and four years, as compared with an overweight and obesity rate of 64 percent in children who were exclusively fed formula (Thomas & Cook, 2005). Very little has been published regarding other aspects of parenting and feeding styles of AI families.

Attitudes

The few studies on weight-related attitudes and behaviors with AI youth have focused primarily on adolescents, and all have indicated that eating disturbances, weight dissatisfaction, and unhealthy weight loss practices are common (Neumark-Sztainer, Story, Resnick, & Blum, 1997; Rosen et al., 1988; Sherwood, Harnack, & Story, 2000; Story et al., 1994). The Pathways Feasibility Study has assessed weight concerns, body size perceptions, weight reduction attempts, and weight loss methods among preadolescent AI youth. Their results illustrate that preadolescent children are concerned about their weight and that weight modification efforts are common among overweight AI children at a young age (Stevens et al., 1999; Story, Stevens, & Evans, 2001), a finding that is echoed in work conducted among urban AI youth (Rinderknecht & Smith, 2002). Yet, to our knowledge, AI parents' perception of childhood weight has been examined in only one study. A focus group study of 77 caregivers from a WIC program in Arizona found that caregivers did not associate over-weight in preschoolers with future health problems (Jossefides-Tomkins & Lujan, 2003).

OBESITY PREVENTION IN CHILDREN AND ADOLESCENTS

Because overweight and obesity arise at early ages in AI/ANs, the development and testing of preventive interventions in childhood are urgently needed. Unfortunately, the literature on randomized controlled trials and other controlled studies on interventions to reduce overweight and obesity in children is small for any population and virtually nonex-istent for AI/AN children. The most recently published Cochrane review on obesity prevention in children and adolescents located only 10 inter-vention trials with long term follow-up (over 1 year). Theer was very limited evidence for the success of any specific intervention strategy in these long-term studies, although the 12 studies with shorter follow-up (under 12 months) provided evidence that some interventions designed to increase activity had an impact on BMI (Summerbell, Waters, Edmunds, Kelly, Brown, et al., 2005). Most of these published studies on childhood obesity interventions have focused on changes in preschool, school, and family environments. A more recent meta-analysis, which included results from less rigorous designs, suggested the impact of prevention programs for children and adolescents was quite small (Stice et al., 2006). Additionally, the U.S. Preventive Services Task Force could not issue a strong recommendation to screen for overweight among children and younger adolescents, in part because few validated treatment approaches exist for children identified in such screenings (Whitlock et al., 2005).

Despite this lack of rigorous research, several aspects of successful interventions have been identified that broadly suggest effective strategies. For example, in an Italian multi-media educational intervention, the effect of written brochures containing nutritional information was augmented by audiovisual aids and trained staff (Simonetti D'Arca et al., 1986). An intervention in the Boston Public Schools to promote physical activity, modify diet, and decrease sedentary behaviors reduced obesity among girls primarily through reductions in sedentary behavior (Gortmaker et al., 1999). Likewise, an intervention in San Jose, California, reduced BMI in children by encouraging reductions in sedentary behaviors (Robinson, 1999), and another in schools in Palo Alto, California, decreased BMI through a physical activity-oriented dance curriculum (Flores, 1995). A successful German study combined a school-based intervention with home-based family counseling to target diet, activity, and sedentary behavior (Müller, Asbeck, Mast, Langnäse, & Grund, 2001). Most recently, results from the CATCH study suggested that a school-based program emphasizing changes in diet and activity slowed increases in childhood overweight in schools where it was implemented (Coleman et al., 2005). A quasi-experimental design, contrasting outcomes from schools that implemented a comprehensive nutrition program with those that did not, also suggested that such programs could help prevent obesity (Veugelers & Fitzgerald, 2005). Furthermore, emerging evidence indicates targeted interventions can affect early childhood behaviors that have been linked to obesity, including increasing breastfeeding (Anderson, Damio, Young, Chapman, & Perez-Escamilla, 2005; Chapman, Damio, Young, & Perez-Escamilla, 2004), decreasing the intake of fat (Talvia et al., 2004), decreasing sedentary activity (Dennison, Russo, Burdick, & Jenkins, 2004), and increasing physical activity (McGarvey et al., 2004).

The need to stem the rising tide of obesity among the young is so urgent that the Institute of Medicine's recent report on preventing childhood obesity has recommended proceeding with intervention trials despite a lack of evidence on their benefit, as long as they are pursued with a careful evaluation strategy (Institute of Medicine, 2005). The report also urged the evaluation and conduct of basic research concurrent with developing and implementing interventions. Specifically, it offered 10 recommendations for future interventions: (1) coordinated leadership on obesity prevention at the national level; (2) actions by industry to promote healthy eating and physical activity; (3) clear and useful nutritional labeling; (4) development of marketing and advertising guidelines to minimize the risk of obesity; (5) multimedia and public relations campaigns focused on obesity prevention; (6) development of community programs; (7) expanded opportunities for physical activity in the built environment; (8) intervention in the health care system to prevent obesity; (9) changes in the school environment to promote healthy eating and activity; and (10) changes in the home environment (Institute of Medicine, 2005).

The literature on obesity interventions in AI/ANs is, not surprisingly, even smaller than that for the general population. In a trial conducted among Southwest tribes, knowledge increased and self-reported behavior improved significantly in intervention schools that received a curriculum on cardiovascular health; however, changes in BMI and skinfold thickness were not reported (Davis, Gomez, Lambert, & Skipper, 1993). The largest trial of a preventive obesity intervention in AI communities was the Pathways study (Byers, 2003; Caballero et al., 2003). This randomized, controlled, school-based trial involved 1,704 children in 41 schools and was conducted from the third to fifth grades, in schools serving AI communities in Arizona, New Mexico, and South Dakota. The trial's objective was to evaluate the effectiveness of a school-based, multicomponent intervention for reducing percentage of body fat. The intervention had four components: (1) change in dietary intake; (2) increase in physical activity; (3) a classroom curriculum focused on healthy eating and lifestyle; and (4) a family-involvement program. Unfortunately, the intervention resulted in no significant reduction in percentage of body fat, which was the primary outcome. The percentage of energy from fat and total energy intake (by 24-hour dietary recall) were significantly reduced in the intervention schools (Himes et al., 2003), but the intervention had no effect on energy intake (by direct observation) and activity levels, as documented by motion sensor data (Going et al., 2003). Some knowledge, attitudes, and behaviors were positively and significantly changed by the intervention (Stevens et al., 2003). Recently reported long-term follow-up on a trial conducted among the Mohawk in the Kahnawake Schools in Quebec was also discouraging, indicating that early gains from an elementary school program were not sustained (Paradis et al., 2005).

OBESITY PREVENTION FOR AMERICAN INDIAN INFANTS AND FAMILIES

The disappointing results from preventive interventions to date, which have occurred in all communities, underscore just how difficult it will be to reverse the dynamics that have shaped the current epidemic of childhood obesity. But here we highlight two promising new approaches with which we have been involved that extend intervention into the earliest years and in relatively comprehensive community-based ways.

Emerging Opportunities for Intervention in Infancy

Drawing on the growing literature that suggest that factors evident in infancy may well predispose children to obesity and overweight, our team at the American Indian and Alaska Native Programs at the University of Colorado at Denver and Health Sciences Center has developed a home-based intervention designed to promote changes in mother's behavior in the areas of feeding and activity for their children. Linked to specific aspects of children's development, and inspired by the example of the Nurse-Family Partnership (Olds, 2002), we will begin working with first-time mothers in a northern plains tribe in the last trimester of their pregnancy, visiting them six times before their child is six months of age. The intervention specifically targets breastfeeding in the early visits before turning to formula or other foods in later visits (or earlier if the mother has decided not to breastfeed), sleep, and finally activity for both the child and family. While we are still in the pilot phase of this intervention, it enjoys broad-based support from our community partners who are discouraged by rates of childhood obesity and overweight that are already apparent in preschool. By using motivational interviewing (Miller & Rollnick, 2002), the intervention also is open to local systems of meaning and values in ways that permit it to enjoy much better local support than a simple educational intervention would.

The Special Diabetes Programs for Indians at the Indian Health Service

The Special Diabetes Program for Indians (SDPI) is a grant program, administered by the Indian Health Service Division of Diabetes Treatment and Prevention, which provides funding for diabetes prevention and treatment services at IHS, tribal, and urban Indian health programs. SDPI has made it possible for AI and AN communities to develop and implement type 2 diabetes primary prevention programs for children and youth—a compelling priority for the future of AI and AN communities. These promising programs are designed to promote healthy lifestyle habits in children and youth to reduce their risk of developing type 2 diabetes and other chronic conditions.

The Special Diabetes Program for Indians grant programs use recommended public health strategies to prevent childhood obesity. One important strategy is breastfeeding promotion. As noted above, breastfeeding plays a particularly important role in preventing both obesity and type 2 diabetes. Other important obesity prevention strategies include encouraging children and youth to increase physical activity, limit television viewing, increase fruit and vegetable intake, control portion sizes, and limit soft drink consumption. The Special Diabetes Program for Indians grant programs have implemented activities to help young children develop physical activity and healthy eating habits. These strategies address the multiple factors that contribute to the development of obesity and subsequent type 2 diabetes, and as a result, are likely to have the greatest impact in preventing type 2 diabetes in youth.

To ensure success, the Special Diabetes Program for Indians grant programs have worked closely with school and community partners to establish policy and environmental changes that support physical activity and healthy eating strategies. For example, grant programs have successfully changed school vending machine and wellness policies, increased the availability of school and community physical activity opportunities, increased access to fitness facilities for children and youth, and built or improved local playgrounds. These programs have created a supportive environment for children and youth to exercise and eat more healthfully, helping to lower their risk for developing diabetes now and in the future.

The Special Diabetes Program for Indians grant programs also have implemented activities and services to support behavior changes for youth and their families. Family involvement in achieving and maintaining a healthy weight for children is essential. Parents need to promote healthy eating behaviors and regular physical activity for their children. They often are responsible for purchasing and offering healthy foods and portion sizes, serving as role models, and making mealtime enjoyable. In addition, one or both parents and other siblings may be overweight or have diabetes, further suggesting that the entire family should be targeted for intervention. Recognizing the key role families play in the health of youth, many grant programs offer weight management, medical nutrition therapy, and behavioral health services for children, adolescents, and their families.

The Special Diabetes Program for Indians grant programs have developed and implemented Indian Health Diabetes Best Practices on preventing obesity and reducing the risk for type 2 diabetes in youth. These Best Practices target women of childbearing age and families to intervene before conception, during the prenatal period, and during the first few years of the child's life. The Special Diabetes Program for Indians grant programs are implementing the elements of these Best Practices through the following actions:

- Reducing in utero exposure to elevated blood sugar levels in gestational diabetes programs

- Promoting breastfeeding of infants for at least two months through awareness campaigns, promotion programs, and policies
- Establishing programs to increase physical activity and improve food choices and eating behaviors early in life
- Intervening earlier with children who are obese and have diabetes and making appropriate referrals.
- Treating youth with type 2 diabetes

The Special Diabetes Program for Indians has brought hope to American Indian and Alaska Native communities that they can reduce the risk for type 2 diabetes in their children and youth. By employing a multi-faceted approach that includes families, schools, the health care system, and other important stakeholders, the Special Diabetes Program for Indians is providing a pathway to health and wellness for children and youth, their families, and future generations.

CONCLUSIONS

As our review of the literature makes clear, the epidemic of childhood overweight and obesity has hit AI/AN communities especially hard. While there is an urgent need for on-going surveillance and epidemiological work on risk and protective factors, there is an even more pressing need to learn these lessons in the context of actual intervention and policy change. AI/AN communities have become increasingly impatient with basic research that continues to document, but does little else to alleviate the health disparities that plague them, and this is especially the case with problems such as those discussed here that affect the next generation (Spicer & Sarche, 2007). Despite a generally discouraging picture regarding the impact of available interventions in the general U.S. population, the AI/AN communities with which we work remain engaged in a wide variety of efforts to begin to address childhood obesity and its related consequences, especially diabetes. We remain optimistic that we have yet to explore all possible avenues for intervention and policy change in AI/AN communities and hope that this chapter points the way to possible additional steps for others.

REFERENCES

Aaron, D. J., Storti, K. L., Robertson, R. J., Kriska, A. M., & Laporte, R. E. (2002). Longitudinal study of the number and choice of leisure time physical activities from mid to late adolescence. *Archives of Pediatric and Adolescent Medicine, 156,* 1075–1080.

Allison, D., Fontaine, K., Manson, J., Stevens, J., & Vanitallie, T. (1999). Annual deaths attributable to obesity in the United States. *Journal of the American Medical Association, 282,* 1530–1538.

Anderson, A., Damio, G., Young, S., Chapman, D., & Perez-Escamilla, R. (2005). A randomized trial assessing the efficacy of peer counseling on exclusive breastfeeding in a predominantly Latina low-income community. *Archives of Pediatric and Adolescent Medicine, 159,* 836–841.

Baughcum, A. E., Burklow, K. A., Deeks, C. M., Powers, S. W., & Whitaker, R. C. (1998). Maternal feeding practices and childhood obesity: A focus group study of low-income mothers. *Archives of Pediatric and Adolescent Medicine, 152,* 1010–1014.

Baughcum, A. E., Chamberlin, L. A., Deeks, C. M., Powers, S. W., & Whitaker, R. C. (2000). Maternal perception of overweight preschool children. *Pediatrics, 106*(6), 1380–1386.

Bell, C., Walley, A., & Froguel, P. (2005). The genetics of human obesity. *Nature Reviews Genetics, 6,* 221–234.

Bergmann, K. E., Bergmann, R. L., von Kries, R., Böhm, O., Richter, R., Dudenhausen, J. W., et al. (2003). Early determinations of childhood overweight and adiposity in a birth cohort study: Role of breast-feeding. *International Journal of Obesity, 27,* 162–172.

Berkowitz, R. I., & Stunkard, A. J. (2002). Development of childhood obesity. In T. A. Wadden & A. J. Stunkard (Eds.), *Handbook of obesity treatment* (pp. 515–531). New York, London: The Guilford Press.

Bernard, L., Lavallee, C., Gray-Donald, K., & Delisle, H. (1995). Overweight in Cree schoolchildren and adolescents: Comparing nonreservation youths with African American and Caucasian peers. *American Journal of Preventive Medicine, 11,* 306–310.

Broussard, B. A., Johnson, A., Himes, J. H., Story, M., Fichtner, R., Hauck, F., et al. (1991). Prevalence of obesity in American Indians and Alaska Natives. *American Journal of Clinical Nutrition, 53,* 1535S–1542S.

Burdette, H. L., Whitaker, R. C., Kahn, R. S., & Harvey-Berino, J. (2003). Association of maternal obesity and depressive symptoms with television-viewing time in low-income preschool children. *Archives of Pediatric and Adolescent Medicine, 157,* 894–899.

Byers, T. (2003). On the hazards of seeing the world through intervention-colored glasses. *American Journal of Clinical Nutrition, 78,* 904–905.

Caballero, B., Clay, T., Davis, S. M., Ethelbah, B., Holy Rock, B., Lohman, T., et al. (2003). Pathways: A school-based, randomized controlled trial for the prevention of obesity in American Indian schoolchildren. *American Journal of Clinical Nutrition, 78,* 1030–1038.

Calle, E. E., & Kaaks, R. (2004). Overweight, obesity, and cancer: Epidemiological evidence and proposed mechanisms. *Nature Reviews Cancer, 4,* 579–591.

Calle, E. E., Rodriguez, C., Walker-Thurmond, K., & Thun, M. J. (2003). Overweight, obesity, and mortality from cancer in a prospectively studied cohort of U.S. adults. *New England Journal of Medicine, 348*(17), 1625–1638.

Carnethon, M. R., Gidding, S. S., Nehgme, R., Sidney, S., Jacobs, D. R., & Liu, K. (2003). Cardiorespiratory fitness in young adulthood and the development of cardiovascular disease risk factors. *Journal of the American Medical Association, 290*(23), 3092–3100.

Centers for Disease Control. (1996). *Inter-tribal heart project: Results from the cardiovascular health survey.* Atlanta, GA: Centers for Disease Control and Prevention.

Centers for Disease Control. (2003a). Diabetes prevalence among American Indians and Alaska Natives and the population—United States 1994–2002. *Morbidity and Mortality Weekly Recommendations and Reports, 52,* 702–704.

Centers for Disease Control. (2003b). Prevalence of physical activity, including lifestyle activities among adults—United States, 2000–2001. *Morbidity and Mortality Weekly Recommendations and Reports, 52*(32), 764–769.

Centers for Disease Control. (2006). Diagnosed diabetes among American Indians and Alaska Natives Aged <35 Years—United States, 1994–2004. *Morbidity and Mortality Weekly Recommendations and Reports, 55,* 1201–1203.

Centers for Disease Control. (2007). Breastfeeding rates by socio-demographic factors, 2005 (Vol. 2007). Atlanta, GA: Centers for Disease Control.

Chan, J. M., Rimm, E. B., Colditz, G. A., Stampfer, M. J., & Willett, W. C. (1994). Obesity, fat distribution, and weight gain as a risk factor for clinical diabetes in men. *Diabetes Care, 17,* 961–969.

Chapman, D. J., Damio, G., Young, S., & Perez-Escamilla, R. (2004). Effectiveness of breastfeeding peer counseling in a low-income, predominantly Latina population. *Archives of Pediatric and Adolescent Medicine, 158,* 897–902.

Cheadle, A., Pearson, D., Wagner, E., Psaty, B. M., Diehr, P., & Koepsell, T. (1994). Relationship between socioeconomic status, health status, and lifestyle practices of American Indians: Evidence from a Plains reservation population. *Public Health Reports, 109*(3), 405–413.

Coates, T., Jeffrey, R., & Wing, R. (1978). The relationship between persons' relative body weights and the quality and quantity of food stored in their homes. *Addictive Behavior, 3,* 179–185.

Coleman, K., Tiller, C., Sanchez, J., Heath, E., Sy, O., Milliken, G., et al. (2005). Prevention of the epidemic increase in child risk of overweight in low-income schools. *Archives of Pediatric and Adolescent Medicine, 159,* 217–224.

Dabelea, D., Hanson, R. L., Bennett, P. H., Roumain, J., Knowler, W. C., & Pettitt, D. J. (1998). Increasing prevalence of type II diabetes in American Indian children. *Diabetologia, 41,* 368–376.

Datar, A., & Sturm, R. (2004). Physical education in elementary school and body mass index: Evidence from the early childhood longitudinal study. *American Journal of Public Health, 94*(9), 1501–1506.

Daviglus, M. L., Liu, K., Yan, L. L., Pirzada, A., Manheim, L., Manning, W., et al. (2004). Relation of body mass index in young adulthood and middle age to Medicare expenditures in older age. *Journal of the American Medical Association, 292*(22), 2743–2749.

Davis, S., Gomez, Y., Lambert, L., & Skipper, B. (1993). Primary prevention of obesity in American Indian children. *Annals of the New York Academy of Sciences, 699,* 167–180.

de Sa Pinto, A., de Barros Holanda, P., Radu, A., Villares, S., & Lima, F. (2006). Musculoskeletal findings in obese children. *Journal of Pediatrics and Child Health, 42*(6), 341–344.

Dennison, B., Edmunds, L., Stratton, H., & Pruzek, R. (2006). Rapid infant weight gain predicts childhood overweight. *Obesity, 14,* 491–499.

Dennison, B. A., Erb, T. A., & Jenkins, P. L. (2002). Television viewing and television in bedroom associated with overweight risk among low-income preschool children. *Pediatrics, 109*(6), 1028–1035.

Dennison, B. A., Russo, T. J., Burdick, P. A., & Jenkins, P. L. (2004). An intervention to reduce television viewing by preschool children. *Archives of Pediatric and Adolescent Medicine, 158,* 170–176.

Drewnowski, A., Darmon, N., & Briend, A. (2004). Replacing fats and sweets with vegetables and fruits—A question of cost. *American Journal of Public Health, 94*(9), 1555–1559.

Ebbeling, C. B., Sinclair, K. B., Pereira, M. A., Garcia-Lago, E., Feldman, H. A., & Ludwig, D. S. (2004). Compensation for energy intake from fast food among overweight and lean adolescents. *Journal of the American Medical Association, 291*(23), 2828–2833.

Eisenmann, J., Katzmarzyk, P., Arnall, D., Kanuho, V., Interpreter, C., & Malina, R. (2002). Growth and overweight of Navajo youth: Secular changes from 1955 to 1997. *International Journal of Obesity, 24*(2), 211–218.

Etelson, D., Brand, D., Patrick, P., & Shirali, A. (2003). Childhood obesity: Do parents recognize this health risk? *Obesity Research, 11,* 1362–1368.

Faith, M. S., Heshka, S., Keller, K. L., Sherry, B., Matz, P. E., Pietrobelli, A., et al. (2003). Maternal-child feeding patterns and child body weight. *Archives of Pediatric and Adolescent Medicine, 157,* 926–932.

Fitzgerald, Shannon, J., Kriska, A. M., Pereira, M. A., & De courten, M. P. (1997). Associations among physical activity, television watching, and obesity in adult Pima Indians. *Medicine and Science in Sports and Exercise, 29*(7), 910–915.

Flores, R. (1995). Dance for health: Improving fitness in African American and Hispanic adolescents. *Public Health Reports, 110*(2), 189–193.

Fontaine, K. R., Redden, D. T., Wang, C., Westfall, A. O., & Allison, D. B. (2003). Years of life lost due to obesity. *Journal of the American Medical Association, 289*(2), 187–193.

Friedlander, S. L., Larkin, E. K., Rosen, C. L., Palermo, T. M., & Redline, S. (2003). Decreased quality of life associated with obesity in school-aged children. *Archives of Pediatric and Adolescent Medicine, 157,* 1206–1211.

Giammattei, J., Blix, G., Marshak, H. H., Wollitzer, A. O., & Pettitt, D. J. (2003). Television watching and soft drink consumption. *Archives of Pediatric and Adolescent Medicine, 157,* 882–886.

Gillman, M. W., Rifas-Shiman, S. L., Camargo, J.C.A., Berkey, C. S., Frazier, A. L., Rockett, H.R.H., et al. (2001). Risk of overweight among adolescents who were breastfed as infants. *Journal of the American Medical Association, 285*(19), 2461–2467.

Goel, M. S., McCarthy, E. P., Phillips, R. S., & Wee, C. C. (2004). Obesity among U.S. immigrant subgroups by duration of residence. *Journal of the American Medical Association, 292*(23), 2860–2867.

Going, S. B., Thompson, J., Cano, S., Stewart, D., Stone, E., Harnack, L., et al. (2003). The effects of the Pathways Obesity Prevention Program on physical activity in American Indian children. *Journal of Preventive Medicine, 37*(1), S62–S69.

Goldberg, H. I., Warren, C. W., Oge, L. L., Helgerson, S. D., Pepion, D. D., LaMers, E., et al. (1991). Prevalence of behavioral risk factors in two American Indian populations in Montana. *American Journal of Preventive Medicine, 7*(3), 155–160.

Gordon-Larsen, P., Adair, L. S., & Popkin, B. M. (2002). Ethnic differences in physical activity and inactivity patterns and overweight status. *Obesity Research, 10*(3), 141–149.

Gordon-Larsen, P., Harris, K. M., Ward, D. S., & Popkin, B. M. (2003). Acculturation and overweight-related behaviors among Hispanic immigrants to the U.S.: the National Longitudinal Study of Adolescent Health. *Social Science and Medicine, 57,* 2023–2034.

Gortmaker, S. L., Peterson, K., Wiecha, J., Sobal, A. M., Dixit, S., Fox, M. K., et al. (1999). Reducing obesity via a school-based interdisciplinary intervention among youth. *Archives of Pediatric and Adolescent Medicine, 153*(4), 409–418.

Gunnarsdottir, I., & Thorsdottir, I. (2003). Relationship between growth and feeding in infancy and body mass index at the age of 6 years. *International Journal of Obesity, 27,* 1523–1527.

Hanley, A., Harris, S., Gittelsohn, J., Wolever, T., Saksvig, B., & Zinman, B. (2000). Overweight among children and adolescents in a Native Canadian community: Prevalence and associated factors. *American Journal of Clinical Nutrition,* 693–700.

Harvey-Berino, J., Wellman, A., Hood, V., Rourke, J., & Secker-Walker, R. (2000). Preventing obesity in American Indian children: When to begin. *Journal of the American Dietetic Association, 100*(5), 564–566.

Hazard, B., & Lee, C. (1996). Understanding youth's health-compromising behaviors in Germany: An application of the risk-behavior framework. *Youth and Society, 30,* 348–366.

Hill, J. O., Wyatt, H. R., Reed, G. W., & Peters, J. C. (2003). Obesity and the environment: Where do we go from here? *Science, 299,* 853–855.

Himes, J. H., Ring, K., Gittelsohn, J., Cunningham-Sabo, L., Weber, J. L., Thompson, J., et al. (2003). Impact of the Pathways intervention on dietary intakes of American Indian schoolchildren. *Preventive Medicine, 37,* S55–S61.

Horowitz, C. R., Colson, K. A., Hebert, P. L., & Lancaster, K. (2004). Barriers to buying healthy foods for people with diabetes: Evidence of environmental disparities. *American Journal of Public Health, 94*(9), 1549–1559.

Hu, F. B., Li, T. Y., Colditz, G. A., Willett, W. C., & Manson, J. E. (2003). Television watching and other sedentary behaviors in relation to risk of obesity and type 2 diabetes mellitus in women. *Journal of the American Medical Association, 289*(14), 1785–1791.

Hu, F. B., Willett, W., Li, T., Stampfer, M. J., Colditz, G. A., & Manson, J. E. (2004). Adiposity as compared with physical activity in predicting mortality among women. *New England Journal of Medicine, 351*(26), 2694–2703.

Huang, Z., Hankinson, S. E., Colditz, G. A., Stampfer, M. J., Hunter, D. J., Manson, J. E., et al. (1997). Dual effects of weight and weight gain on breast cancer risk. *Journal of the American Medical Association, 278,* 1407–1411.

Huang, Z., Willett, W. C., Manson, J. E., Rosner, B., Stampfer, M. J., Speizer, F. E., et al. (1998). Body weight, weight change, and risk for hypertension in women. *Annals of Internal Medicine, 128,* 81–88.

Indian Health Service. (1999). *Regional Differences in Indian Health.* Washington, DC: Department of Health and Human Services.

Institute of Medicine. (2005). *Preventing Childhood Obesity: Health in the Balance.* Washington, DC: National Academies Press.

Jackson, J., Strauss, C., Lee, A., & Hunter, K. (1990). Parents' accuracy in estimating child weight status. *Addictive Behavior, 15,* 65–68.

Jackson, M. (1993). Height, weight, and body mass index of American Indian schoolchildren, 1990–1991. *Journal of the American Dietetic Association, 93*(10), 1136–1140.

Jago, R., Baranowski, T., Watson, K., Baranowski, J. C., Nicklas, T., & Zakeri, I. F. (2004). Relationship between maternal and child cardiovascular risk factors. *Archives of Pediatric and Adolescent Medicine, 158,* 1125–1131.

Jain, A., Sherman, S. N., Chamberlin, L. A., Carter, Y., Powers, S. W., & Whitaker, R. C. (2001). Why don't low-income mothers worry about their preschoolers being overweight? *Pediatrics, 107*(5), 1138–1146.

Jeffery, A. N., Voss, L. D., Metcalf, B. S., Alba, S., & Wilkin, T. J. (2005). Parents' awareness of overweight in themselves and their children: cross sectional study within a cohort (EarlyBird 21). *British Medical Journal, 330,* 23–24.

Jossefides-Tomkins, M., & Lujan, C. (2003). Perceptions of American Indian caregivers towards overweight in preschool children. *IHS Primary Care Provider, 28,* 149–154.

Katz, M. L., Gordon-Larsen, P., Bentley, M. E., Kelsey, K., Shields, K., & Ammerman, A. (2004). "Does skinny mean healthy?" Perceived ideal, current, and healthy body sizes among African-American girls and their female caregivers. *Ethnicity and Disease, 14,* 533–541.

Knowler, W. C., Pettitt, D. J., Saad, M. F., Charles, M. A., Nelson, R. G., Howard, B. V., et al. (1991). Obesity in the Pima Indians: Its magnitude and relationship with diabetes. *American Journal of Clinical Nutrition, 53,* 1543s–1551s.

Kvaavik, E., Tell, G. S., & Klepp, K. I. (2003). Predictors and tracking of body mass index from adolescence into adulthood. *Archives of Pediatric and Adolescent Medicine, 157,* 1212–1218.

Lakka, H. M., Laaksonen, D. E., Lakka, T. A., Niskanen, L. K., Kumpusalo, E., Tuomilehto, J., et al. (2002). The metabolic syndrome and total and cardiovascular disease mortality in middle-aged men. *Journal of the American Medical Association, 288*(21), 2709–2716.

Lee, E. T., Howard, B. V., Savage, P. H., Cowan, L. D., Fabsitz, R. R., Oopik, A. J., et al. (1995). Diabetes and impaired glucose tolerance in three American Indian populations aged 45–74 years: The Strong Heart Study. *Diabetes Care, 18,* 599–610.

Lee, E. T., Welty, T. K., Cowan, L. D., Wang, W., Rhoades, D. A., Devereux, R., et al. (2002). Incidence of diabetes in American Indians of three geographic areas. *Diabetes Care, 25*(1), 49–54.

Maynard, L. M., Galuska, D. A., Blank, H. M., & Serdula, M. K. (2003). Maternal perceptions of weight status of children. *Pediatrics, 111,* 1226–1231.

McGarvey, E., Keller, A., Forrester, M., Williams, E., Seward, D., & Suttle, D. E. (2004). Feasibility and benefits of a parent-focused preschool child obesity intervention. *American Journal of Public Health, 94*(9), 1490–1495.

Mendlein, J. M., Freedman, D. S., Peter, D. G., Allen, B., Percy, C. A., Ballew, C., et al. (1997). Risk factors for coronary heart disease among Navajo Indians: Findings from the Navajo Health and Nutrition Survey. *Journal of Nutrition, 127,* 2099S–2105S.

Michels, K. B., Willett, W. C., Graubard, B. I., Viadya, R. L., Cantwell, M. M., Sansbury, L. B., et al. (2007). A longitudinal study of infant feeding and obesity throughout the lifecourse. *International Journal of Obesity, 31*(7), 1078–1085.

Miech, R., Kumanyika, S., Stettler, N., Link, B., Phelan, J., & Chang, V. (2006). Trends in the associations of poverty with overweight among U.S. adolescents, 1971–2004. *Journal of the American Medical Association, 295,* 2385–2393.

Miller, W. R., & Rollnick, S. (2002). *Motivational Interviewing: Preparing People for Change.* (2nd Ed.). New York: Guilford Press.

Mokdad, A. H., Ford, E. S., Bowman, B. A., Dietz, W. H., Vinicor, F., Bales, V. S., et al. (2003). Prevalence of obesity, diabetes, and obesity-related health risk factors, 2001. *Journal of the American Medical Association, 289*(1), 76–79.

Molina, J., & Campos-Outcalt, D. (1991). Coronary artery disease risk factors in Yaqui Indians and Mexican Americans. *Journal of the National Medical Association, 8312,* 1075–1080.

Moum, K. R., Holzman, G. S., Harwell, T. S., Parsons, S. L., Adams, S. D., Oser, C. S., et al. (2004). Increasing rate of diabetes in pregnancy among American Indian and white mothers in Montana and North Dakota, 1989–2000. *Maternal and Child Health Journal, 8*(2), 71–75.

Müller, M. J., Asbeck, I., Mast, M., Langnäse, K., & Grund, A. (2001). Prevention of obesity—more than an intention. Concept and first result of the Kiel Obesity Prevention Study (KOPS). *International Journal of Obesity,* *25*(suppl1), S66–S74.

Must, A., Jacques, P. F., Dallal, G. E., Bajema, C. J., & Dietz, W. H. (1992). Longterm morbidity and mortality of overweight adolescents: A follow-up of the Harvard Growth Study of 1922–1935. *New England Journal of Medicine,* *327,* 1350–1355.

Must, A., Spadano, J., Coakley, E., Field, A., Colditz, G., & Dietz, W. (1999). The disease burden associated with overweight and obesity. *Journal of the* *American Medical Association, 282,* 1523–1529.

Mustillo, S., Worthman, C., Erkamli, A., Keeler, G., Angold, A., & Costello, E. J. (2003). Obesity and psychiatric disorder: Development trajectories. *Pediatrics, 111,* 851–859.

Neumark-Sztainer, D., Story, M., Resnick, M., & Blum, R. (1997). Psychosocial concerns and weight control behaviors among overweight and nonoverweight Native American adolescents. *Journal of the American Dietetic Association,* *97,* 598–604.

Newby, P. K., Peterson, K. E., Berkey, C. S., Leppert, J., Willett, W. C., & Colditz, G. A. (2003). Dietary composition and weight change among low-income preschool children. *Archives of Pediatric and Adolescent Medicine, 157,* 759–764.

Ogden, C., Carroll, M., Curtin, L., McDowell, M., Tabak, C., & Flegal, K. (2006). Prevalence of overweight and obesity in the United States, 1999–2004. *Journal of the American Medical Association, 295,* 1549–1555.

Olds, D. L. (2002). Prenatal and infancy home visiting by nurses: From randomized trials to community replication. *Prevention Science, 3*(3), 153–172.

Owen, C., Martin, R., Whincup, P., Smith, G., & Cook, D. (2005). Effects of infant feeding on the risk of obesity across the life course: A quantitative review of published evidence. *Pediatrics, 115,* 1367–1377.

Paradis, G., Levesque, L., Macauley, A., Cargo, M., McComber, A., Kirby, R., et al. (2005). Impact of a diabetes prevention program on body size, physical activity, and diet among Kanien'keha:ka (Mohawk) children 6–11 years old: 8-year results from the Kahnawake Schools Diabetes Prevention Project. *Pediatrics, 115,* 333–339.

Patrick, K., Norman, G. J., Calfas, K. J., Sallis, J. F., Zabinski, M. F., Rupp, J., et al. (2004). Diet, physical activity, and sedentary behaviors as risk factors for overweight in adolescence. *Archives of Pediatric and Adolescent Medicine,* *158,* 385–390.

Pettitt, D. J., Forman, M. R., Hanson, R. L., Knowler, W. C., & Bennett, P. H. (1997). Breastfeeding and the incidence of non-insulin dependent diabetes mellitus in the Pima Indian population. *Lancet, 350,* 166–168.

Pettitt, D. J., Moll, P. P., Knowler, W. C., Mott, D. M., Nelson, R. G., Saad, M. F., et al. (1993). Insulinemia in children at low and high risk for NIDDM. *Diabetes Care, 16,* 608–615.

Plagemann, A., Harder, T., Kohlhoff, R., Rohde, W., & Dorner, G. (1997). Overweight and obesity in infants of mothers with long-term insulin-dependent diabetes or gestational diabetes. *International Journal of Obesity, 21,* 451–456.

Rinderknecht, K., & Smith, C. (2002). Body-image perceptions among urban Native American youth. *Obesity Research, 10*(5), 315–327.

Robinson, T. N. (1999). Reducing children's television viewing to prevent obesity: A randomised controlled trial. *Journal of the American Medical Association, 282*(16), 1561–1567.

Rosen, L., Shafer, C., Drummer, G., Cross, L., Deuman, G., & Malmberg, S. (1988). Prevalence of pathogenic weight-control behaviors among Native American women and girls. *International Journal of Eating Disorders, 7,* 807–811.

Schulze, M. B., Manson, J. E., Ludwig, D. S., Colditz, G. A., Stampfer, M. J., Willett, W. C., et al. (2004). Sugar-sweetened beverages, weight gain, and incidence of type 2 diabetes in young and middle-aged women. *Journal of the American Medical Association, 292*(8), 927–934.

SEARCH for Diabetes in Youth Study Group. (2006). The burden of Diabetes Mellitus among U.S. youth: Prevalence estimates from the SEARCH for Diabetes in Youth Study. *Pediatrics, 118,* 1510–1518.

Serdula, M., Ivery, D., Coates, R., Freedman, D., Williamson, D., & Byers, T. (1993). Do obese children become obese adults?: A review of the literature. *Preventive Medicine, 22,* 167–177.

Sherwood, N. E., Harnack, L., & Story, M. (2000). Weight-loss practices, nutrition beliefs, and weight-loss program preferences of urban American Indian women. *Journal of the American Dietetic Association, 100*(4), 442–446.

Simonetti D'Arca, A., Tarsitani, G., Cairella, M., Siani, V., De Filippis, S., Mancinelli, S., et al. (1986). Prevention of obesity in elementary and nursery school children. *Public Health, 100,* 166–173.

Spicer, P., & Sarche, M. (2007). Culture and community in research with American Indian and Alaska Native infants, toddlers, and families. *Zero to Three, 27*(5), 55–56.

Stettler, N., Zemel, B., Kumanyika, S., & Stallings, V. (2002). Infant weight gain and childhood overweight status in a multicenter, cohort study. *Pediatrics, 109,* 194–199.

Stevens, J., Story, M., Becenti, A., French, S. A., Gittlesohn, J., Going, S. B., et al. (1999). Weight-related attitudes and behaviors in fourth grade American Indian children. *Obesity Research, 7*(1), 34–42.

Stevens, J., Story, M., Ring, K., Murray, D. M., Cornell, C. E., Juhaeri, et al. (2003). The impact of the Pathways intervention on psychosocial variables related to diet and physical activity in American Indian schoolchildren. *Journal of Preventive Medicine, 37*(1), S70–S79.

Stice, E., Shaw, H., & Marti, C. (2006). A meta-analytic review of obesity prevention programs for children and adolescents: The skinny on interventions that work. *Psychological Bulletin, 132,* 667–691.

Story, M., Evans, M., Fabsitz, R. R., Clay, T. E., Holy Rock, B., & Broussard, B. (1999). The epidemic of obesity in American Indian communities and the need for childhood obesity-prevention programs. *American Journal of Clinical Nutrition, 69*(Suppl.), 747S–754S.

Story, M., Hauck, F., Broussard, B., White, L., Resnick, M., & Blum, R. (1994). Weight perceptions and weight control practices in American Indian and Alaska Native adolescents: A national survey. *Archives of Pediatric and Adolescent Medicine, 148,* 567–571.

Story, M., Stevens, J., & Evans, M. (2001). Weight loss attempts and attitudes toward body size, eating, and physical activity in Native American children: Relationship to weight status and gender. *Obesity Research, 9,* 356–363.

Strauss, R. (2000). Childhood obesity and self-esteem. *Pediatrics, 105,* e15.

Summerbell, C. D., Waters, E., Edmunds, L. D., Kelly, S., Brown, T., & Campbell, K. J. (2005). Interventions for preventing obesity in children. *Cochrane Database of Systematic Reviews, 3.*

Talvia, S., Lagstrom, H., Rasanen, M., Salminen, M., Rasanen, L., Salo, P., et al. (2004). A randomized intervention since infancy to reduce intake of saturated fat. *Archives of Pediatric and Adolescent Medicine, 158,* 41–47.

Thomas, S. L., & Cook, D. (2005). Breastfeeding duration and prevalence of overweight among 4- and 5-year olds. *The IHS Primary Care Provider, 30*(4), 100–102.

Toschke, A. M., Grote, V., Koletzko, B., & von Kries, R. (2004, May). Identifying children at high risk for overweight at school entry by weight gain during the first two years. *Archives of Pediatric and Adolescent Medicine, 158,* 449–452.

Trifonopoulos, M. (1995). *Anthropometry and diet of Mohawk schoolchildren in Kahnawake.* Unpublished MSc thesis, McGill University, Montreal.

Uzark, K., Becvker, M., Dielman, T., Rocchini, A., & Kastch, V. (1988). Perceptions held by obese children and their parents: Implications for weight control intervention. *Health Education Quarterly, 15,* 185–198.

Vandewater, E., Shim, M., & Caplovitz, A. (2003). Linking obesity and activity level with children's television and video game use. *Journal of Adolescence, 27,* 71–85.

Veugelers, P., & Fitzgerald, A. (2005). Effectiveness of school programs in preventing childhood obesity: A multilevel comparison. *American Journal of Public Health, 95,* 432–435.

von Kries, R., Toschke, A.M., Wurmser, H., Sauerwald, T., & Koletzko, B. (2002). Reduced risk for overweight and obesity in 5- and 6-y- old children by duration of sleep: A cross-sectional study. *International Journal of Obesity, 26,* 710–716.

Wang, G., & Dietz, W. (2002). Economic burden of obesity in youths aged 6 to 17 years: 1979–1999. *Pediatrics, 109,* 1–6.

Weinstein, A. R., Sesso, H. D., Lee, I. M., Cook, N. R., Manson, J. E., Buring, J. E., et al. (2004). Relationship of physical activity vs. body mass index with type 2 diabetes in women. *Journal of the American Medical Association, 292*(10), 1188–1194.

Weiss, R., Dziura, J., Burget, T. S., Tamborlane, W. V., Taksali, S. E., Yeckel, C. W., et al. (2004). Obesity and the metabolic syndrome in children and adolescents. *New England Journal of Medicine, 350*(23), 2362–2374.

Welty, T. K. (1991). Health implications of obesity in American Indians and Alaska Natives. *American Journal of Clinical Nutrition, 53,* 1616s–1620s.

Welty, T. K., Lee, E. T., Yeh, J., Cowan, L. D., Go, O., Fabsitz, R. R., et al. (1995). Cardiovascular risk factors among American Indians: The Strong Heart Study. *American Journal of Epidemiology, 142*(3), 269–287.

Whitaker, R., Wright, J., Pepe, M., Kristy, D., & Dietz, W. (1997). Predicting obesity in young adulthood from childhood and parental obesity. *New England Journal of Medicine, 37,* 869–873.

Whitlock, E., Williams, S., Gold, R., Smith, P., & Shipman, S. (2005). Screening and interventions for childhood overweight: A summary of evidence for the U.S. Preventive Services Task Force. *Pediatrics, 116,* 125–144.

Wing, R., Epstein, L., & Neff, D. (1980). Accuracy of parents' reports of height and weight. *Journal of Behavioral Assessment, 2,* 105–110.

Wing, R. R., & Jeffrey, R. W. (1995). Effect of modest weight loss on changes in cardiovascular risk factors: Are there differences between men and women or between weight loss and maintenance. *International Journal of Obesity, 19,* 67–73.

Witteman, J.C.M., Willett, W. C., Stampfer, M. J., Colditz, G. A., Sacks, F. M., Speizer, F. E., et al. (1989). A prospective study of nutritional factors and hypertension among U.S. women. *Circulation, 80,* 1320–1327.

Wolf, A., & Colditz, G. (1998). Current estimates of the economic cost of obesity in the United States. *Obesity Research, 6,* 97–106.

Young, T. K. (1991). Prevalence and correlates of hypertension in a subarctic Indian population.*Preventive Medicine, 20,* 474–485.

Young-Hyman, D., Herman, L., Scott, D., & Schlundt, D. (2000). Caregiver perception of children's obesity-related health risk: a study of African American families. *Obesity Research, 8,* 241–248.

Zephier, E., Himes, J., & Story, M. (1999). Prevalence of overweight and obesity in American Indian school children and adolescents in the Aberdeen area: A population study. *International Journal of Obesity, 23*(Suppl. 2), S28–S30.

Zephier, E., Himes, J., Story, M., & Zhou, X. (2006). Increasing prevalences of overweight and obesity in northern plains American Indian children. *Archives of Pediatric and Adolescent Medicine, 160,* 34–39.

Zhang, Q., & Wang, Y. (2004). Socioeconomic inequality of obesity in the United States: Do gender, age, and ethnicity matter? *Social Science and Medicine, 58,* 1171–1180.

Chapter 8

OBESITY IN AFRICAN AMERICANS AND LATINO AMERICANS

Helen D. Pratt, Manmohan Kamboj, and Robin Joseph

Childhood obesity has been described as epidemic, pandemic, and pervasive in the United States. Childhood overweight as a public health concern is important because childhood obesity/overweight is a strong predictor of adult obesity. Childhood overweight can lead to increased risk of adult complications of overweight and obesity (Weiss et al., 2004). Childhood overweight has also been linked to several medical disorders (hepatic steatosis, hyperlipidemia, cholelithiasis, and childhood hypertension), metabolic syndrome, type 2 diabetes in children, increased stress on joints, and early puberty. Some acute complications may include sleep apnea (Dietz & Robinson, 2005). In addition to physical complications several socio-behavioral and psychosocial adjustment arise, including that fact that obesity is a predictor of perpetrating or being a victim and of bullying behavior (Buhs, Ladd, & Herald, 2006; Falkner et al., 2001; Weiss et al., 2004).

The issues of preventable morbidity and mortality in children and adolescents makes identification of overweight an essential component to quality health care and the first step towards implementing therapeutic measures in the reduction or prevention of such complications in our youth (Anderson & Butcher, 2006; Janssen, Craig, Boyce, & Pickett, 2004; Nesbitt et al., 2004). This is especially true for African and Latino Americans who disproportionately affected by overweight and obesity (Murray, Kulkarni, & Ezzati, 2005). Significant disparities in access to and the delivery of health care to ethnic minorities also exist in the United States. (Anderson &

Butcher, 2006). Concerns for the prevalence of obesity in ethnic minorities and the resultant morbidity and mortality, combined with these has caused researchers to issue a call to action to evaluate overweight ethnic children for improved screening for overweight and its potential consequences. This is especially true for cardiovascular risk (Murray et al., 2005; Nesbitt et al, 2004).

This chapter will focus on issues affecting African American and Latino youth in the United States. Other topics on physical activity, school achievement, peer relations, self esteem, obesity, American Indians, environmental influences, media, food systems, prevention, intervention, and ethics are covered in detail in the other chapters of this text.

DEFINITIONS OF OBESITY

Obesity refers to the presence of excessive body fat. Body mass index (BMI) has been increasingly used in pediatrics as a measure of obesity (Deurenburg, Weststrate, & Seidell, 1991). Using the Centers for Disease Control (CDC) growth charts, BMI between the 85th and 95th percentiles indicates overweight and tendency towards obesity (Dietz & Robinson, 2005; Deurenberg et al., 1991; Baker et al., 2005; Barlow & Dietz, 1998). The terms obese and overweight are commonly used to describe adults who are considered to be at a weight that places them at risk for medical risks.

$$BMI = \frac{\text{weight in KgO}}{(\text{height in meters})^2}$$

DEFINITIONS OF OVERWEIGHT IN CHILDREN AND ADOLESCENTS

A BMI of higher than the 95th percentile (age and sex matched) is considered to be consistent with obesity in children and adolescents, except in very muscular athletes. And the term overweight historically was used to describe youth whose BMI is between the 85th and 95th percentile. While the criteria for inclusion as overweight and obese remain the same, the terminology changes when describing youth as overweight or obese. The changes in terminology *at-risk-of-overweight* instead of *overweight* and *overweight* instead of *obesity* are suggested to avoid the potential negative connotations associated with the terms *obesity*, and *overweight* when discussing the weights of children and adolescents (U.S. Department of Health and Human Services [USDHS], 2005). The term at-risk of-overweight should be used to refer to children and adolescents (2 to 20 years of age) whose body mass index (BMI)-for-age between the 85th and the 95th percentiles. The term *overweight* should be used to refer to youth whose BMI-for-age is at or above the 95th percentile and whose excess body weight could pose medical risks (USDHS, 2005).

PREVALENCE OF AT-RISK-FOR-OVERWEIGHT AND OVERWEIGHT AMONG AFRICAN AMERICAN AND LATINO YOUTH IN THE UNITED STATES

According to Third National Health and Nutrition Examination Survey (NHANES III), 17 percent of children aged 2 to 19 years were at risk for overweight, with BMI between 85th and 95th percentiles for their age and sex, while 11 percent were overweight with BMI over the 95th percentile, matched for age and sex (Ogden et al., 1997). The prevalence of overweight was shown to increase two-fold between 1974 and 1994 (Ogden et al., 2006). Between 1980 and 1994, children and adolescents considered to be overweight (BMI-for-age > 95th percentile) increased by 100 (USDHS, 2005). Between one-quarter to slightly more than one-third of youth between the ages of 2 and 19, in the United States are at risk for overweight or overweight.

African American and Latino youth have higher prevalence of being at risk for being at risk for overweight (see table 8.1), overweight, and statistically they exercise less often than their non-Hispanic Caucasian peers and have lower rates of engaging in compensatory behaviors to maintain or lose excess weight (see tables 8.1 and 8.2) (Eaton et al., 2006).

African American Youth

African American ages 12–19 have slightly higher rates of overweight than Latino American youth, while both groups have rates two times higher than non-Hispanic Caucasians (Eaton et al., 2006). Although overweight has increased among all adolescents over past 30 years, it has increased 150 percent in African American girls compared to 40 percent in Euro-American girls (Troiano, Flegal, Kuemarski, Campbell, & Johnson, 1995; Neff, Sargent, McKeown, Jackson, & Valois, 1997). All groups showed more obesity among males than females except for African Americans, in which there was a 27 percent in males and a 34 percent in females (Popkin & Udry, 1997).

Table 8.1
At Risk for overweight and overweight from a nationwide survey of high school students (Grades 9 to 12).

	All Students	Males				Females			
		All	White	Black	Hispanic	All	White	Black	Hispanic
At risk for becoming overweight									
	15.7	15.8	15.2	16.7	16.5	15.5	13.8	22.6	16.8
Overweight									
	13.1	16.0	15.2	15.9	21.3	10.0	8.2	16.1	12.1
Described themselves as being overweight									
	35.5	25.1	24.7	17.6	32.0	38.1	37.7	36.3	42.4

Adapted from. Eaton, D. K., Kann, L., Kinchen, S., Ross, J. Hawkins, J., Harris, W.A., et al. (2006).Youth Risk Behavior Surveillance—United States, 2005. *MMWR Surveillance Summaries* 55(SS05):1–108. http://www.cdc.gov/mmwr/preview/mmwrhtml/ss5505a1.htm

Latino American Youth

Latino American youth ages 2 to 5 and 12 to 11 years of age have higher rates of overweight than Caucasian and African American youth of the same age (USDHS, 2005). Latino adolescents born in the United States are more than twice as likely to be obese as are their first generation parents and peers who immigrate to the United States (Popkin &

Table 8.2
Daily physical activity in a physical education class from a nationwide survey of high school students (Grades 9 to 12).

	All	Males				Females			
		All	White	Black	Hispanic	All	White	Black	Hispanic
Attended									
	54.2	60.0	—	—	—	48.3	—	—	—
Attended daily									
	33.0	37.1	37.6	37.5	—	29.0	26.6	31.6	—
Exercised or played sports 20 minutes or more during an average class									
	54.2	87.2	89.3	83.8	85.0	80.3	82.5	73.1	77.5
Played on one or more sports teams									
	56.0	61.8	61.5	64.6	62.0	50.2	53.9	43.6	43.8

Adapted from. Eaton, D. K., Kann, L., Kinchen, S., Ross, J. Hawkins, J., Harris, W.A., et al. (2006).Youth Risk Behavior Surveillance—United States, 2005. *MMWR Surveillance Summaries* 55(SS05):1–108. http://www.cdc.gov/mmwr/preview/mmwrhtml/ss5505a1.htm

Udry, 1998; Markowitz & Cosminsky, 2005). The first anthropometric study in over 20 years was published in 2005. The study evaluated the growth of children (aged 2 to 18) of migrant Latino agricultural workers; these children were previously not included in the National Health and Nutrition Examination studies, because of their transience (Markowitz & Cosminsky, 2005). The researchers examined the links between BMI/sex/ age percentile, height/sex/age percentile, and the prevalence of stunting, at-risk-for-overweight and overweight children in southern New Jersey. They assessed using anthropometric measurements of height, weight, and skinfold thickness with reference to the NHANES Guidelines 1999–2000. Results showed that 20 percent of their subjects were overweight. This percentage in 2–5-year olds equaled or exceeded the rate of obesity that was previously found among settled Latino Americans. Even thought Latino American youth who were born in the United States are taller than their immigrant parents, one-fifth of them are overweight (Markowitz & Cosminsky, 2005). Another study of 3,176 Latino Americans and 1,841 non-Hispanic Caucasians found that Latino Americans were more likely to be overweight than the comparison group (Stern et al., 1990).

CAUSE OF OBESITY

Most researchers support that obesity is the result of an imbalance between the amount of caloric intake ingested and amount of caloric expenditure. Multiple factors may be responsible for this imbalance (USDHS, 2005; Gungor & Arslanian, 2002). Other factors that must be considered include the interaction between (a) caloric intake and inges-tion, (b) caloric expenditure, and (c) underlying genetic predisposition with environmental factors (such as, nutritional intake, physical activity, and psychosocial factors). These factors are also affected by hormonal and metabolic function. It is important to realize that specific underly-ing etiology or hormonal disorders account for only a small proportion of patients with obesity. The bio-psychosocial factors that maintain high caloric intake and low activity are complex and uniquely individual. Being at-risk-of-overweight or overweight has also been linked to some youth experiencing problems with academic performance, self-esteem, peer relationships, and emotional well-being (Falkner et al., 2001).

ENERGY INTAKE AND ENERGY EXPENDITURE

No single factor has led to increases in overweight in children or adolescents. Several controversial views have been put forth (Eaton et al.,

2006; Fitzgibbon & Stolley, 2004. Rather current views hold that when children and adolescents gain weight, many complementary changes have simultaneously increased the individual's energy intake and decreased the energy expenditure. Caloric restriction and leisure-time physical activity are not routine in minority communities (Eaton et al., 2006). Some researchers offer that in minority populations, those who do not maintain normal weight outnumber those who do; thus, overweight has often become the community norm. Some researchers contend that because of the increase in access to food and decrease in jobs that require significant amounts of energy expenditure, upwardly mobile ethnic minorities have become increasingly obese. They further offer that the high fat intake eating habits of both African and Latino Americans are currently obsolete (high fat intake), because they were developed during a more physically active era (Eaton et al., 2006).

PHYSICAL ACTIVITY

In one study, researchers concluded that regardless of gender, maturation, and body composition, African and Latino American youth have lower aerobic fitness levels than Caucasian youth (Shaibi, Ball, & Goran, 2006). Results from a national survey of high school students (9th–12th grades) examined the overall prevalence rates for physical activity for all students. The results showed that 57.8 percent of Caucasian students played on more than one sports team, whereas the rate for African Americans was 53.7 percent and 53.0 percent for Latino American students (Eaton et al., 2006). Gender specific data are shown in table 8.2.

TELEVISION WATCHING

Poor minority youth watched more television than youth who are not poor and have fewer alternatives for physical activity; therefore they are exposed to more media concepts and advertisements about food (Kumanyika & Grier, 2006; Crespo et al., 2001). This increased sedentary lifestyle is proposed as one of the possible causes of the increased rates of obesity among poor minority youth. Data from a national survey of high school students yielded that 37.2 percent of all students watched three or more hours of television (TV) per day, with African American adolescents having the highest rates of television viewing (Eaton et al., 2006).

For many families that have single mothers employed outside of the home, having their children stay inside and watch TV is a safer and less costly alternative to having them exposed to potential dangers in their communities. The physical impact may result in increased at–risk-of-overweight or overweight, but in the short term the positive outcome is decreased by later increases in morbidity and mortality.

POVERTY

The prevalence of obesity is significantly higher in poor communities than in affluent communities. Since the 1970s and 1980s obesity has become more prevalent in low income and minority youth. Obesity rates are about 50 percent higher in families below the poverty line when compared to youth whose family income is at or above the poverty line. These rates are higher for ethnic females, African Americans, Hispanics, and Native Americans than among whites (Wickrama, Wickrama, & Bryant, 2006; Yerkel, Poston, Reeves, & Forey, 2005; Gordon-Lassen, Adair, & Popkin, 2003).

Wickrama et al. (2006) conducted a study of the link between obesity and socioeconomic status (SES). The authors looked at community influences on adolescent obesity and racial and ethnic differences; when they analyzed their data they looked at those adolescents who had remained in their same environments and only experienced changes in their family income and parental education; the effect on the disparities in overweight prevalence was limited. The researchers had several conclusions: (a) Community poverty had a greater influence on Caucasian adolescents than minority adolescents; (b) Race/ethnicity moderated the influences of community poverty on the prevalence of obesity; and (c) Unlike Caucasians, minorities may not benefit from increased resources that Caucasians may use to lower their body weights. For example, as income increases, the prevalence of overweight decreases among Caucasian, Latino, and Asian American females but remains elevated and even increases among African American females. The authors offer that efforts to reduce overweight disparities between ethnic groups must look beyond income and education and focus on other factors, such as environmental, contextual, biological, and sociocultural factors (Wickrama et al., 2006).

CONSEQUENCES OF OVERWEIGHT

Another study supporting that ethnic minorities were disproportionately affected by overweight was conducted by Nesbitt et al. (2004). This work group study is a part of the efforts of the Children Are Our Messengers: Changing the Health, Message initiative sponsored by the International

Society on Hypertension in Blacks. The authors of this report reviewed the literature about overweight in children and adolescents, as related to ethnicity, risk factors, clinical disease, and determinates of overweight and clinical trials with ethnic children. They concluded that obesity is one of the chronic diseases that have resulted in an excess of young people dying, including, among African Americans in the U.S., African American males in this country have highest mortality rate in the world (Murray et al., 2005). Poor African Americans living in middle America, the rural South, and those living in high-risk urban environments experience higher mortality rates than all other Americans. Their rates of mortality are two times higher than the rate of people live in very poor under developed regions of the world. These are individuals who live in one of the richest countries in the world.

PSYCHOSOCIAL ISSUES

At risk for overweight and overweight youth may face developmental challenges as they develop. Some of those experiences include: (a) behavioral and learning problems, (b) being victims or perpetrators of bullying teasing and physical fighting, (c) social discrimination and exclusion, (d) negative self-image, and (e) parental neglect. Such experiences during the developmental years and transition into adulthood can leave chronic problems (depression, school avoidance, and academic underachievement) that often persist into adulthood (Denny, Clark, Fleming, & Wall, 2004; Zeller & Modi, 2006; Buhs et al., 2006; Falkner et al., 2001).

SPECIAL ISSUES

Asthma and Overweight

African- (17%) and Latino-American (78%) youth were studies to determine the relationship between the diagnosis of asthma and age-sex adjusted BMI (Gennuso, Epstein, Paluch, & Cerny, 1948). Results indicated that 30.6 percent of the youth were overweight, 28.3 percent of subjects had asthma and were overweight, but only 12 percent of their controls met criteria for both conditions. The researchers concluded that asthma is a risk factor for overweight but overweight was not linked to the severity of asthma.

Dietary Habits

Obesity and dieting are common among youth in the United States. If one conceptualized obesity as an eating disorder, then the data on obesity among youth in the United States indicates that the predominate eating disorder would occur more frequently among African and Latino Americans. Table 8.3 shows the prevalence of compensatory behaviors employed by high school youth.

In research on adolescent girls and obesity, Neff et al. (1997) and Nichter (2000) concluded that Caucasian adolescents were more likely to diet and to engage in unhealthy weight management practices than African American adolescents because Caucasian adolescents were more likely to see themselves as overweight. In her research on adolescent girls and how their mother's perceived obesity found that the mothers of the African American subjects were less concerned about their daughter's weight than about their personal characteristics (Nichter, 2000). Nichter also found that 48 percent of African American girls said they had not tried to lose weight in the last year while 39 percent of Caucasian girls gave the same response. Only 30 percent of all the girls in the study said they had tried to lose weight one or two times in the past year, and 11 percent said they were always trying to lose weight (see table 8.2) (Eaton et al., 2006). The Center for Disease Control uses the prevalence of eating fruits and vegetables five or more times a day as one indicator of healthy eating behavior. The rates of eating fruits and vegetables fiver or more times a day were higher among African and Latino American girls (22.1% and 23.2%, respectively) than for Caucasian girls (21.8%).

Body Mass Index

Striegel-Moore et al. (2000) studied adolescent females who took part in the National Heart, Lung, and Blood Institute Growth and Health Study and found that African American girls were heavier, had higher body mass index (BMI) scores, and were more advanced in terms of sexual maturation than Caucasian girls; but had lower body dissatisfaction and drive for thinness scores. Studies on eating disorders show that African American adolescents have a low tolerance for thinness, which Striegel-Moore and colleagues concluded was noteworthy, given the higher prevalence of obesity and the low prevalence of anorexia nervosa among African Americans.

Distribution of Body Fat

Fat distribution for Mexican Americans has been reported to be different from fat distribution among non-Hispanic Caucasians. This caused one research group to conclude that the tables of ideal weights derived from non-Hispanic populations are not applicable to Latino Americans. Additionally,

Table 8.3
Weight loss and weight control practices from a nationwide survey of high school students (Grades 9 to12).

Based on 30 days before survey	All	Males				Females			
		All	White	Black	Hispanic	All	White	Black	Hispanic
Tried to lose weight	45.6	29.9	28.8	24.4	38.6	61.7	63.5	52.7	64.1
Restricted intake or ate low fat foods	40.7	26.8	26.4	22.0	31.5	54.8	58.8	39.6	53.2
Exercised	60.0	52.9	51.2	51.6	63.0	64.4	69.8	56.5	68.9
Did not eat for 24 or more hours	12.3	7.6	7.5	8.6	7.4	17.0	17.6	14.0	17.7
Took diet pills, powders, or liquids with out a doctors advice	6.3	4.6	4.2	—	5.7	8.1	9.2	4.9	7.5
Vomited or took laxatives	4.5	2.8	2.3	—	3.9	6.2	6.7	4.0	6.8

Adapted from. Eaton, D. K., Kann, L., Kinchen, S., Ross, J., Hawkins, J., Harris, W. A., et al. (2006). Youth Risk Behavior Surveillance—United States, 2005. *MMWR Surveillance Summaries* 55(SS05):1–108. http://www.cdc.gov/mmwr/preview/mmwrhtml/ss5505a1.htm

Latino American appeared to tolerate higher body weights without an adverse impact on their mortality experience (Kumanyika, 1993).

Special attention must be given to obesity as it occurs in and affects ethnic minorities (especially, African and Latino Americans) in the United States. In her research on obesity, Kumanyika (1993) contends that a high-risk body fat distribution (upper body or central obesity) occurs to a greater extent in some minority populations than in whites. Recognition of this factor when evaluating overweight in minority groups seems to be an important in addition to overall obesity because of the suggested changes in insulin-glucose homeostasis with central obesity (Freedman et al., 1987).

Another research who examined Latino Americans suggested that conventional tables, derived from non-Hispanic-populations tables of ideal weight probably underestimate the ideal weight range for Latino Americans; therefore, new tables should be generated based on information derived from prospective data specific to Latino American and other minority populations (Graziano, Jensen-Campbell, Shebilske, & Lundgren, 1993). The current authors suggest that the same consideration should be given to developing new tables based on information derived from prospective data specific to African American populations.

BEAUTY, BODY SIZE, AND THE WESTERN IDEAL

In Western or industrialized countries, being overweight or obese has negative connotations and may result in social or prejudicial biases. Such negative perceptions may affect hiring and promotion practices, peer relationships, dating opportunities, self-esteem, stigmatizing experiences, and dieting (Neumark-Sztainer, Story, & Faibisch, 1998). In Western cultures and in the United States in particular, thinness is associated with attractiveness, fitness, and health, whereas obesity is associated with poor health, lack of will power or self-control, and unattractiveness (Stunkard, 1996). Female adolescents in particular are more likely to be affected and influenced by other women's views of attractiveness (Graziano et al., 1993).

Ethnic girls are keenly aware of differences in the ideal of beauty between African Americans and Caucasians (Nichter, 2000). African American girls generally describe beauty in terms of personality traits instead of physical attributes. Among these girls beauty, is defined by intelligence, social skills, altruism, grooming, and having a good sense of humor. This perception of beauty is counter to the media portrayals of the Western ideal. Nichter (2000) described African American girls perceptions of beauty as flexible, fluid, and exceeding physical characteristics; beauty was judged on the basis of how one moved rather than how much one weighed.

Over one-quarter (26.7%) of the adolescent girls in one study reported high body satisfaction (Kelly et al., 2005). Highest satisfaction was among African American girls (40.1%) and underweight girls (39.0%). In adjusted analyses, girls with high body satisfaction were more likely to report parental and peer attitudes that encouraged healthy eating and exercising to be fit (versus dieting) and were less likely to report personal weight-related concerns and behaviors. The immediate subculture in which adolescent girls exists may play an important role in fostering high body satisfaction.

Another research team compared levels of body dissatisfaction between Latino, Asian American, and Caucasian adolescents (sixth and seventh grades) (Robinson et al., 1996). Latino and Asian American participants who were among the leanest 25 percent of girls reported significantly more body dissatisfaction than did the Caucasian participants. Caucasian girls who were shorter in height and Asian American girls who were taller in height than their peers were also more likely to be unhappy with their body type. Parents' education level and socioeconomic status (SES) were not significantly associated with body dissatisfaction. The authors concluded that BMI was the strongest independent predictor of increased body dissatisfaction in for all subjects.

Baskin, Ahluwalia, and Resnicow (2001) offered that the positive body images of African American girls need not be viewed as problematic or abnormal. In fact, it could be argued that majority culture has a dysfunctional view of body image and obesity. Thus, the researchers state that rather than holding whites and majority culture as the ideal, it may be important to incorporate the positive elements of black culture regarding body image and food rather than attempting to shift their values toward those of European Americans.

Some groups in non-Western countries have a greater acceptance of higher body weights. In many of these countries fatness or plumpness may be considered a sign of beauty. In recent times, the blending of what constitutes beauty across different socioeconomic levels, different cultures, different races, and different ethnic groups may make plumpness less desirable in all regions of the world (Cunningham et al., 1995). Slimness or being thin is not considered important for attractiveness and fatness or plumpness is accepted more easily and even encouraged among some ethnic groups and cultures in the non-Western world. Since obesity has been defined as a medical problem and since some behaviors that contribute to obesity have been labeled as a mental health problem (e.g., bulimia), obesity becomes a symptom of pathology.

MEDIA INFLUENCES

Views of beauty and body size are generally of skinny or very thin Caucasian females with thin noses, with long torsos and legs. Overweight youth are generally portrayed as food-obsessed or as clowns. As more people of substance (people who do not fit the ideal body size) obtain access to making media portrayals of larger individuals, more positive images are presented. Movies such as *Phat Gilrz* (Likké, 2006), *Sisterhood of the Traveling Pants* (Kwapis, Brashares, & Ephron, 2005) and *Real Women have Curves* (Cardoso, Lopez, & LaVoo, 2002) portray more substantial females as human beings with all the same needs and desires as perfect or thin people. In the movie *Phat Gilrz,* one major issue is repeatedly reinforced: full figured women are more desirable in many other parts of the world. These messages and images are essential for young women and men who have larger body types, are healthy, and not walking examples of medical- or psycho-pathology.

It is important that clinicians remember that there are other standards of beauty and body size among ethnic groups and other cultures. Recent research has shown that not all African Americans and Latinos who are not thin are unhealthy or exhibiting medical or mental pathology. However, the acceptance of Western ideals of thinness as the only form of beauty can create conflicting cultural demands for people from varied ethnic backgrounds that can result in increased manifestation of disordered patterns of eating, body dissatisfaction, poor self esteem, and feelings of cultural isolation. Additionally, as people of color move in this direction, the incidence of disordered eating among these groups will increase (Littlewood, 1995; Speiser et al., 2005).

ASSESSMENT OF OVERWEIGHT CHILDREN AND ADOLESCENTS

Some assessment guidelines for specific age groups of children and adolescents are offered in table 8.4, with a caution that clinicians should evaluate any underlying treatable causes and co-morbidities. All assessments should also be designed to be culturally and ethnically sensitive. Components of the assessment should include: medical history, family history (including eating disorders metabolic disorders), dietary assessment (detailed information about dietary history including eating patterns of the family; food choices of the person concerned, as well as, the family concerned; portion sizes and methods of meal preparation should be inquired about in detail). Physical activity assessment (time spent in physical activity in the form of walking, gym, after school and weekend activities) should also be evaluated. Screen-time should be assessed as many studies have linked the incidence of obesity to screen-time (the time spent in television viewing or video games) (Littlewood, 1995; Speiser et al., 2005).

Once a young person is identified as overweight, an in-depth assessment is required to determine if that individual is truly overfat and at increased risk for health complications related to overweight. This type of assessment provides a basis for management plans as shown in table 8.5. Among children over seven years, practitioners should pay particular attention to family history and secondary complications of overweight, such as hyperlipidemia and hypertension. The child's or adolescent's concern about his or her own weight should also be taken into consideration before beginning a weight loss program.

Laboratory testing in obese patients has not been standardized but it is recommended that evaluation include assessment of fasting glucose and insulin levels, along with a lipid profile and ALT liver enzyme levels. ALT is useful to detect non-alcoholic fatty liver disease (NFLD) in

Table 8.4
Considerations when screening for at risk for and overweight youth.

Infants and children under the age of two years

Plot the weight-for-length, weight-for-age, and length-for-age using the CDC Growth Charts. Overweight, does not pose the same risk among infants as it does among children two years and older.

Children 24 to 36 months of age

CDC recommends measuring stature for children two years and older who are able to stand on their own, calculating BMI and plotting it on the BMI-for-age chart. Whether the child's length or stature is measured determines which growth chart will be used.

Adolescents

Adolescence represents the period of greatest risk for developing adult obesity (Whitaker, 1997). Measures of weight relative to stature, like BMI-for-age, are influenced by pubertal status. For early or late maturing children, these indices should be interpreted with caution.

Adapted from United States Department of Health and Human Services, Centers for Disease Control and Prevention, National Center for Chronic Disease Prevention and Health Promotion: Division of Nutrition and Physical Activity. 2005. Overweight children and adolescents screen and manage. Author http://www.cdc.gov/nccdphp/dnpa/growthcharts/training/modules/module3/text/contents.htm.

these patients with levels which may be two to three times normal. Any hyperlipidemias/dyslipidemias detected should be treated because of the increased risk of atherosclerosis. Other investigations may be indicated depending on underlying cause, for example, hypothyroidism, polycystic ovarian syndrome, Cushings syndrome, and sleep apnea (Speiser et al., 2005). Appropriate imaging may be indicated to assess for cholelithiasis, NFLD, ovarian/uterine status, type 2 diabetes mellitus, slipped capital femoral epiphysis, Blount's disease, sleep apnea, and obesity hypoventilation syndrome. Referral and follow-up by the concerned subspecialists may offer more aggressive, effective, and specific care and should be encouraged.

Children and adolescents aged 2 to 20 years identified as overweight require an in-depth medical assessment and weight management that might include a family history, the family's and/or the patient's concern about weight, blood pressure, and total cholesterol screening, and determination of any recent, large changes in BMI-for-age. Further assessment will help verify excess body fat and determine if complications such as hyperlipidemia or hypertension are present, indicating a need for weight loss. If no risk factors are identified, re-screen in one year. This is true except in the case of infants; overweight infants may not be at increased risk of being overweight in adulthood, and they do not have the medical risks associated with overweight in childhood (Whitaker et al., 1997).

Weight-for-age and stature-for-age are useful indices to help monitor growth and to interpret changes in BMI-for-age. However, they are incomplete screening indices by themselves and need to be used in combination with BMI-for-age. Weight-for-age reflects body mass relative to chronological age. Short-term changes, such as an increase in weight-for-age, may result in a change in the BMI-for-age. Likewise, changes in stature also affect BMI-for-age. The following examples demonstrate the advantages of using BMI-for-age in combination with weight-for-age and stature-for-age to screen for overweight.

TREATMENT OPTIONS

General Treatment Options

There is no specific treatment for obesity. Comprehensive therapeutic treatment options offering a multi-pronged approach to address the complex issue of obesity includes life style modification with diet and exercise; possible pharmacologic therapy; and behavioral therapy and counseling, which must include nutrition education, family involvement, portion control caloric restrictions, increased physical activity, structured and individualized program of exercise, and strategies for dealing with crises and stress. Strategies used in a management plan are based on information obtained from the assessment. Weight loss is recommended if complications such as hyperlipidemia or hypertension are identified, and for children seven years or older with a BMI-for-age above the 95th percentile. Otherwise, weight maintenance is recommended.

All treatment intervention are designed to decrease consumption of high calorie, less-nutritious foods, to control caloric intake, and more importantly, to increase muscle mass.

SPECIAL CONSIDERATIONS FOR AFRICAN AMERICAN AND LATINO YOUTH

Because of situational and cultural factors, effective obesity prevention and treatment approaches may need to be defined on an ethnicity-specific basis. Increased attention to obesity as it occurs in and affects diverse ethnic groups can help to address critical health issues in minority communities. Such efforts can also broaden and enrich aspects of obesity research for which models based on white populations are inappropriate or limited (Kumanyika, 1993).

Anderson and Butcher (2006) concluded that African and Latino American children do not receive the same level of care as their white counterparts. They receive fewer screenings for blood pressure (29% vs. 47.7%, respectively), and for diet and exercise counseling. The researchers further stated that access and type of care varied by age, insurance type, and clinician type. Exercise counseling occurred half as often in physician office visit for African American children. The researchers suggest that more African and Latino obesity specialists, nutritionists, and exercise physiologists are needed to provide care and increase awareness of these problems.

Baskin et al. (2001) stated that often, researchers and clinicians generally view the African American community from a deficit model with African Americans viewed as having less desirable health practices and a higher disease risk. However, in developing interventions for African Americans, it is important to keep in mind positive aspects of black culture as they relate to obesity (Cunningham et al., 1995).

Effective Treatments

Unfortunately evidence from previous research on the management of overweight and at risk for overweight in children and adolescents supports

Table 8.5
Recommendations for weight management of overweight children and adolescents.

Infants and children up to age 2 years

- Weight loss is generally not recommended However, health care providers may determine that follow up is appropriate in certain circumstances (e.g., delayed motor development due to excess body weight) and refer children younger than two years to a pediatric obesity center.

Children age 2 to 7 years

- *Weight maintenance* For those with no identified complications, maintenance of current weight is recommended. Prolonged maintenance will allow a gradual decline in BMI units (and BMI-for-age percentile) as children grow in height.
- *Weight loss* If complications are identified and BMI-for-age is ≥ 95th percentile, gradual weight loss is recommended. Weight loss in children should be recommended with caution and should generally be no more than one pound per month.

Children age 7 years and older

- *Weight maintenance* For those at risk of overweight with no identified complications, weight maintenance is recommended.
- *Weight loss* For those overweight and those at risk of overweight with complications, weight loss is indicated. An appropriate final goal for all children and adolescents who are overweight or at risk of overweight is a BMI-for-age below the 85th percentile. The rate of weight loss should be based on health risks and balancing the costs and benefits of loss versus those risks.

COMPLICATIONS

- For those with complications, improvement or resolution of the condition is an important goal. Acute complications should be referred the appropriate specialists.

Individualized Recommendations

- Recommendations for change must consider the family's readiness for change, family support, financial concerns, and neighborhood characteristics (including access to play areas and grocery stores).
- Treatment should begin early, involve the family, and institute permanent changes in a stepwise manner. Parenting skills are the foundation for successful intervention.

Adapted from United States Department of Health and Human Services, Centers for Disease Control and Prevention, National Center for Chronic Disease Prevention and Health Promotion: Division of Nutrition and Physical Activity. 2005. Overweight children and adolescents screen and manage. Author http://www.cdc.gov/nccdphp/dnpa/growth-charts/training/modules/module3/text/contents.htm.

that the positive effects of any combination of these therapies is not lasting for a great number of participants of treatment programs (Martul, Rica, Vela, & Aguaya, 2005).

CONCLUSION

The issues of preventable morbidity and mortality in children and adolescents makes identification of overweight an essential component to quality health care and the first step towards implementing therapeutic measures in the reduction or prevention of such complications in our youth. This is especially true for African and Latino Americans who are disproportionately affected by overweight and obesity. Significant disparities in access to and the delivery of health care also exist in the United States, for these ethnic youth.

Fat distribution for African and Latino Americans is different than for their non-Hispanic Caucasian. The tables of ideal weights derived from non-Hispanic populations are not applicable to African and Latino Americans. Research suggests that Latino Americans appeared to tolerate higher body weights without an adverse impact on their mortality experience and therefore support the notion that new tables should be derived from prospective data specific to minority populations (especially, black Americans, Hispanic Americans) in the United States. Assessment and treatment interventions should also take into account the cultural and ethnic issues related to providing health care that meets the general and specific needs of these populations.

REFERENCES

Anderson, P. M., & Butcher, K. F. (2006). Childhood Obesity: Trends and potential causes. *The Future of Children, 16*, 19–46.

Baker, S., Barlow, S., Cochran, W., Fuchs, G., Klish, W., Krebs, N., et al. (2005). Overweight children and adolescents: A clinical report of the North American Society for Pediatric Gastroenterology, Hematology and Nutrition. *Journal Pediatric Gastroenterology Nutrition, 40*, 533–543.

Barlow, S. E., & Dietz, W. H. (1998). Obesity evaluation and treatment: Expert Committee recommendations. The Maternal and Child Health Bureau, Health Resources and Services Administration and the Department of Health and Human Services. *Pediatrics, 102*, E29.

Baskin, M. L., Ahluwalia, H. K., & Resnicow, K. (2001). Obesity intervention among African-American children and adolescents. *Pediatric Clinics of North America, 48*(4),1027–1039.

Buhs, E. S., Ladd, G. W., & Herald, S. L. (2006). Peer exclusion and victimization: Processes that mediate between peer group rejection and children's classroom engagement and achievement? *Journal of Educational Psychology, 98,* 1–13.

Cardoso, P. (Director), Lopez, J. (Writer), & LaVoo, G. (Writer). (2002). *Real Women have Curves* [Motion Picture]. United States: HBO Independent Productions.

Crespo C. J., Smit, E., Troiano, R. P., Bartlett, S. J., Macera, C. A., & Andersen, R. E. (2001). Television watching, energy intake, and obesity in U.S. children: Results from the third National Health and Nutrition Examination Survey, 1988–1994. *Archives Pediatrics Adolescent Medicine, 155,* 360–365.

Cunningham, M. R., Roberts, A. R., Barbee, A. P., Druen, P. B., & Wu, C. H. (1995). Their ideas of beauty are, on the whole, the same as ours: Consistency and variability in the cross-cultural perception of female physical attractiveness. *Journal of Personality and Social Psychology, 68,* 261–279.

Denny, S., Clark, T. C., Fleming, T., & Wall, W. (2004). Emotional resilience: Risk and predictive factors for depression among alternative education students in New Zealand. *American Journal of Orthopsychiatry, 74,* 137–149.

Deurenberg P., Weststrate, J. A., & Seidell, J. C. (1991). Body mass index as a measure of body fatness: age- and sex-specific prediction formulas. *British Journal of Nutrition, 65,* 105–114.

Dietz, W. H., & Robinson, T. N. (2005). Clinical practice: Overweight children and adolescents. *New England Journal of Medicine, 352,* 2100–2109.

Eaton, D. K., Kann, L., Kinchen, S., Ross, J., Hawkins, J., Harris, W. A., et al. (2006). Youth Risk Behavior Surveillance—United States, 2005. *Morbidity and Mortality Weekly Report: Surveillance Summaries, 55,* (SS05),1–8. Retrieved from http://www.cdc.gov/mmwr/preview/mmwrhtml/ss5505a1.htm.

Falkner, N. H., Neumark-Sztainer, D., Story, M., Jeffery, R. W., Beuhring, T., & Resnick, M. D. (2001). Social, educational, and psychological correlates of weight status in adolescents. *Obesity Research, 9,* 32–42.

Fitzgibbon, M. L., & Stolley, M. R. (2004). Environmental Changes: May be needed for prevention of overweight in minority children. *Pediatric Annals, 33,* 45–49.

Freedman, D. S., Srinivasan, S. R., Burke, G. L., Harsha, D. W., Webber, L. S., & Berenson, G. S. (1987). Relation of body fat distribution to hyperinsulinemia in children and adolescents: The Bogalusa Heart Study. *American Journal of Clinical Nutrition, 46,* 403–410.

Gennuso, J., Epstein, L. H., Paluch, R. A., & Cerny, F. (1998). Relationship between asthma to obesity with minority children and adolescents. *Archives of Pediatrics and Adolescent Medicine, 152,* 1197–1200.

Gordon-Larsen, P., Adair, L. S., & Popkin, B. M. (2003). The relationship of ethnicity, socioeconomic factors, and overweight in U.S. adolescents. *Obesity Research, 11*(1), 121–129.

Graziano, W. G., Jensen-Campbell, L. A., Shebilske, L. J. & Lundgren, S. R. (1993). Social influence, sex differences, and judgments of beauty putting the interpersonal back in interpersonal attraction. *Journal of Personality and Social Psychology, 65*, 522–531.

Gungor, N., & Arslanian, S. (2002). Nutritional disorders—Integration of energy metabolism and its disorders in childhood. In M. A. Sperling (Ed.), *Pediatric Endocrinology* (2nd ed., pp. 689–724). Philadelphia: Saunders.

Janssen, I., Craig, W. M., Boyce, W. F., & Pickett, W. (2004). Associations between overweight and obesity with bullying behaviors in school-aged children. *Pediatrics, 113*, 1187–1194.

Kelly, A. M., Wall, M., Eisenberg, M. E., Story, M., & Neumark-Sztainer, D. (2005). Adolescent girls with high body satisfaction: who are they and what can they teach us? *Journal of Adolescent Health, 37*, 391–396.

Kumanyika, S. K. (1993). Special issues regarding obesity in minority populations. *Annals of Internal Medicine Volume, 119*, 650–654.

Kumanyika, S., & Grier, S. (2006). Targeting Interventions for ethnic minority and low-income populations. *The Future of Children, 16*, 187–207.

Kwapis, K. (Director), Brashares, A. (Writer), & Ephron, D. (Writer). (2005). *The Sisterhood of the Traveling Pants* [Motion picture]. United States: Alcon Entertainment.

Likké, N. (Writer/Director). (2006). *Phat Girlz* [Motion Picture]. United States: Outlaw Productions and Fox Searchlight Pictures. http://www2.foxsearchlight.com/phatgirlz/main.php

Littlewood, R. (1995). Psychopathology and Personal Agency: Modernity, culture change and eating disorders in South Asian societies. *British Journal of Medical Psychology, 68*, 45–63.

Markowitz, D. L., & Cosminsky, S. (2005). Overweight and stunting in migrant Hispanic children in the United States. *Economics and Human Biology, 3*, 215–240.

Martul, P., Rica, L., Vela, A., & Aguaya, A. (2005). Clinical evaluation and Healthcare in children and adolescents. *Journal of Pediatrics Endocrinology and Metabolism, 18*, 1207–1213.

Murray, C.J.L., Kulkarni, S., & Ezzati, M. (2005). Eight Americas: New perspectives on U.S. health disparities. *American Journal of Preventive Medicine, 29* (5, Suppl.), 4–10.

Neff, L. J., Sargent, R. G., McKeown, R. E., Jackson, K. L., & Valois, R. F. (1997). Black-white differences in body size perceptions and weight management practices among adolescent females. *The Journal of Adolescent Health, 20*, 459–465.

Nesbitt, S. D., Ashaye, M. O., Stettler, N., Sorof, J. M., Goran, M. I., Parekh, R. et al. (2004). Overweight as a risk factor in children: A focus on ethnicity. *Ethnicity and Disease, 14*, 94–110.

Neumark-Sztainer, D., Story, M., & Faibisch, L. (1998). Perceived stigmatization among overweight African-American and Caucasian adolescent girls. *Journal of Adolescent Health, 23*, 264–270.

Nichter, M. (2000). *"Fat talk": What girls and their parents say about dieting.* Cambridge: Harvard University Press.

Ogden, C. L., Carroll, M. D., Curtin, L. R., McDowell, M. A., Tabak, C. J., & Flegal, K. M. (2006). Prevalence of overweight and obesity in the United States, 1999–2004. *Journal of the American Medical Association, 295,* 1549–1555.

Ogden, C. L., Troiano, R. P., Briefel, R. R., Kuczmski, R. J., Flegal, K. M., & Johnson, C. L. (1997). Prevalence of overweight among preschool children in the United States, 1971 through 1994. *Pediatrics, 99,* E1.

Popkin, B. M., & Udry, J. R. (1998). Adolescent obesity increases significantly in second and third generation U.S. immigrants: The National Longitudinal Study of Adolescent Health. *Journal of Nutrition, 128,* 701–706.

Robinson, T. N., Killen, J. D., Litt, I. F., Hammer, L. D., Wilson, D. M., Haydel, et al. (1996). Ethnicity and body dissatisfaction: Are Hispanic and Asian girls at increased risk for eating disorders. *Journal of Adolescent Health, 19,* 384–393.

Shaibi, G. Q., Ball, G. D., & Goran, M. I. (2006). Aerobic fitness among Caucasian, African-American, and Latino youth. *Ethnicity and Disease, 16,* 120–125.

Speiser P. W., Rudolf, M. C., Anhalt, H., Camacho-Hubner, C., Chiarelli, F., Eliakim, A., et al. (2005). Obesity consensus working group: Childhood obesity. *Journal of Clinical Endocrinology and Metabolism, 90,* 1871–1887.

Stern, M. P., Patterson, J. K., Mitchell, B. D., Haffner, S. M., & Hazuda, H. P., (1990). Overweight and mortality in Mexican Americans. *International Journal of Obesity, 14,* 623–629.

Striegel-Moore, R. H., Schreiber, G. B., Lo, A., Crawford, P., Obarzanek, E., & Rodin, J. (2000). Eating disorder symptoms in a cohort of 11- to 16-year-old black and white girls: The NHLBI Growth and Health Study. *International Journal of Eating Disorders, 27,* 49–66.

Stunkard, A. I. (1996). Current views on obesity. *The American Journal of Medicine, 100,* 230–236.

Troiano, R. P., Flegal, K. M., Kuczmarski, R. J., Campbell, S., & Johnson, C. L. (1995). Overweight prevalence and trends for children and adolescents. *Archives of Pediatric Adolescent Medicine, 149,* 1085–1091.

U.S. Department of Health and Human Services, Centers for Disease Control and Prevention, National Center for Chronic Disease Prevention and Health Promotion: Division of Nutrition and Physical Activity. (2005). *Overweight children and adolescents screen and manage.* Atlanta: Centers for Disease Control and Prevention.

Weiss, R., Dziura, J., Burgert, T., Tamborlane, W., Taksali, S., Yeckel, K., et al. (2004). Obesity and the metabolic syndrome in children and adolescents. *New England Journal of Medicine, 350,* 2362–2374.

Whitaker, R. C., Wright, J. A., Pepe, M. S., Seidel, K. D. & Dietz, W. H. (1997). Predicting obesity in young adulthood from childhood and parental obesity. *New England Journal of Medicine, 37,* 869–873.

Wickrama, K. A. T., Wickrama, K. A. S., & Bryant, C. M. (2006). Community influence on adolescent obesity: Race/ethnic differences. *Journal of Youth and Adolescence, 35*, 647–657.

Yerkel, L. A., Poston, W. S. C., Reeves, R. S., & Forey, J. P. (2005). Behavioral interventions for obesity. *Journal of the American Dietetic Association, 105* (5 Suppl.), S35–S43.

Zeller, M. H. & Modi, A. C. (2006). Predictors of health-related quality of life in obese youth. *Obesity,* 14, 122–113.

Part III

PREVENTION AND INTERVENTION

Chapter 9

MANAGING THE OVERWEIGHT CHILD

Ihuoma Eneli and Karah Daniels Mantinan

Within the last four decades, the prevalence of obesity in the United States has increased threefold, with a disproportionate rise in low socioeconomic and minority populations (Ogden et al., 2006). Between 2003 and 2004, 32.2 percent of adults and 17.1 percent of children 2 to19 years old were obese. Paralleling this trend is an increase in serious weight-related medical complications and a rising economic burden. Medical complications previously seen only in adults now occur more frequently in children. In 2000, the overall cost of obesity in America was estimated at $117 billion, rivaling medical expenditures attributable to smoking. Expenses for obesity-related hospitalizations in children tripled from $35 million to $127 million from 1979–1981 to 1997–1999 (Wang & Dietz, 2002). Most compelling is that obese children are likely to become obese adults at risk for increased morbidity and mortality (Whitaker, Wright, Pepe, Seidel, & Dietz, 1997). Thus there is urgency for effective weight loss interventions for the child who is already overweight, within the wider scope of socio-ecological preventive efforts.

The primary goal for any childhood obesity intervention is to maintain the balance between caloric intake and energy expenditure without jeopardizing growth and development. To effectively achieve this goal, several factors must be considered such as age, psychological maturity, presence or absence of complications, pubertal stage, family structure and dynamics, socioeconomic status, family history of obesity, ethnicity, and physical environment. Successful outcomes for addressing childhood obesity rest on three pillars: establishing healthy dietary and physical activity behaviors early in childhood, family participation, and public health policy. The initial step for any clinical intervention is to evaluate the child for psychological or medical complications associated with their unhealthy weight (table 9.1). Thus in the next section, we provide an overview of medical complications seen in overweight children.

PSYCHOLOGICAL SEQUELAE

Overweight children face discrimination, teasing, bullying, low self-esteem, peer rejection, and abnormal eating behaviors (Dietz, 1998; Strauss, 2000). Low self-esteem in these children increases the likelihood they will engage in high-risk behaviors such as smoking or using alcohol. In addition, accelerated growth and early physical maturation seen often

Table 9.1
Medical and psychological consequences of childhood obesity.

Psychological
  Depression
  Low self esteem
  Teasing, bullying
Metabolic
  Type 2 diabetes
  Impaired glucose tolerance
  Metabolic syndrome
  Polycystic ovarian disease
  Elevated uric acid
Orthopedic
  Slipped capital femoral epiphysis
  Blount's disease
Cardiovascular
  Dyslipidemia
  Hypertension
  Left ventricular hypertrophy
  Atherosclerosis
Neurological
  Pseudotumor cerebri
Hepatic
  Nonalcoholic steatohepatitis
  Gall bladder disease
Pulmonary
  Obstructive sleep apnea
  Asthma

in the overweight child distorts societal expectations, placing increased pressures on the child and family.

The risk for psychological problems increases as the child gets older, and is occurs more often in girls than boys (Reilly et al., 2003). Overweight children are more likely to be teased or bullied by their peers with deleterious effects persisting five years later (Eisenberg, Neumark-Sztainer, Haines, & Wall, 2006; Haines, Neumark-Sztainer, Eisenberg, & Hannan, 2006). In a population-based sample of adolescents, 63 percent obese girls were teased about their weight, followed by 58 percent of obese boys (Neumark-Sztainer et al., 2002). While overweight children are more likely than average weight children to be the victims of bullying, they are also more likely to bully other children (Janssen, Craig, Boyce, & Pickett, 2004). This bi-directional pattern of bullying behavior is related in part to low-self esteem and exclusion from peer social groups and activities.

Even among 10 to 11 year olds, overweight children were rated the least desirable to have as friends. More recently, a nationally representative population sample of 90,118 seventh to twelfth graders enrolled in the National Longitudinal Study of Adolescent Health, found that overweight adolescents were less popular than their non-overweight peers. These findings were more prominent among non-Hispanic whites compared with their African American or Hispanic counterparts (Strauss & Pollack, 2003) reflecting differences frequently noted in studies on obesity, stigma, and ethnicity. Minority populations appear to be more tolerant of larger sizes. As early as the fourth grade, black female selections for ideal body size were significantly larger than those of white girls (Thompson, Corwin, & Sargent, 1997). Finally, obese children are at increased risk for negative body image and disordered eating. In a review of the literature, a consistent relationship between BMI and body dissatisfaction, especially among girls has been reported (Ricciardelli & McCabe, 2001). In another report, binge eating disorder (BED) in older morbidly obese girls occurred in 30 percent of patients, comparable to the prevalence of BED in obese adult women.

Social and Economic Consequences

Overweight during adolescence has been associated with negative social and economic consequences. Women who were overweight in early adolescence completed fewer years of advanced education, had a lower family income, higher poverty rate, and were less likely to get married by early adulthood, compared with the women who had not been obese during adolescence (Gortmaker, Must, Perrin, Sobol, & Dietz, 1993). Men who were overweight in adolescence were less likely to be married in adulthood. A study conducted in Great Britain did not find a relationship between obesity in childhood and adult social class, income, years of schooling, relationships, or psychological morbidity (Viner & Cole, 2005). However, when childhood obesity persisted into adulthood, women had a higher risk of never having been gainfully employed (odds ratio = 1.9) and not involved in a current relationship.

MEDICAL SEQUELAE

Obesity is associated with serious health consequences such as hypertension, coronary artery disease, stroke, type-2 diabetes, sleep apnea, cancer, and osteoarthritis. A single unit rise in body mass index (BMI) over 22 is associated with a 25 percent increase in risk for diabetes. Morbidly obese males (BMI > 40kg/m) have a 10-fold increase in risk of death compared to their normal weight peers (BMI = 25.5–29) (Bray & Gray, 1988). For most of these complications, the process starts early. Autopsy studies of overweight children and young adults who died of traumatic causes show early atherosclerotic lesions in the aorta and coronary arteries.

Early Maturation

Childhood obesity is associated with early puberty and advanced bone age. Because of earlier closure of the growth plates, overweight children tend to be taller than their non-overweight peers during childhood, but achieve shorter heights in adulthood. Higher prepubertal BMI and early puberty have also been associated with higher BMI and hip and waist circumference in adulthood.

Cardiovascular Disease

Overweight children are at higher risk for developing high blood pressure, dyslipidemia, abnormalities in endothelial function and glucose metabolism, and high insulin levels and/or insulin resistance. These factors increase the likelihood of developing coronary heart disease (CHD). In a recent study, 61 percent of obese children ages 5 to 10 years already had at least one cardiovascular risk factor (Freedman, Dietz, Srinivasan, & Berenson, 1999). Obese children were more likely to have high total cholesterol (OR 2.4), elevated diastolic blood pressure (OR 2.4), high triglycerides levels (OR 7.1), and fasting insulin (OR 12.6). The odds that an overweight child would have two or three risk factors for cardiovascular disease compared with a normal weight child were 9.7 and 43.5 respectively. In a separate study, 29 percent of 12 to 19 year old obese children had metabolic syndrome (a syndrome comprised of obesity, insulin resistance, and high waist circumference) compared with only 0.1 percent of children with a BMI below the 85th percentile (Cook, Weitzman, Auinger, Nguyen, & Dietz, 2003).

Type 2 Diabetes

Once considered primarily an adult disease, type 2 diabetes is emerging as an epidemic among children, paralleling trends in rising obesity. Type 2 diabetes is a well-known risk factor for cardiovascular disease. Native Americans, African Americans, and Hispanics have a greater susceptibility towards developing type 2 diabetes. Currently, 4.1 in 1,000 U.S. adolescents have type 2 diabetes (American Diabetes Association, 2000). The Centers for Disease Control and Prevention estimates that, if current rates of obesity continue, one in three children born in 2000 will eventually develop type 2 diabetes (Narayan, Boyle, Thompson, Sorensen, & Williamson, 2003).

Fatty Liver or Non-Alcoholic Steatohepatitis (NASH)

In the early 1980s, liver damage similar to that found in alcoholics but without exposure to alcohol, was reported almost exclusively in overweight children (Baldridge, Perez-Atayde, Graeme-Cook, Higgins, & Lavine, 1995; Kinugasa et al., 1984; Moran, Ghishan, Halter, & Greene, 1983). NASH is now thought to be the most common cause of liver disease in children, and some researchers link it to the metabolic syndrome of hypertension, hyperlipidemia, and diabetes mellitus (Lavine & Schwimmer, 2004; Mager & Roberts, 2006). Approximately 10–25 percent of overweight children have elevated liver enzymes, and a majority may have evidence of NASH on ultrasound or CT scans. Although some children with NASH present with an enlarged liver or right abdominal pain, the vast majority are asymptomatic. While the natural course of this disease is not well known, progression to greater liver damage with elevated liver enzymes has been documented.

Other Complications

Other medical sequelae include sleep apnea, slipped capital femoral epiphysis, pseudotumor cerebri, and polycystic ovarian disease. Children with obstructive sleep apnea have difficulty sleeping at night, snoring, restless sleep, daytime sleepiness, or morning headaches and usually will need a sleep study for evaluation. Orthopedic complications include slipped capital femoral epiphysis and Blount's disease. These disorders present with leg or hip pain, limited hip range of motion on exam, or bowing of the lower extremities. Symptoms of pseudotumor cerebri include persistent headaches and changes in vision caused by increased intracranial pressure.

INTERVENTIONS FOR THE OVERWEIGHT CHILD

Obesity is a multifactorial health condition best approached using a socio-ecological model. The socio-ecological model evolves outward, starting with the individual at the center. At this level, there are internal or *intrapersonal* factors that affect an individual's weight, such as attitudes, knowledge, and skills related to nutrition and physical activity. At next level of the model, positive and negative external forces not under the direct control of the individual influence their weight and behaviors. Examples of external forces include: (a) interpersonal (e.g., family members or peer groups that influence attitudes and beliefs about diet or physical activity habits); (b) community (e.g., neighborhood advocacy groups to improve playground safety); (c) organizations (e.g., schools that enact policies banning soda machines in schools); and (d) society (e.g., state legislation or county policies). Since most children do not have complete autonomy over their food and physical activity choices, a significant interpersonal external force is the parent or caregiver.

Obesity interventions can be dietary, physical activity, behavioral, pharmacologic, and surgical, as well as combinations of these methods. Interventions are carried out in a variety of settings, such as schools, family units, healthcare settings, group and individual counseling sessions, and within community health centers. To evaluate the efficacy of interventions, changes in weight, BMI, skin folds measurements, and percentage body fat are commonly used.

Recently, clinical programs that target the individual child and their family have been increasingly reported in the literature. Table 9.2 summarizes studies on clinical interventions that lasted for six months or longer, were randomized clinical trials or had a control group, with obesity treatment as a primary focus. At their core is a multidisciplinary approach delivered by a team of professionals, usually consisting of a nutritionist, health educator, exercise physiologist, and a psychologist or behaviorist. The role of the physician has either been indirect; where

Table 9.2
Characteristics and results of randomized controlled trials of behavioral child and adolescent treatment studies in clinic-based settings.

Study Reference	Study Population Country	Subject ages (y), gender	Intervention	Length of intervention, duration of follow up	Outcome measures	Results at last follow up
Brownell (Brownell, Kelman, & Stunkard, 1983)	42, USA	12–16 21.4% male	All subjects received a program that included behavior modification, nutrition education, exercise instruction, and social support. Group 1. Mother and child attended separate weekly sessions (n=14). Group 2. Mother and child attended sessions together (n=15). Group 3. Mothers did not take part in any sessions (n=13).	16 weeks, 1 year	Change in weight (kg)	Group 1. −7.7 kg Group 2. +2.9 kg Group 3. +3.2 kg
Duffy and Spence(Duffy & Spence, 1993)	27, Australia	7–13 21% male	All subjects received 8 weeks of 90 minute behavioral therapy sessions and were encouraged to participate in aerobic exercise and avoid 'red light foods'. Group 1. Cognitive self management training (n=9). Group 2. Relaxation training (control) (n=8).	8 weeks, 3 and 6 months	Percent over-weight change	Group 1. −8.9% Group 2. −9.2%

(Continued)

Table 9.2 *(Continued)*

Study Reference	Study Population Country	Subject ages (y), gender	Intervention	Length of intervention, duration of follow up	Outcome measures	Results at last follow up
Ebbeling (Ebbeling, et al., 2003)	16, USA	13–21 31% male	Group 1. Ad libitum reduced glycemic load diet (n=7). Group 2. Conventional reduced fat diet (n=7).	6 months, 1 year	Absolute change in BMI	Group 1. −1.3 kg/m^2 Group 2. −0.7 kg/m^2
Epstein (Epstein, et al., 1985)	41 families, USA	8–12 40% male	All subjects received 8 weekly sessions of treatment and 10 monthly maintenance sessions which included behavior modification and a 1200 kcal/day diet based on the Traffic Light Diet. Group 1. Diet plus programmed aerobic exercise (n=13). Group 2. Diet plus lifestyle exercise (n=12). Group 3. Diet plus callisthenic exercise (n=10).	1 year, 2 years	Percent overweight change	Group 1. −41% (31.5 % at 1 year) Group 2. −30.3% (32.2% at 1 year) Group 3.−40.8% (30.5% at 1 year)
Epstein (1985)	23, USA	8–12 all female	All subjects received 8 weekly sessions of treatment and 10 monthly maintenance sessions. Sessions included diet and nutrition education and behavior management techniques. Group 1. Diet plus exercise 3 x weeks for the first 6 weeks of the intervention. Group 2. Diet without exercise.	1 year, 2 years	Change in weight (kg)	Group 1. −3.86 kg (at 1 year) Group 2. −1.36 kg (at 1 year)

Epstein (1985)c	24, USA	5–80% male	All subjects received 6 weekly meetings and 9 monthly maintenance sessions that included the same diet and exercise. Group 1. Behavioral management including parent management techniques and social learning principles (n=8). Group 2. Control (n=11).	1 year, none	Percent over-weight change	Group1. –26.3% Group 2. –11.2%
Epstein (Epstein, et al., 1994)	44 families, USA	8–12 26% male	All subject received 26 weeks of treatment and 6 monthly follow up sessions up to 2 years. Sessions included instruction on Traffic Light Diet, behavioral modification, and exercise. Group 1. Mastery of behavioral skills. Praise for mastery and weight loss (n=17). Group 2. No requirement for mastery of skills and no praise (n=22).	6 months, 18 months	Percent over-weight change	Group1. –15.4% Group 2. –10.6%

(Continued)

Table 9.2 (Continued)

Study Reference	Study Population Country	Subject ages (y), gender	Intervention	Length of intervention, duration of follow up	Outcome measures	Results at last follow up
Epstein (Epstein et al., 1995)	61 families, USA	8–12 27% male	All subjects received 4 months of weekly treatment and bimonthly follow ups up to 1 year. The Traffic Light Diet (1000–1200 kcal/day) was used. Group 1: Reinforcing decreased sedentary behavior. Group 2. Reinforcing increased physical activity (control 1). Group 3. Reinforcing reduced sedentary behavior and increased physical activity (control 2).	4 months, 1 year	Percent overweight change	Group1. –18.7% Group 2. –10.3% Group 3. –8.7%
Epstein (Epstein, et al., 2000)	67, USA	Age range mean 10.3 48% male	All groups received a 6-month family-based behavioral weight control program. Group 1. Problem solving taught to parent and child (n=17). Group 2. Problem solving taught to child (n=18). Group 3. Standard family-based treatment (n=17).	6 months, 1 and 2 years	Change in weight (kg)	1 year follow up Group1. –1.2 kg Group 2. –2.4 kg Group 3. –1.3 kg

| Epstein (Epstein, Paluch, Gordy, & Dorn, 2000) | 90 families, USA | 8–12 32% male | All subjects received 16 weekly meetings followed by 2 biweekly and 2 monthly meetings. The Traffic Light Diet was used. Group 1: Low dose (10 hours per week) increased physical activity (n=18). Group 2: High dose (20 hours per week) increased physical activity (n=19). Group 3: Low dose (10 hours per week) reduced sedentary time (n=19). Group 4: High dose (20 hours per week) reduced sedentary time (n=20). | 6 months, 2 years | Percent overweight change | Group1. –12.4% Group 2. –13.2% Group 3. –11.6% Group 4. –14.3% |
| Epstein (Epstein, Paluch, Kilanowski, & Raynor, 2004) | 72 families, USA | 8–12 37% male | All subjects had 16 weekly meetings, followed by 2 biweekly meetings, and 2 monthly meetings where 4 main components were emphasized: weight control and monitoring, Traffic Light Diet, behavior change techniques, and maintenance of behavior change. Group 1. Reinforcement group. Positive reinforcement for reducing sedentary behaviors. Group 2. Stimulus control group. Positive reinforcement for recording sedentary behaviors. | 6 months, 1 year | Change in z-BMI score | Group 1. –0.6 Group 2. –0.9 |

(Continued)

Table 9.2 (*Continued*)

Study Reference	Study Population Country	Subject ages (y), gender	Intervention	Length of intervention, duration of follow up	Outcome measures	Results at last follow up
Figueroa-Colon (Figueroa-Colon, von Almen, Franklin, Schuftan, & Suskind, 1993)	19, USA	7–17 43% male	All subjects received exercise, behavioral, and parental involvement components. Group 1. Protein sparing modified fast (PSMF) 600-800 kcal/day for 10 weeks, followed by a hypocaloric diet (1000-1200 kcal/day) up to 1 year.(n=10). Group 2. Hypocaloric balanced diet (HBD) 800-1000 kcal/day for 10 weeks, followed by a hypocaloric diet (1000-1200 kcal/day) up to 1 year (n=9).	10 weeks, 1 year	Percent of overweight change	Mean weight for both groups returned to baseline levels at 1 year follow up.
Flodmark (Flodmark, Ohlsson, Ryden, & Sveger, 1993)	94, Sweden	10–11 48% male	Group 1. Family therapy and conventional treatment (diet, counseling, encouragement to exercise) (n=25). Group 2. Conventional treatment (control, n=19).Group 3. Untreated control (n=50).	14–18 months, 1 year post-intervention	Change in BMI	Group 1. +1.1 kg/m^2 Group 2. +1.6 kg/m^2 Group 3. +2.8 kg/m^2

Study	N, location	Age, sex	Intervention	Follow-up	Outcome	Results
Golan (Golan, Fainaru, & Weizman, 1998)	60, Israel	6–11 38% male	Group 1. Behavior modification where the parents are the primary agents of change (n=30). Group 2. Behavior modification where children are primary agents of change (n=30).	1 year	Percent of over-weight change	Group 1. −14.6% Group 2. -8.4%
Golan (Golan, Kaufman, & Shahar, 2006)	32 families, Israel	6–11 46% male	All subjects received a comprehensive educational and behavioral program for a healthy lifestyle. Parents were encouraged to use authoritative parenting style. Group 1. Parents alone. Group 2. Parents and children together.	6 months, 1 year	Percentage of over-weight change	Group 1. −9.5% Group 2. −2.4%
Graves (Graves, Meyers, & Clark, 1988)	40, USA	6–12 Not reported	Group 1.Training in behavioral weight loss methods. Group 2. Training in behavioral weight loss methods and parent problem solving exercises associated with children's weight control Group 3. Instructional-only group, with additional 15 minutes of exercise during sessions.	8 weeks, 6 months	Percent of over-weight change	Group 1. −10.2% Group 2. −24.4% Group 3. −9.3%

(Continued)

Table 9.2 (*Continued*)

Study Reference	Study Population Country	Subject ages (y), gender	Intervention	Length of intervention, duration of follow up	Outcome measures	Results at last follow up
Israel (1985)	33, USA	8–12 30% male	Group 1. Weight Reduction Only group: multicomponent behavioral weight loss program. Parents and children attend 9 weekly 90-minute sessions (n=12). Group 2. Parent training group: parents attend 9 weekly 90-minute sessions of weight reduction program and two 1-hour sessions to develop skills in behavioral child management (n=12). Group 3. Waiting list control (n=9).	9 weeks, 1 year	Percent of overweight change	Group 1. −1.3% Group 2. −10.2% Group 3. Not reported.
Israel (Israel, Guile, Baker, & Silverman, 1994)	36 families, USA	8–13 Not reported	Parents and children met separately for 8 sessions of 90 minutes each, followed by 9 biweekly sessions. Group 1. Standard treatment, with emphasis on parental responsibility for motivation of children (n=18). Group 2. Enhanced child involvement, with less emphasis on parental responsibility (n=16).	26 weeks, 3 years	Percent of overweight change	Group 1. +6.4% Group 2. −4.8%

Study			Intervention			Results
Mellin (Mellin, Slinkard, & Irwin, 1987)	66, USA	12–18 21% male	Group 1. SHAPEDOWN program (cognitive, behavioral, and affective techniques aimed at making small, sustainable changes to diet, exercise, communication, and affect). Fourteen 90-minute sessions, 2 parent sessions, and intervention fees (n=37). Group 2. No treatment control, exempt from fees (n=29).	3 months, 1 year	Percent of over-weight change	Group 1. –9.9% Group 2. –0.1%
Nemet (Nemet et al., 2005)	54, Israel	6–16 57% male	Group 1. Diet and exercise program (4 sessions with parents, 6 sessions with a dietitian, and exercise training twice per week for one hour per session) (n=20). Group 2. Ambulatory nutrition clinic referrals once per week and instruction to be physically active at least three days per week (control) (n=20).	3 months, 1 year	Change in weight (kg), change in body mass index (BMI)	Group 1. +0.6 kg, –1.7 kg/m^2 Group 2. +5.3 kg, +0.6 kg/m^2

(Continued)

Table 9.2 (Continued)

Study Reference	Study Population Country	Subject ages (y), gender	Intervention	Length of intervention, duration of follow up	Outcome measures	Results at last follow up
Rolland-Cachera (Rolland-Cachera et al., 2004)	121, France	11–16 26% male	All subjects lived in an obesity treatment center and were instructed to follow a diet of the same energy level (1750 kcal/day) and fat content (31%) and participated in 7 hours/week vigorous activity. Group 1. 15% protein, 54% carbohydrate (n=53). Group 2. 19% protein, 50% carbohydrate (n=46).	9 months, 2 years	Change in body mass index (BMI)	Results at 9 months- Group 1. −11.9 kg/m^2 Group 2. −12.4 kg/m^2
Schwingshandl (1999)	30, Australia	6–16 43% male	Group 1. Physical training program (60-70 minutes 2 x week) and dietary advice (n=14). Group 2. Dietary advice only (n=16).	12 weeks, 1 year	Change in fat free mass	12 week results Group 1. 2.7 Group 2. 0.4

Reference		Age (% male)	Intervention groups	Follow-up	Outcome measure	Results
Saelens (Saelens et al., 2002)	44, USA	12–16, 59% male	Group 1. Healthy Habits intervention: multicomponent behavioral weigh control intervention (n=23). Group 2. Typical Care: single session of physician weight counseling (n=21).	4 months, 7 months	Percent of overweight change, change in BMI (statistical analyses on BMI z scores)	Group 1. −2.4%, +0.1 kg/m^2 Group 2. +4.1%, +1.4 kg/m^2
Senediak and Spence (1985)	45, Australia	6–13, 66% male	Group 1. Behavioral program on a rapid schedule (8 sessions twice weekly for 4 weeks) (n=9). Group 2. Behavioral program on a schedule of gradually decreasing frequency (8 sessions with increasingly extended time periods over 15 weeks) (n=10). Group 3. Non-specified procedure control (n=7). Group 4. Waiting list control.	4–15 weeks, 6 months	Percent of weight change	Group 1. −13% Group 2. −19.3 Group 3. −5.9% Group 4. Data not reported

(Continued)

Table 9.2 (Continued)

Study Reference	Study Population Country	Subject ages (y), gender	Intervention	Length of intervention, duration of follow up	Outcome measures	Results at last follow up
Wadden (Wadden et al., 1990)	47, USA	12–1 60% male	Sixteen week behavioral weight control program based on manual for Weight Reduction and Pride (WRAP) program. Parental involvement varied in three ways: Group 1. Child alone. Group 2. Mother and child together. Group 3. Mother and child separately.	16 weeks	Change in weight (kg)	Group 1. −1.6 kg Group 2. −3.7 kg Group 3. −3.1 kg
Warsch-burger (Warschburger, Fromme, Petermann, Wojtalla, & Oepen, 2001)	197, Germany	9–19 Not reported	Group 1. 'Obesity training': 3-part program that included a cognitive behavioral component, a calorie-reduced diet, and an exercise program (n=121). Group 2. Same diet and exercise program as Group 1. Received relaxation training instead of behavioral component (n=76).	6 weeks, 6 months and 1 year	Percent of weight change	Group 1. 14.3% Group 2. 15.7%

they refer to these programs without ongoing input; or direct, where the physician is a key member of the multidisciplinary team.

In 1998, a multidisciplinary group of experts convened by the U.S. Department of Health and Human Services developed guidelines for evaluation and treatment of the overweight child (table 9.3). These guidelines are derived from our understanding of factors that increase the likelihood of successful outcomes, as there are no known effective, generalizable, evidence-based treatments. These factors include (1) interventions that are applied over six months to one year; (2) interventions that promote nutrition education and physical activity with behavior modification; (3) parental involvement in treatment; (4) reduction in sedentary behaviors; and (5) regular follow up.

DIETARY APPROACHES

The American Dietetic Association (ADA) categorizes dietary interventions based on proportion of macronutrients (carbohydrates, protein, and fat) in the diet using the Institute of Medicine (IOM) Dietary Reference Intakes as a guide. The IOM Dietary Reference Intakes recommends: "Adults should get 45 percent to 65 percent of their calories from carbohydrates, 20 percent to 35 percent from fat, and 10 to 35 percent from protein. Acceptable ranges for children are similar to those for adults, except that infants and younger children need a slightly higher proportion of fat (25%–40%)." (Institute of Medicine [IOM], 2007). When the macronutrient is within the recommended range, the intervention is a balanced macronutrient diet. Examples include individualized lifestyle dietary recommendations, the traffic-light diet, and food guide pyramid diets. In the second category, the macronutrient content is

Table 9.3
Guidelines for effective pediatric obesity intervention.

Pediatric expert committee (Barlow & Dietz, 1998)	1. Early intervention
	2. Assess readiness to change
	3. Assess and educate on medical complications
	4. Family participation
	5. Small gradual changes
	6. Lifestyle changes
	7. Multidisciplinary team
	8. Weight goal based on age and presence of complications
	9. Improve parenting skills

altered, using various methods, including some very low calorie diets (VLCD), or low carbohydrate or low glycemic index or high protein diets such as Atkins.

Balanced Macronutrient Diet

The traffic light diet is a popular diet used as a part of a pediatric multidisciplinary obesity programs. This diet supplies approximately 900 to 1,500 kilocalories per day and is structured to meet recommendations of the food guide pyramid. It has been used predominantly in young children ages 6 to12 years. (see table 9.3) Foods are classified into three groups: red-foods usually high fat, high sugar foods-intake of these foods is limited; yellow-foods to be eaten in moderation with portion control; and green-foods such as vegetables, which can be consumed freely. Epstein, Wing, Penner, and Kress, (1985) in a randomized clinical trial of 53 obese children aged 8 to 12 years used the traffic light diet. Three study groups, with an average of 18 children per group, were assessed. Group 1 received dietary intervention and exercise, group 2 received only dietary intervention, and group 3, the control group, had no intervention. Following a six-month intervention period, there was mean decline of 9 percent in overweight status in groups 1 and 2 compared to an increase of 3 percent in the control group. Other studies using the traffic light diet are summarized in table 9.3. Although the same group of investigators has carried out most published studies using the traffic light diet, their results suggest that the diet is effective for weight management in children.

Altered Macronutrient Diets

Altered macronutrient diets, such as low carbohydrate diets, have not been thoroughly evaluated for the treatment of childhood obesity. One study compared a low fat diet compared to a low carbohydrate diet in a clinical trial with overweight 12 to 18 year old adolescents (Sondike, Copperman, & Jacobson, 2003). The study design was a randomized, controlled, non-blinded trial conducted over a 12-week period with subjects referred from an atherosclerosis prevention center. Subjects assigned to the low carbohydrate diet consumed less than 20 grams of carbohydrate for two weeks and less than 40 grams of carbohydrate for 10 weeks, while subjects in the low fat group were instructed to consume a diet with less than 30 percent calories from fat (<40 grams/day). After 12 weeks, adolescents assigned to the low carbohydrate group lost more weight than the adolescents assigned to the low fat group, with mean decreases in weight of 9.9 kg and 4.9 kg respectively.

Another low carbohydrate diet was tested in randomized controlled trial with 16 obese adolescents ages 13 to 21 years. Subjects assigned to the treatment group consumed a diet of 30–35 percent fat and 45–50 percent carbohydrate, while the controls received a traditional low fat diet consisting of 25–30 percent fat and 55–60 percent carbohydrate. These diets were followed for six months. Six months after treatment ended, mean BMI in the low carbohydrate load group was reduced 1.7 kg/m^2, while the mean BMI for the low fat group increased 0.7 kg/m^2. It is unclear whether the modest weight changes noted in these studies can be attributed to the low carbohydrate content alone. In all the studies, the participants on a low carbohydrate diet consumed fewer calories. Thus the weight loss reported may be due to a caloric deficit rather than the reduced carbohydrate content of the diets.

The use of a high protein, low calorie diet, also called a protein sparing modified fast (PSMF), has been described in adolescents. High protein, low fat diets are thought to be effective for weight loss by increasing and maintaining a sense of satiety and preserving lean muscle mass, while burning fat mass. The PSMF diet must be used under close medical supervision. PSMF is initially formulated to provide 600–800 kcal/day, 2 grams of protein/kg of body weight up to 100 grams, with minimal carbohydrate intake, and mineral and vitamin supplementation. Typically, the PSMF is used for a limited number of weeks and then the caloric intake is liberalized over time to include at least 1,400–1,500 kcal/day. PSMF promotes up to 1 kg/week of weight loss, while sparing the breakdown of lean muscle mass for metabolic fuel. During the fast, the participants check for the presence of ketones in their urine daily. A positive result indicates compliance with the treatment regimen.

In a 36 week program using a PSMF followed by a balanced macronutrient diet, moderate intensity exercise, and behavior modification sessions, all the adolescents maintained their weight loss six months after the program ended (Suskind et al., 2000). Another study evaluated a low fat, protein sparing diet in six obese adolescents aged 12 to 15 years with body weights above 200 percent of their ideal body weight (Willi, Oexmann, Wright, Collop, & Key, 1998). All participants in this study consumed a diet that was low in carbohydrate (25 grams), fat (25 grams), and calories (650–725 calories/day). After eight weeks, participants added additional carbohydrate to their diet for 12 weeks. At the end of the first phase of the diet, subjects had lost 15.4 kg. After the second phase, an additional 2.3 kg were lost. Over the entire period of the intervention, BMI, body fat, and cholesterol were significantly reduced. Although use of the PSMF showed weight loss with improvement in lipid levels, patients must be closely monitored to prevent complications. PSMF remains a diet used mainly in research settings or as a component of a medically monitored multidisciplinary obesity program.

Finally, dietary interventions that target eating patterns can successfully affect weight gain. Eating patterns refers to a how often meals and snacks are served, where meals are eaten, and what drives our need to eat-physiological (from short term energy depletion) or psychological hunger (eating when not hungry). Strong family connectedness can have a strong positive influence on their child's diet and food-related behaviors, which affects diet, physical activity, and health and social risk behaviors.

Other Dietary Interventions

A common assumption is that restricting dietary intake of an overweight child is helpful in controlling future weight gain and, if pursued rigorously, will lead to weight loss. However, a number of studies suggest restricting intake (dieting), which is our current standard nutritional intervention in children, leads to later onset of obesity, inappropriate hunger and satiety cues, and eating disorders. The poor success rate of our current dietary restriction for the overweight child provides an impetus for a new nutritional paradigm.

One such paradigm is the trust model proposed by Satter (2005; 1986). The trust model focuses on division of feeding responsibility, regular eating patterns, and trust in the child's ability to self-regulate food intake by recognizing hunger and satiety cues. The model deemphasizes portion sizes, calorie counting, external restriction of intake, and reliance on low fat or low calorie food options. The trust model is comparable with a new approach called intuitive eating, which, designed for obese adults, is gaining greater acceptance among dietitians and the public. Intuitive eating is comprised of three interrelated components: (a) unconditional permission to eat when hungry and when food is desired; (b) eating for physical rather than emotional reasons; and (c) reliance on internal hunger and satiety cues to determine when and how much to eat. Intuitive eating has shown encouraging short- and long-term weight loss for overweight adults and teenagers. Further research incorporating the elements of the trust model is needed before this approach can be advocated for overweight children.

PHYSICAL ACTIVITY APPROACHES

Energy expenditure is part of the energy balance equation and has therefore been a target of many pediatric obesity interventions. Physical activity (PA) reduces fat stores and increases lean muscle mass, resulting in increased resting energy expenditure. Thus PA accelerates weight loss and improves maintenance of weight changes. Physical activity, even independent of weight loss, may reduce the risk of metabolic and cardiovascular complications. While dietary modification based on caloric restriction alone may indeed facilitate weight loss, few interventions focusing solely on caloric restriction have provided positive results. Increasing physical activity, in addition to modifying dietary intake, has been more successful.

Some studies have promoted physical activity without a nutrition education component. A community study, Stanford GEMS Pilot Study, conducted with African American girls consisted of after school dance classes and a family-based intervention to reduce TV viewing time (Robinson et al., 2003). Results from the study found no change in BMI, but did show a reduction in TV time, a risk factor for childhood obesity.

Reducing sedentary behaviors (e.g., time spent on television viewing, using computers, and playing videogames) can lead to weight loss. In another study, researchers conducted a physical activity intervention with obese youth age 8 to 12 years. The intervention compared three different activity regiments of: (a) increased exercise, (b) decreased sedentary behavior, and (c) both increased exercise and decreased sedentary activities. At one year, youth whose intervention targeted reducing sedentary behavior experienced a greater decrease in percent overweight (-18.7%) than the combined group (-10.3%) or the exercise group (-8.7%). In 2000, Epstein reported on another intervention with obese 8 to 12 year olds that evaluated decreased sedentary behavior versus increased physical activity with varying doses of each. Significant decreases in percent overweight, body fat, and improved aerobic fitness were noted in both groups. Interestingly, decreasing sedentary behavior appears to have an effect not only on physical activity, but also on energy intake in both overweight and non-overweight children (Epstein, Paluch, Gordy, & Dorn, 2000).

BEHAVIORAL APPROACHES

Theories on behavior change conceptualize variables that mediate behavior change, hence improving our understanding of why, how, and when individuals make choices. Different behavior change theories have been used for obesity treatments, most commonly are the social cognitive theory (SCT), social learning theory, and the transtheoretical model of change.

The SCT revolves around self-efficacy, modeling behavior, and the expectation of an outcome when a targeted behavior is adopted. First developed by Bandura in the 1960s, SCT describes three components affecting behavior: the personal characteristics of the person performing the behavior (including expectations, beliefs, and self-perceptions), the environment, and the qualities of the behavior itself. Inherent to the theory is the notion of *self-efficacy,* the tendency to repeat behavior based on one's a priori expectation that one will achieve a successful outcome. Self-efficacy, the conviction that one can successfully execute the behavior can predict change in fat intake, quality of diet, and physical activity, although some studies report a stronger correlation with intention than with actual behavior change. Also important is *observational learning,* the idea that one can learn by observing others without having to perform a behavior by oneself. These concepts have been widely used to develop successful interventions in the public health field, both in adults and in children.

Unlike SCT and other models that emphasize external influences on behavior, the transtheoretical model of change (TTM) focuses on the internal decision-making process of the individual. The central construct of this model is the stages of change. Rather than seeing behavior change as a single point in time, TTM views it as a process. With regards to a particular behavior change, an individual can be placed in one of six categories: precontemplation, contemplation, preparation, action, maintenance, and termination. Individuals can move from one stage to another (forward or backward) over time. By correctly classifying an individual in a stage, one can more accurately target treatment toward those in whom it will be most effective. Although applied most frequently in smoking cessation, TTM has been applied to many health problems crossing geographical boundaries and age groups.

Behavior modification is focused on changing behaviors that are related to diet and physical activity to promote weight loss. Behavioral treatment can help obese youth to build confidence, change diet and physical activity habits, and set realistic goals for improving their lifestyle. Important components of behavioral therapy programs include self-monitoring, stimulus control, problem solving, and cognitive restructuring. Identifying events and factors that precipitate inappropriate eating, exercise, or thoughts related to food, exercise, and weight can assist in restructuring eating and physical activity habits.

Few studies have examined the effect of behavioral interventions alone. In a study of 67 families who received six-month family-based behavioral weight control program and were randomized to receive either problem-solving methods taught to the parent and child, to the child only, or standard treatment with no problem solving (Epstein, Paluch, Gordy, Saelens, & Ernst, 2000). The standard therapy group had greater decreases in BMI than the parent and child combined group. The group concluded that problem solving did not add an additional benefit beyond standard family-based behavioral therapy.

In a six-week in-patient program, the treatment group received a cognitive behavioral therapy program and the comparison group received a program without psychological intervention (Warschburger, Fromme, Petermann, Wojtalla, & Oepen, 2001). Both groups were assigned to a reduced calorie diet and participated in an exercise program. Average BMI in the treatment group was 31.1 at admission, 28.6 at discharge, 29.2 six months later, and 30.4 one year later. The mean BMI in the comparison group was 31.7 at admission, 28.8 at discharge, 29 six months later, and 30.1 one year later. Although the mean percentage of overweight decreased following the intervention in both groups, the results were similar in both groups. Further research is needed to determine the optimum behavior approach for children.

Pharmacologic Treatment

Pharmacotherapy is a more intense approach to weight loss that is sometimes used in adolescents when lifestyle interventions fail repeatedly. In adults, the effect of adding pharmaceutical agents to treatment is an additional 2–10 kg of weight loss, which is usually achieved in the first four to six months of treatment. Although some pharmaceutical agents may produce modest weight loss in adolescents, their safety and long-term effectiveness has not been proven. Thus in the United States, these medications are usually used within research settings (table 9.4).

The appetite suppressant sibutramine works by simultaneously inhibiting the re-uptake of serotonin in the central nervous system while increasing the level of norepinehrine in the brain by the same mechanism. Berkowitz, Wadden, Tershakovec, and Cronquist (2003) conducted a randomized controlled trial of sibutramine, in addition to caloric restriction and a comprehensive family-based behavioral program. The study population was composed of 82 adolescents with a BMI between 32 and 44 kg/m . The addition of sibutramine to the behavioral therapy produced

Table 9.4

Characteristics and results of randomized controlled trials of child and adolescent pharmacologic treatment studies in clinic-based settings.

Study Reference	Number of subjects Country	Subject ages (y), gender	Intervention description (number remaining in group at last follow up)	Length of intervention	Outcome measures	Results at last follow up (−) weight loss (+) weight gain
Berkowitz (Berkowitz, Wadden, Tershakovec, & Cronquist, 2003)	82, USA	13–17 33% male	Group 1. Behavioral therapy and sibutramine (increased to 15 mg at 7 weeks) for 12 months. Group 2. Behavioral therapy and placebo for 6 months, followed by sibutramine for 6 months.	12 months	Change in mean weight (kg), change in mean body mass index percentage	Results at 6 months Group 1. -7.8 kg, –8.5% Gain of 0.8 kg body weight at 12 months Group 2. –3.2 kg, –4.0%Loss of 1.3 kg body weight at 12 months
Berkowitz (Berkowitz et al., 2006)	498, USA	12–16 34.2% male	All subjects received site-specific behavior therapy program. Group 1. 10 mg sibutramine (n=281). Group 2. Placebo (n=80). At 6 months, subjects in both groups were uptitrated to 15 mg sibutramine or placebo if they had not lost 10% of their initial BMI.	1 year	Change in mean body mass index (BMI)	Group 1. −2.9 kg/m^2 Group 2. –0.3 kg/m^2

Study	N, Location	Age, % male	Intervention	Duration	Outcome	Results
Chanoine (Chanoine, Hampl, Jensen, Boldrin, & Hauptman, 2005)	539, USA and Canada	12–16, 29% male	All subjects received general instructions for behavioral therapy, mildly hypocaloric diet (30% calories from fat), and exercise. Group 1. 120 mg orlistat three times daily (n=232). Group 2. Placebo (n=117).	54 weeks	Change in mean weight (kg), change in mean body mass index (BMI)	Group 1. +0.53 kg, −0.55 kg/m^2 Group 2. +3.14 kg, +0.31 kg/m^2
Ozkan (Ozkan, Bereket, Turan, & Keskin, 2004)	42, Turkey	10–16, 33% male	All subjects received a lifestyle modification program that included diet (20% reduction in calories based on age and sex) and increased physical activity (at least 30 minutes of moderate activity per day). Group 1. 120 mg orlistat three times daily and a daily multivitamin preparation (n=15). Group 2. Control (n=15).	5–15 months	Change in mean weight (kg), percent change in weight, change in mean body mass index (BMI)	Group 1. −6.27 kg, −7.65%, −4.09 kg/m^2 Group 2. +4.16 kg, +5.7%, +0.11 kg/m^2

(Continued)

Table 9.4. *(Continued)*

Study Reference	Number of subjects- Country	Subject ages (y), gender	Intervention description (number remaining in group at last follow up)	Length of intervention	Outcome measures	Results at last follow up (–) weight loss (+) weight gain
Srinivasan (Srinivasan et al., 2006)	28, Australia	9–18 46% male	Subjects received 1 g metformin twice daily for 6 months and placebo for 6 months, each with a 2-week washout period. Group 1. Metformin then placebo (n=10). Group 2. Placebo then metformin (n=12).	6 months	Change in mean weight (kg), change in mean body mass index (BMI)	Metformin. –4.35 kg, –1.26 kg/m^2 Results from placebo not reported

significantly greater weight loss than the placebo, 6.8 percent reduction versus 5.4 percent reduction respectively. Despite promising results, no additional weight loss occurred in the subsequent six months for individuals taking sibutramine, and significantly adverse effects such as hypertension and tachycardia were noted.

Orlistat is a drug that inhibits pancreatic lipase, an enzyme that breaks down dietary fat leading to decreased fat absorption on the gut. In a trial of obese adolescents, Orlistat combined with lifestyle intervention reduced weight 4.4–4.6 kg over a three-month period. Because there is increased loss of fat in the stool, common side effects of Orlistat are greasy stools and flatulence. Both conditions have made Orlistat less desirable among teenagers. Orlistat also reduces the absorption of fat-soluble vitamins A, D, E and K, so vitamin supplementation is recommended during therapy. In January 2006, the Federal Drug Administration (FDA) gave initial approval for the sale of low dose Orlistat without a prescription.

Metformin has been studied as a weight loss drug, although its primary use is in patients with type 2 diabetes. Metformin is thought to act by increasing the sensitivity of the cells to insulin, thus reducing insulin resistance, decreasing glucose absorption from the gut and glucose production in the liver. Metformin was evaluated in obese adolescents with high insulin levels, but who did not yet have type 2 diabetes. Over an eight-week trial period, 24 adolescents ages 13 to 17 years treated with metformin lost on average 6.1 kg compared with 3.2 kg in participants who received a placebo. Recent trials on the efficacy of metformin show promising preliminary results. Metformin has also been used off-label for polycystic ovary disease and NASH, two conditions in which insulin resistance plays a role in their pathogenesis.

A new drug, Rimonabant, is a selective cannabinoid receptor inhibitor and has shown some promise in adult trials. Inhibition of the cannabinoid receptor in animals decreases appetite, and liver and fat cell production of lipids. This drug leads to moderate weight loss and decrease in waist circumferences, while lowering triglyceride levels and increasing high-density lipoprotein (HDL) levels. Thus, preliminary studies show Rimonabant improves the cardiometabolic risk profile in obese individuals. Rimonabant not yet been studied in children and adolescents.

Surgical Treatment

Surgical treatment is a last resort for obese adolescents who have been unsuccessful in achieving weight loss and are morbidly obese.

The rationale for this type of intensive treatment is to reduce morbidity and mortality related to obesity, which can sometimes present greater risk to the child than the surgery itself. In adults, bariatric surgery has been shown to improve 15-year survival rates. Criteria for surgery candidates are (1) at least six months of failure at organized, non-surgical weight loss attempts, (2) severe obesity (defined by the World Health Organization as a BMI greater than 40 kg/m^2, or 100 pounds overweight, or 100 percent above ideal body weight), (3) majority of skeletal maturity (generally >13 years of age for girls and >15 years of age for boys) is complete, and (4) presence of comorbidities related to obesity that have potential to be improved through bariatric surgery (Inge et al., 2004). Most importantly, these adolescents must demonstrate decisional capacity.

In general, bariatric procedures result in a 25 to 35 percent reduction in body weight. This is achieved through procedures that lead to decreased caloric intake and/or malabsorption. Two procedures, the Roux-en-Y, a gastric bypass technique, and adjustable gastric banding (the Lap-Band), are used in children and are effective in treating obesity-related comorbidities. In gastric bypass surgeries, the surgeon creates a small pouch from the upper portion of the stomach. This pouch is surgically separated from the lower portion of the stomach. A part of the intestine called the jejunum is then attached to the pouch. That way, food travels directly from the pouch to the small intestine. For the lap-band, the procedure is much less invasive and surgery is performed laparascopically. A small band made of silicone is placed around the upper part of the stomach. A small port placed underneath the skin can control the opening between the upper and lower part of the stomach. Both surgeries create a sense of fullness with very small amounts of food. Since adolescents are still experiencing growth, timing of these procedures is important in order to maintain adequate nutrition and avoid compromise of linear growth. More severe outcomes, including death, are also possible.

Preliminary data from bariatric surgery procedures show mean body fat decreasing from 47 percent to 37 percent and mean BMI from 59 to 38 at one year post-operatively (Inge, Zeller, Lawson, & Daniels, 2005). In a study of 33 adolescents who underwent gastric bypass, all individuals lost weight, but five had regained some or all of their body weight in the subsequent 5 to 10 years following surgery. It is estimated that up to 15 percent of patients will regain weight. The long-term effectiveness of bariatric surgery among adolescents continues to be investigated.

SUMMARY

Interventions within the pediatric population have shown better long-term results than adult obesity programs, suggesting intervening early in the life span will provide greater benefits. In addition, parental participation in pediatric obesity programs improve weight loss, and changes in dietary habits and compliance with the program. Normalizing a child's relationship with food, while increasing physical activity behaviors leads to sustainable lifestyle changes. These changes, although not always measurable in the short term in terms of weight loss, produce cost effective benefits in quality of life, less use of medical services, and greater attainment goals as the child grows. Overall, treatment options that involve decreasing sedentary behavior, increasing physical activity, adopting healthy dietary options, and use of behavior therapy, have improved various measures of obesity.

REFERENCES

American Diabetes Association. (2000). Type 2 diabetes in children and adolescents. American Diabetes Association. *Pediatrics, 105*(3 Pt. 1), 671–680.

Baldridge, A. D., Perez-Atayde, A. R., Graeme-Cook, F., Higgins, L., & Lavine, J. E. (1995). Idiopathic steatohepatitis in childhood: A multicenter retrospective study. *Journal of Pediatrics, 127*(5), 700–704.

Berkowitz, R. I., Fujioka, K., Daniels, S. R., Hoppin, A. G., Owen, S., Perry, A. C., et al. (2006). Effects of sibutramine treatment in obese adolescents: a randomized trial. *Annals of Internal Medicine, 145*(2), 81–90.

Berkowitz, R. I., Wadden, T. A., Tershakovec, A. M., & Cronquist, J. L. (2003). Behavior therapy and sibutramine for the treatment of adolescent obesity: A randomized controlled trial. *Journal of the American Medical Association, 289*(14), 1805–1812.

Bray, G., & Gray, D. (1988). Obesity. Part I—pathogenesis. *West Journal of Medicine, 149,* 429–441.

Brownell, K. D., Kelman, J. H., & Stunkard, A. J. (1983). Treatment of obese children with and without their mothers: Changes in weight and blood pressure. *Pediatrics, 71*(4), 515–523.

Chanoine, J. P., Hampl, S., Jensen, C., Boldrin, M., & Hauptman, J. (2005). Effect of orlistat on weight and body composition in obese adolescents: a randomized controlled trial. *Journal of American Medical Association, 293*(23), 2873–2883.

Cook, S., Weitzman, M., Auinger, P., Nguyen, M., & Dietz, W. H. (2003). Prevalence of a metabolic syndrome phenotype in adolescents: Findings from the third National Health and Nutrition Examination Survey, 1988–1994. *Archives of Pediatric and Adolescent Medicine, 157*(8), 821–827.

Dietz, W. H. (1998). Health consequences of obesity in youth: Childhood predictors of adult disease. *Pediatrics, 101*(3 Pt. 2), 518–525.

Duffy, G., & Spence, S. H. (1993). The effectiveness of cognitive self-management as an adjunct to a behavioural intervention for childhood obesity: A research note. *Journal of Child Psychology and Psychiatry, 34*(6), 1043–1050.

Ebbeling, C. B., Leidig, M. M., Sinclair, K. B., Hangen, J. P., & Ludwig, D. S. (2003). A reduced-glycemic load diet in the treatment of adolescent obesity. *Archives of Pediatrics Adolescent Medicine, 157*(8), 773–779.

Eisenberg, M. E., Neumark-Sztainer, D., Haines, J., & Wall, M. (2006). Weight-teasing and emotional well-being in adolescents: Longitudinal findings from Project EAT. *Journal of Adolescent Health, 38*(6), 675–683.

Epstein, L. H., McKenzie, S. J., Valoski, A., Klein, K. R., & Wing, R. R. (1994). Effects of mastery criteria and contingent reinforcement for family-based child weight control. *Addictive Behaviors, 19*(2), 135–145.

Epstein, L. H., Paluch, R. A., Gordy, C. C., & Dorn, J. (2000). Decreasing sedentary behaviors in treating pediatric obesity. *Archives of Pediatric and Adolescent Medicine, 154*(3), 220–226.

Epstein, L. H., Paluch, R. A., Gordy, C. C., Saelens, B. E., & Ernst, M. M. (2000). Problem solving in the treatment of childhood obesity. *Journal of Consulting and Clinical Psychology, 68*(4), 717–721.

Epstein, L. H., Paluch, R. A., Kilanowski, C. K., & Raynor, H. A. (2004). The effect of reinforcement or stimulus control to reduce sedentary behavior in the treatment of pediatric obesity. *Health Psychology, 23*(4), 371–380.

Epstein, L. H., Valoski, A. M., Vara, L. S., McCurley, J., Wisniewski, L., Kalarchian, M. A., et al. (1995). Effects of decreasing sedentary behavior and increasing activity on weight change in obese children. *Health Psychology, 14*(2), 109–115.

Epstein, L. H., Wing, R. R., Penner, B. C., & Kress, M. J. (1985). Effect of diet and controlled exercise on weight loss in obese children. *Journal of Pediatrics, 107*(3), 358–361.

Figueroa-Colon, R., von Almen, T. K., Franklin, F. A., Schuftan, C., & Suskind, R. M. (1993). Comparison of two hypocaloric diets in obese children. *American Journal of Diseases in Childhood, 147*(2), 160–166.

Flodmark, C. E., Ohlsson, T., Ryden, O., & Sveger, T. (1993). Prevention of progression to severe obesity in a group of obese schoolchildren treated with family therapy. *Pediatrics, 91*(5), 880–884.

Freedman, D. S., Dietz, W. H., Srinivasan, S. R., & Berenson, G. S. (1999). The relation of overweight to cardiovascular risk factors among children and adolescents: The Bogalusa Heart Study. *Pediatrics, 103*(6 Pt. 1), 1175–1182.

Golan, M., Fainaru, M., & Weizman, A. (1998). Role of behaviour modification in the treatment of childhood obesity with the parents as the exclusive agents of change. *International Journal Obesity and Related Metabolic Disorders, 22*(12), 1217–1224.

Golan, M., Kaufman, V., & Shahar, D. R. (2006). Childhood obesity treatment: targeting parents exclusively v. parents and children. *British Journal of Nutrition, 95*(5), 1008–1015.

Gortmaker, S. L., Must, A., Perrin, J. M., Sobol, A. M., & Dietz, W. H. (1993). Social and economic consequences of overweight in adolescence and young adulthood. *New England Journal of Medicine, 329*(14), 1008–1012.

Graves, T., Meyers, A. W., & Clark, L. (1988). An evaluation of parental problem-solving training in the behavioral treatment of childhood obesity. *Journal of Consulting and Clinical Psychology, 56,* 246–250.

Haines, J., Neumark-Sztainer, D., Eisenberg, M. E., & Hannan, P. J. (2006). Weight teasing and disordered eating behaviors in adolescents: Longitudinal findings from Project EAT (Eating Among Teens). *Pediatrics, 117*(2), e209–215.

Inge, T. H., Krebs, N. F., Garcia, V. F., Skelton, J. A., Guice, K. S., Strauss, R. S., et al. (2004). Bariatric surgery for severely overweight adolescents: Concerns and recommendations. *Pediatrics, 114*(1), 217–223.

Inge, T. H., Zeller, M. H., Lawson, M. L., & Daniels, S. R. (2005). A critical appraisal of evidence supporting a bariatric surgical approach to weight management for adolescents. *Journal of Pediatrics, 147*(1), 10–19.

Institute of Medicine (IOM) 2007. *Dietary Reference Intakes for Energy, Carbohydrate, Fiber, Fat, Fatty Acids, Cholesterol, Protein, and Amino Acids.* Retrieved on January 10, 2007 from http://www.iom.edu/CMS/3788/4576/4340. aspx.

Israel, A. C., Guile, C. A., Baker, J. E., & Silverman, W. K. (1994). An evaluation of enhanced self-regulation training in the treatment of childhood obesity. *Journal of Pediatric Psychology, 19*(6), 737–749.

Israel, A. C., Stolmaker, L., & Andrian, C. A. G. (1985). The effects of training parents in general child management skills on a behavioral weight loss program for children. *Behavior Therapy, 16,* 169–180.

Janssen, I., Craig, W. M., Boyce, W. F., & Pickett, W. (2004). Associations between overweight and obesity with bullying behaviors in school-aged children. *Pediatrics, 113*(5), 1187–1194.

Kinugasa, A., Tsunamoto, K., Furukawa, N., Sawada, T., Kusunoki, T., & Shimada, N. (1984). Fatty liver and its fibrous changes found in simple obesity of children. *Journal of Pediatric Gastroenterology and Nutrition, 3*(3), 408–414.

Lavine, J. E., & Schwimmer, J. B. (2004). Nonalcoholic fatty liver disease in the pediatric population. *Clinical Liver Disease, 8*(3), 549–558, viii–ix.

Mager, D. R., & Roberts, E. A. (2006). Nonalcoholic Fatty liver disease in children. *Clinical Liver Disease, 10*(1), 109–131.

Mellin, L. M., Slinkard, L. A., & Irwin, C. E., Jr. (1987). Adolescent obesity intervention: Validation of the SHAPEDOWN program. *Journal of the American Dietetic Association, 87*(3), 333–338.

Moran, J. R., Ghishan, F. K., Halter, S. A., & Greene, H. L. (1983). Steatohepatitis in obese children: a cause of chronic liver dysfunction. *American Journal of Gastroenterology, 78*(6), 374–377.

Narayan, K. M., Boyle, J. P., Thompson, T. J., Sorensen, S. W., & Williamson, D. F. (2003). Lifetime risk for diabetes mellitus in the United States. *Journal of the American Medical Association, 290*(14), 1884–1890.

Nemet, D., Barkan, S., Epstein, Y., Friedland, O., Kowen, G., & Eliakim, A. (2005). Short- and long-term beneficial effects of a combined dietary-behavioral-physical activity intervention for the treatment of childhood obesity. *Pediatrics, 115*(4), e443–449.

Neumark-Sztainer, D., Falkner, N., Story, M., Perry, C., Hannan, P. J., & Mulert, S. (2002). Weight-teasing among adolescents: correlations with weight status and disordered eating behaviors. *International Journal of Obstetric Related Metabolism Disorders, 26*(1), 123–131.

Ogden, C. L., Carroll, M. D., Curtin, L. R., McDowell, M. A., Tabak, C. J., & Flegal, K. M. (2006). Prevalence of overweight and obesity in the United States, 1999–2004. *Journal of the American Medical Association, 295*(13), 1549–1555.

Ozkan, B., Bereket, A., Turan, S., & Keskin, S. (2004). Addition of orlistat to conventional treatment in adolescents with severe obesity. *European Journal of Pediatrics, 163*(12), 738–741.

Reilly, J. J., Methven, E., McDowell, Z. C., Hacking, B., Alexander, D., Stewart, L., et al. (2003). Health consequences of obesity. *Archives of the Diseases of Childhood, 88*(9), 748–752.

Ricciardelli, L. A., & McCabe, M. P. (2001). Children's body image concerns and eating disturbance: A review of the literature. *Clinical Psychology Review, 21*(3), 325–344.

Robinson, T. N., Killen, J. D., Kraemer, H. C., Wilson, D. M., Matheson, D. M., Haskell, W. L., et al. (2003). Dance and reducing television viewing to prevent weight gain in African-American girls: The Stanford GEMS pilot study. *Ethnic Diseases, 13*(1 Suppl. 1), S65–S77.

Rolland-Cachera, M. F., Thibault, H., Souberbielle, J. C., Soulie, D., Carbonel, P., Deheeger, M., et al. (2004). Massive obesity in adolescents: Dietary interventions and behaviours associated with weight regain at 2 y follow-up. *International Journal of Obesity and Related Metabolic Disorders, 28*(4), 514–519.

Saelens, B. E., Sallis, J. F., Wilfley, D. E., Patrick, K., Cella, J. A., & Buchta, R. (2002). Behavioral weight control for overweight adolescents initiated in primary care. *Obesity Research, 10*(1), 22–32.

Satter, E. M. (1986). The feeding relationship. *Journal of the American Dietetics Association, 86*(3), 352–356.

Satter, E. M. (2005). *Your child's weight: helping without harming.* Madison, WI: Kelcy Press.

Schwingshandl, J., Sudi, K., Eibl, B., Wallner, S., & Borkenstien, M. (1999). Effect of an individualized training program during weight reduction on body composition: a randomized trial. *Archives of Disease in Childhood, 81,* 426–428.

Senediak, C., & Spence, S. H. (1985). Rapid versus gradual scheduling of therapeutic contact in a family-based behavioral weight control program for children. *Behavioral Psychotherapy, 13,* 265–287.

Sondike, S. B., Copperman, N., & Jacobson, M. S. (2003). Effects of a low-carbohydrate diet on weight loss and cardiovascular risk factor in overweight adolescents. *Journal of Pediatrics, 142*(3), 253–258.

Srinivasan, S., Ambler, G. R., Baur, L. A., Garnett, S. P., Tepsa, M., Yap, F., et al. (2006). Randomized, controlled trial of metformin for obesity and insulin resistance in children and adolescents: improvement in body composition and fasting insulin. *Journal of Clinical Endocrinology and Metabolism, 91*(6), 2074–2080.

Strauss, R. S. (2000). Childhood obesity and self-esteem. *Pediatrics, 105*(1), e15.

Strauss, R. S., & Pollack, H. A. (2003). Social marginalization of overweight children. *Archives of Pediatric and Adolescent Medicine, 157*(8), 746–752.

Suskind, R. M., Blecker, U., Udall, J. N., Jr., von Almen, T. K., Schumacher, H. D., Carlisle, L., et al. (2000). Recent advances in the treatment of childhood obesity. *Pediatric Diabetes, 1*(1), 23–33.

Thompson, S. H., Corwin, S. J., & Sargent, R. G. (1997). Ideal body size beliefs and weight concerns of fourth-grade children. *International Journal of Eating Disorders, 21*(3), 279–284.

Viner, R. M., & Cole, T. J. (2005). Adult socioeconomic, educational, social, and psychological outcomes of childhood obesity: A national birth cohort study. *British Medical Journal, 330*(7504), 1354.

Wadden, T. A., Stunkard, A. J., Rich, L., Rubin, C. J., Sweidel, G., & McKinney, S. (1990). Obesity in black adolescent girls: a controlled clinical trial of treatment by diet, behavior modification, and parental support. *Pediatrics, 85*(3), 345–352.

Wang, G., & Dietz, W. H. (2002). Economic burden of obesity in youths aged 6 to 17 years: 1979–1999. *Pediatrics, 109*(5), E81–81.

Warschburger, P., Fromme, C., Petermann, F., Wojtalla, N., & Oepen, J. (2001). Conceptualization and evaluation of a cognitive-behavioral training programme for children and adolescents with obesity. *International Journal of Obstetric Related Metabolic Disorders, 25*(Suppl 1), S93–S95.

Whitaker, R. C., Wright, J. A., Pepe, M. S., Seidel, K. D., & Dietz, W. H. (1997). Predicting obesity in young adulthood from childhood and parental obesity. *New England Journal of Medicine, 337*(13), 869–873.

Willi, S. M., Oexmann, M. J., Wright, N. M., Collop, N. A., & Key, L. L., Jr. (1998). The effects of a high-protein, low-fat, ketogenic diet on adolescents with morbid obesity: body composition, blood chemistries, and sleep abnormalities. *Pediatrics, 101*(1 Pt. 1), 61–67.

Chapter 10

PARENTS AS THE PRIMARY TARGET FOR HEALTHY EATING AMONG YOUNG CHILDREN

Mildred A. Horodynski, Kami J. Silk, and Michelle Henry

Childhood obesity is a major problem in the United States with the number of overweight and obese children increasing significantly each year. The impact of childhood obesity has finally captured the attention of the public, and policy makers are expressing a need for action. In 2004, the Institute of Medicine (IOM) identified the prevention of childhood obesity as a national priority. The IOM noted the serious health problems related to childhood obesity and the spiraling economic costs for treating children with obesity-related conditions. Although there are many risk factors and a variety of interventions, no one strategy is consistently effective in combating the problem of childhood obesity. It is critical that effective programs and policies, which target parents/caregivers and young children, are developed and implemented. This chapter addresses the current understanding and the problem of childhood obesity. Specifically, it provides information, guidelines, and theoretical models related to nutrition and prevention strategies that target parents of young children. The chapter is organized to present: (1) an overview of the problem, (2) nutrition guidelines and recommendations, (3) nutrition interventions, (4) theories to inform prevention approaches, and (5) directions for future research.

OVERVIEW OF OBESITY: DEFINITION AND ASSESSMENT PARAMETERS

Obesity is the most common nutrition problem in the United States, and this is especially true for children. Childhood obesity is difficult to define or diagnose because of the rapid changes in height and weight that occur during this time. Various indicators are used to define overweight and obesity for different age groups. The Centers for Disease Control and Prevention (CDC) and others have referred to children at or above the 85th percentile of the weight-for-height growth chart (see figures 10.1 and 10.2) as being at risk for overweight, and those at or above the 95th percentile as being overweight(National Center for Health Statistics, 2000). In this chapter, we will use the labels *overweight* and *obese* to be consistent with the adult definitions of overweight and obesity and will refer to childhood obesity as meaning both overweight and obesity in young children.

Facts and Figures about Childhood Obesity, History, and Etiology

The incidence of childhood obesity in the United States has increased dramatically over the last three decades. It is estimated that over 15 percent of children, ages 6–19, are overweight and another 15 percent of this age group is at risk for becoming overweight. The increased prevalence of overweight is evident even in preschool children. Rates have doubled in two- to five-year-olds, and even in the youngest age group (6–23 months), there has been a significant increase since the 1970s (Dewey, 2003). Experts believe that pediatric obesity is under diagnosed, and moreover, under treated (Plourde, 2006). Childhood obesity is taking a heavy toll on the health of our children. Many obesity-related health conditions, such as type 2 diabetes and high blood pressure, are now seen in children, where previously these conditions were almost exclusively adult-related health problems.

Physical inactivity is a major contributing factor for the recent increase in childhood obesity. The time children spend each day watching television and playing with computers contributes to the sedentary lifestyle. Many research studies have shown that children who spend more time watching TV are more likely to be overweight (Blass et al., 2006; Davison, Marshall, & Birch, 2006). The current recommendation is to limit children's television viewing to less than two hours per day for children over two years of age; for toddlers less than two years of age it is recommended that television viewing be discouraged altogether (Prochaska & Diclemente, 1983). Children need at least 60 minutes of physical activity every day.

As childhood obesity has increased throughout the last decades in the United States, the kinds of foods eaten by children and the context in which

Figure 10.1

Centers for Disease Control Growth Chart: United States: Birth to 36 Months for Girls, Length for Age, Weight for Age Percentiles

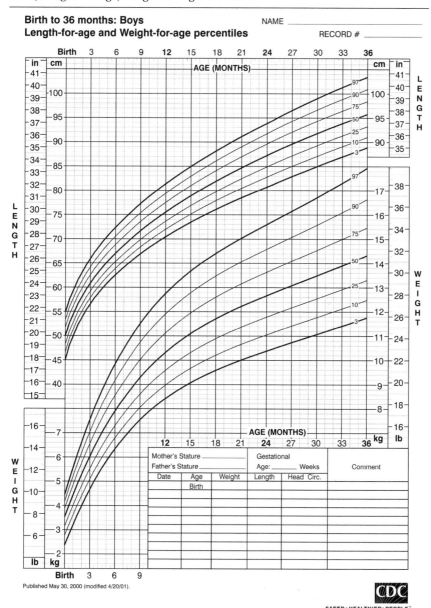

Birth to 36 months: Boys
Length-for-age and Weight-for-age percentiles

NAME _____

RECORD # _____

Published May 30, 2000 (modified 4/20/01).

CDC
SAFER · HEALTHIER · PEOPLE™

Source: Developed by the National Center for Health Statistics in collaboration with the National Center for Chronic Disease Prevention and Health Promotion (2000). http://www.cdc.gov/growthcharts

Figure 10.2

Centers for Disease Control Growth Chart: United States: Birth to 36 months for Boys, Length for Age, Weight for Age Percentiles

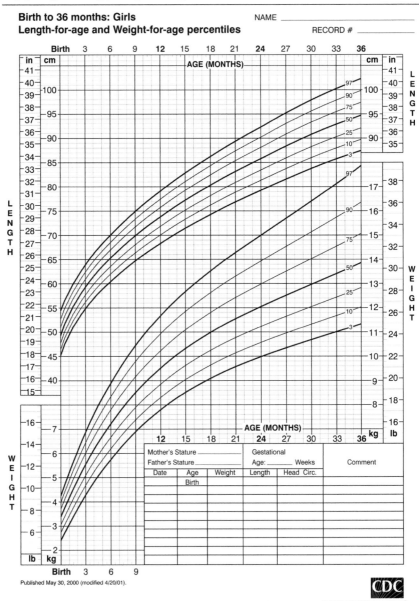

Source: Developed by the National Center for Health Statistics in collaboration with the National Center for Chronic Disease Prevention and Health Promotion (2000). http://www.cdc.gov/growthcharts

they are consumed have also undergone significant changes. A growing body of research indicates that among the biggest culprits in the obesity trend is the increasing frequency and energy density in snacks consumed by children (Adair & Popkin, 2005; Jackson, Romo, Castillo, & Castillo-Duran, 2004; Jahns, Siega-Riz, & Popkin, 2001). Between 1989 and 1996, the prevalence of snacking increased in all age groups of children 2–18 years old (Jahns et al., 2001). The most significant problems are seen in low-income populations and those with the least education (Drewnowski & Specter, 2004; North, Emmett, & ALSPAC Study Team, 2000). This is likely influenced by an inverse relation between energy density and food cost, in addition to the fact that high energy density usually means higher palatability and results in higher energy intake (Drewnowski & Specter, 2004; Jackson et al., 2004). Monetary considerations often dominate food choices (Furst, Connors, Bisogni, Sobal, & Falk, 1996).

Another significantly influential factor in food choice is convenience, both in terms of time and in ease of access or preparation (Furst et al., 1996). Unfortunately, convenience foods also tend to be those high in sugar and fat, and throughout the past decades, the nutrient contribution of snacks decreased in nutrient density while increasing in energy density (Jahns et al., 2001). Nearly a third of children aged 7 to 24 months do not consume vegetables or fruits on a daily basis, and the vegetable most commonly consumed by 15- to 18-month-old toddlers is french fries. Toddlers also consume unnecessary calories from sugar-sweetened beverages (Fox, Reidy, Novak, & Ziegler, 2006). These trends contribute to an increased availability and consumption of energy-dense foods and beverages, which can lead to obesity in children.

Children from low-income families and from ethnic minority groups are at risk for obesity (Kumanyika & Grier, 2006). Recent research has revealed an alarmingly high rate of obesity and obesity-related health problems in low-income African American and Hispanic schoolchildren. This trend may be related to culture and home environment. Low-income mothers from a minority group often identified the influence of their own culture as a contributor to obesity and recognized that a barrier to physical activity for them was the lack of a safe place to walk or run (Chatterjee, Blakely, & Barton, 2005). Among low-income children, programs like WIC have already proven beneficial in improving diet behaviors, including lower incidence of snacking and positive effects on fat, carbohydrate, added sugar, and fruit intakes, compared with children of the same age not receiving WIC (Siega-Riz et al., 2004).

Children with obese parents are also at high risk for becoming obese. In fact, parental obesity more than doubles the likelihood that a young child will become an obese adult (Rolfes, Whitney, & Pinna, 2006). This may be due in part to genetics, but is also a result of the fact that obese parents tend to overfeed their children. Obese preschool children consumed significantly more fat and calories on a daily basis than non-obese children of the same age. Obesity even in very young children is correlated with higher rates of obesity in adulthood. Over half of children who are obese between the ages of 3 and 6 are obese at age 25 (Whitaker, Wright, Pepe, Seidel, & Dietz, 1997).

Appropriate Growth and Weight Gain: Infancy to Age Six

While growth is very rapid throughout childhood, the rate of growth varies greatly during this time period, especially during the early years. Infancy is a period of rapid growth, such that by 6 months of age, an infant's birth weight is usually doubled, and by 12 months of age, infants usually weigh three times their birth weight. Tripling birth weight before one year of age, however, is associated with an increased risk for obesity. After one year of age, toddlers' growth rate progressively declines. In the second year, the usual weight gain is 7–10 lb; and in each year thereafter, it is 4–7 lb, until the child reaches six years of age (Escott-Stump, 2002; Rolfes et al., 2006).

Parents need to know that by one year of age, children's appetites begin to decrease, coinciding with a decrease in their rapid growth rates. Weight gains that are out of proportion with growth may indicate overeating and inactivity, two of the most significant factors leading to childhood obesity.

NUTRITION GUIDELINES AND RECOMMENDATIONS IN INFANCY AND TODDLERHOOD

During the first six months of life, the greatest factors affecting the infant's nutritional status include the type of feeding the infant receives (breast milk or formula), and at what age solid foods are introduced (Rolfes et al., 2006). Because of the nutrition and health benefits conferred to the infant through the mother's milk, the American Academy of Pediatrics (AAP) and American Dietetic Association (ADA) strongly advocate breastfeeding for full-term infants (American Academy of Pediatrics [AAP], 2005; American Dietetic Association [ADA], 2005). Both organizations recommend exclusive breastfeeding for the first 6 months of life, followed by breastfeeding with the addition of complementary foods until 12 months of age. Complementary foods are defined as any food other than breast milk or formula that is given to an infant when developmentally ready. The nutrient composition of breast milk is nearly perfect for meeting all of the infant's nutritional needs, with two exceptions: it is low in vitamin D and iron. Full term infants usually have sufficient iron stores to last until six months of age, when iron-fortified cereal can be introduced into the diet. Infants who are exclusively breastfed for the first six months and rarely exposed to the sun may need a vitamin D supplement, usually prescribed by a pediatrician.

Once the infant is developmentally ready to accept complementary foods, it is important to make the right food choices. The AAP recommends that complementary foods may be introduced between 4 and 6 months. Examples of appropriate complimentary foods include iron-fortified cereals and mashed fruits and vegetables. Concentrated sweets, such as sugar-sweetened beverages and baby food desserts provide no beneficial nutrients and can lead to extra calorie intake. Fruit juices need to be limited to 4–6 oz per day and served diluted, in a cup, rather than a bottle (Sherry, 2005). While it is important to help children make healthy food choices, it is also important that over-concerned parents do not over-restrict their children's diets. For this reason, nutrition labels on foods meant for children under two years of age do not include fat content. Fat intake is extremely important for growth and development during the early years of life, and it could be detrimental to a child's health if parents try to restrict fat intake. Therefore, it is recommended that whole (cow's) milk is served as an infant is weaned from breast milk or formula (Rolfes et al., 2006). Two to three-and-a-half cups of milk per day is sufficient to meet an infant's needs and portions should not greatly exceed this amount. Milk consumption in excess of three-and-a-half cups per day can displace important iron-rich foods in an infant's diet, leading to milk-induced anemia (Baptist & Castillo, 2002).

Dietary recommendations for toddlers, one to three years of age, include foods from each of the five food groups every day and include: (1) milk/dairy, (2) meat/beans, (3) vegetables, (4) fruit, and (5) grains. Daily amount of food from each food groups include: (1) 2 cups milk/dairy; (2) 1.5–2 ounce equivalents lean meat/beans; (3) 1 cup vegetables (2 servings); (4) 1 cup fruit (2 servings), and (5) 2–3 ounce equivalents of grains per day (U.S. Department of Agriculture, 2005).[1]

NUTRITION INTERVENTIONS FOR CHILDHOOD OBESITY

In childhood obesity, the goal is to reduce the rate of weight gain as the child continues to grow. Parents play the most important role in helping to prevent and reduce childhood obesity for infants and toddlers. The most frequently used strategies for curbing childhood obesity include: encouraging children to eat when they are hungry and stop when they are full—never force a child to clean his or her plate; teaching children how to make healthy food choices, and offering healthy foods for meals and snacks; limiting sugar-sweetened beverages; discouraging eating while watching TV; discouraging sedentary activity; and encouraging increased physical activity (see table 10.1).

Children begin to assert independence in the second year, which can lead to conflict between parent and child, especially around feeding and

Table 10.1
Strategies for curbing childhood obesity—healthy feeding of infants and toddlers.

Person Responsible	Strategy/Behavior
Parental Role Model (Parent Provides)	• Offer food in a happy environment. Children like foods associated with fun. • Turn off the TV. Talk to your child during meals and snacks. • Offer new foods many times. It can take 10–20 tries before food becomes familiar and child accepts the food. • Eat the same food as your child. Children are more likely to try a food when others at the table enjoy the food. • Do not insist that your child eat all of the food and do not reward or bribe children for eating everything. • Serve meals and snacks at a regular time every day.
Child Eating Behaviors (Child Decides)	• Children have small stomachs, about the size of their fist; serve appropriate portion sizes (small portions on small plates). • Provide variety of nutritious foods and let the child decide if the child wants to eat and how much to eat. • Allow children to help prepare the meal or set the table as appropriate to the age of child. • Serve small portions of food and allow child to ask for more if wanted. • Remove uneaten food without comment. • Do not ever try to force a toddler to eat! It can cause choking and make the child dislike the food. • Accept that mealtimes may be messy as toddlers learn to feed themselves. • Allow toddler to use a fork and spoon to eat.

mealtimes. Parents typically believe they know what is best for the child, even during mealtimes, which includes how much the parent thinks the child should eat. It is important that children determine their own food intake. Coercion, bribery, and threatening in order to get children to eat according to the parent's knowledge of what is best can be detrimental to the child's future eating behavior, decreasing the child's attention to internal hunger and satiety cues. By age three or four, eating is no longer driven by these internal cues, but more by external influences, such as being presented with larger portion sizes. Rather than control, parents need to serve as role models for their children, demonstrating healthy food choices and eating behaviors, and creating a positive eating environment.

The Role of Parents in Preventing Childhood Obesity

Parents play a pivotal role in preventing childhood obesity. They purchase, prepare, and feed infants and toddlers their meals and snacks. They are typically the key role models in children's young lives, informing children's perceptions of what is good or not good, too little or too much, and what behavior is easy or difficult to perform. In other words, parents serve as primary role models of behavior for healthy diets and lifestyles. Thus, parents comprise an important target audience for health campaign prevention messages about childhood obesity.

Prevention Efforts for Childhood Obesity

The source of the problem of childhood obesity has been defined at the genetic, individual, family, organizational, and societal levels, indicating the multi-causal nature of the epidemic. Efforts to target obesity at these different levels include individual weight loss regimens, national media campaigns, community-based programs, school health promotions, environmental changes, and lifestyle intervention. However, despite these efforts the problem of childhood obesity continues to grow. Behavior change and health campaigns generally have small effects that result in some knowledge gain and awareness, slight attitude change, and even less behavior change. To improve the effectiveness of efforts targeted to parents it is critical that theory be incorporated into intervention design and campaign strategies. One reason for this is the unrealistic expectation that knowledge alone will ultimately result in behavior change.

Additionally, parents themselves may find these theories insightful as they initiate or change eating behaviors or activities to improve their own and their children's health. The next section of this chapter will discuss two theories, the transtheoretical model (Prochaska & Velicier, 1997) and the theory of planned behavior (Ajzen, 1991). Explanations of the two theories are provided along with examples to illustrate their application. The focus of the examples will be to illustrate the relevance of the theories for individuals seeking to design an obesity intervention or campaign as well as to parents and providers who are attempting to change eating behaviors in children.

THEORIES TO INFORM PREVENTIVE APPROACHES FOR CHILDHOOD OBESITY

Transtheoretical Model

The transtheoretical model (TTM) explains stages for individuals' readiness to change a behavior. People can be in the precontemplation, contemplation, preparation, action, or maintenance stages in terms of their readiness to change a behavior (see table 10.2). People who do not believe a problem exists would be in the *precontemplation* stage. These individuals have no serious intention to change and likely do not believe that there is a problem. Individuals in the *contemplation* stage are aware that there is a weight problem and have thought about doing something about it, but have made no serious commitment to make a change. Individuals in the *preparation* stage intend to take action to change and may seek information about how to facilitate the behavior change. In the *action* stage, people have begun to address their weight problem by adopting a new behavior and/or ceasing a problem behavior. When individuals engage in the healthy behavior change for at least six months, they have entered the *maintenance* stage. Relapse occurs when individuals revert back to old behaviors that are not recommended or healthy. Although the stages are presented in a linear fashion, they do not necessarily occur consecutively. In other words, individuals can skip stages or revert back to a previous stage. Additionally, people continually go through a decisional balance, examining the pros and cons associated with engaging in healthful practices. Self-efficacy is fundamental to successful behavior change because it is essential for people to have the confidence in their ability to maintain the behavior to avoid relapse.

The TTM explains stages for parents' readiness to change a behavior related to feeding their infant or toddler. Parents may be in either precontemplation, contemplation, preparation, action, or maintenance stages in terms of their readiness to change their behavior related to feeding their infants and toddlers. Parents who do not believe a problem exists would

Table 10.2
Stages of the transtheoretical model.

Stage	Description
Pre-contemplation	Unaware problem exists. No serious intention of changing. *Example: Alice is unaware that her toddler is obese.*
Contemplation	Aware problem exists. Thinking about taking action. *Example: The doctor informs Alice her toddler is obese. She begins to worry about her child's health.*
Preparation	Intends to take action soon. Considers possibilities. *Example: Alice identifies new physical activities for her child and looks for healthier snack options.*
Action	Actively engaging in behavior change strategies. *Example: Alice takes her toddler to the park on a daily basis and serves fruit slices for snack time.*
Maintenance	Engaging in the behavior without relapse for six months. *Example: Alice continues to find active play and games as well as healthy food options for her toddler.*
Relapse	Engaging in so-called old or not recommended behavior. *Example: Alice becomes very busy with other things and goes back to so-called quick snacks like cookies.*

be in the precontemplation stage. These parents have no serious intention to change how they feed their children and likely do not believe that feeding toddlers foods such as french fries is unhealthy for their toddlers. Parents in the contemplation stage are aware that they should not give their toddlers french fries and have thought about giving their toddlers something else to eat, but have made no serious commitment to stop giving their toddlers french fries when they dine in restaurants. Parents in the preparation stage intend to take action to change and may seek information to help them facilitate feeding their toddlers healthy foods. They might talk with their pediatrician, go online to find nutrition information, or talk with other parents about what they feed their children. In the action stage, parents have begun to address the issue by providing an alternate food choice instead of the french fries. When the parents continue to engage in the healthy behavior change for at least six months (e.g., consistently choosing healthy food options for the child), parents have entered the maintenance stage.

The TTM also accounts for the likelihood that people will relapse at times. A relapse can be a one-time event or it can be more significant, resulting in a person completely returning to unhealthy behaviors. For example, over the holiday season parents might find it difficult to maintain the same diet and activity schedule that they were maintaining for their young children. They may get back on track as soon as their schedule returns to normal or they may continue to maintain unhealthy practices into the New Year. Parents continually go through a decisional balance, examining the pros and cons associated with engaging in healthful feeding practices with their infants and toddlers. As long as the pros continue to outweigh the cons, parents are likely to maintain healthy feeding practices. Self-efficacy is also important for parents because they need to have confidence in their ability to maintain healthy feeding practices with their child to avoid relapse into unhealthy behavior.

There are processes of change that people use to progress through the six stages of change. The 10 activities or change processes associated with the different stages that can help move parents through the behavior change progression include: consciousness raising, social liberation, dramatic relief, self-reevaluation, self-liberation, counter-conditioning, stimulus control, contingency management, helping relationships, and environmental reevaluation (see table 10.3). These processes of change provide parents with strategies to encourage healthy feeding and eating practices. For example, consider a new mother and her attempt to delay the early introduction of solid foods based on AAP recommendations (AAP, 2005).

The AAP recommends that babies should be fed exclusively breastmilk or formula until six months of age because infants are not developmentally ready to begin solid foods until they are four to six months of age. Mothers face the dilemma of when to start feeding their baby anything other than breast milk or formula. Often mothers think it is good to feed their babies solid foods early (before they are developmentally ready, before the baby is almost six months old) because it will help them grow or that giving the baby cereal will help the baby sleep through the night. Table 10.3 provides an example of the change processes of the TTM. The example is how a mother might think about changing her feeding behavior with her infant, along with strategies for health professionals and others who are helping mothers with infants to change their feeding behaviors.

The TTM acknowledges that people are at different stages of readiness to make changes. Strategies for healthy behavior change, therefore, need to be tailored to the needs of different audiences, and in the current case, the target audiences are parents/caregivers of infants and toddlers as well as the children themselves. The TTM provides a tool for selecting appropriate activities and messages designed to influence attitudes and behaviors of parents and caregivers about feeding young children.

Table 10.3
Processes of change in the transtheoretical model[a]

Change process	Definition	Application to Healthy Feeding Practices
Consciousness-raising	Increasing awareness about healthy behavior change.	Increase understanding of what constitutes a so-called solid food.[1]
Social liberation	Realizing that social norms are changing to support the healthy behavior change.	Increase understanding of guidelines for infant feeding.[2]
Dramatic relief	Experiencing negative emotions that go along with unhealthy feeding choices.	Recognizing that following feeding guidelines might be challenging, but you will feel good about their benefits for your baby.
Self-reevaluation	Taking a look at current practices and assessing them.	Understanding that your baby is not an exception to recommended practices.
Self-liberation	Making a firm commitment to change.	Mothers can write down their goal to only breastfeed for the first six months
Counter-conditioning	Substituting healthy behaviors for unhealthy behaviors.	Instead of immediately feeding a crying baby, try other strategies to calm baby, such as talking softly.
Stimulus control	Removing cues for unhealthy behavior and adding cues for healthy behavior.	Do not purchase baby food or feeding alternatives before the baby is at least 6 months old.
Contingency management	Using rewards and punishments.	Give yourself credit for every week you delay the early introduction of solid foods.
Helping relationships	Using social support for the healthy behavior change.	Talk with other mothers who are trying to engage in healthy feeding practices.
Environmental re-evaluation	Examining the impact of the behavior on social and physical environments.	Talk with your baby during feeding time to create a healthy environment for the baby.

Note [a] How mothers think about feeding their infants was developed using data from focus groups done with mothers of 0–12 months of age. [1] Solid Foods (for infants) are any food or liquid other than breast milk or formula. [2] The American Academy of Pediatrics (2005) states that an infant may be physically ready to accept solid foods sometime between four and six months.

Theory of Planned Behavior

Another theory helpful in considering how to address the obesity epidemic for parents and children is the theory of planned behavior (TPB). An extension of the theory of reasoned action (Ajzen & Fishbein, 1980), TPB argues that behavioral intention is the most important predictor of future behavior. The theory assumes individuals to be rational decision-makers who consider options and implications of a behavior before actually engaging in the behavior. Behavioral intention refers to whether or not a person plans to perform a particular behavior. The greater a person's behavioral intention to perform a specific behavior, the greater the likelihood the person will actually perform that behavior. For example, if a person intends to eat healthy food, he or she will be more likely to do it than if he or she had intended to eat unhealthy selections. According to the TPB, behavioral intention is predicted by three determinants: attitudes, subjective norms, and perceived behavioral control (see figure 10.3 for a conceptual model).

Attitudes

Attitudes are comprised of behavioral beliefs that have outcome evaluations associated with them (Conner, Warren, Close, & Sparks, 1999; Fishbein & Ajzen, 1975). Behavioral beliefs refer to the consequences or outcomes of a behavior, while the outcome evaluations refer to the positive or negative value assigned to each of the associated behavioral

Figure 10.3
The Theory of Planned Behavior

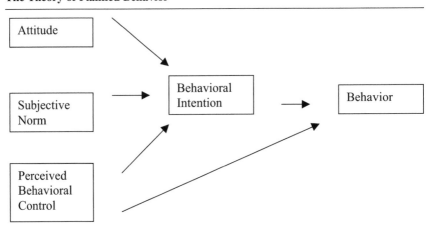

beliefs. An individual attitude toward a behavior is determined by the sum of the beliefs about performing the behavior, weighted by the evaluations of the beliefs. In general, behaviors that are thought to produce a favorable outcome have positive attitudes associated with them, while behaviors that are thought to produce negative outcomes have negative attitudes associated with them. For example, if parents believe that eating fruits and vegetables will result in a positive outcome like stronger bones, they will likely make greater efforts to provide healthy foods for their toddler than if they thought otherwise. As infants and toddlers continue to get older, their own attitudes will influence their food choices and eating behavior. For example, if a young child thinks that eating healthy will result in a positive outcome, such as the mother or father being pleased with the child, the child is likely to have a positive attitude toward eating healthy.

Subjective Norms

Subjective norms are defined as a person's beliefs about certain individuals' or groups' (referents) evaluations about performing a given behavior (Conner et al., 1999). Subjective norms are a function of different types of normative beliefs and are determined by the sum of the products of normative beliefs and one's motivation to comply. Normative beliefs are the individual beliefs that underlie subjective norms; they involve specific individuals (e.g., wife, parent, or pastor) or groups (e.g., church, sorority, athletic team) that may influence how individuals perceive a particular behavior (Ajzen & Fishbein, 1980). Motivation to comply with normative beliefs can range from nonexistent to very high, depending on the importance and influence of the referent(s). In the family system, parents are key role models for how children learn to value healthy eating practices. If parents perceive that the norm is important to provide healthy foods so their child will choose and eat healthy foods, they are more likely to do so. Parents who do not perceive the need to provide healthy foods or do not perceive certain foods to be unhealthy are less likely to choose and eat healthy foods. These norms are also learned by the child. For example, a child who perceives it is normative to make healthy food selections will be more likely to eat healthy foods than if he or she perceives the behavior is not normative in the family. In addition, if children do not believe their referents (i.e., parents) value healthy eating, they will be less likely to eat healthy food.

Perceived Behavioral Control

Perceived behavioral control refers to the perception that performance of a specific behavior is within a person's volitional control (Ajzen &

Fishbein, 1980), which can be seen as a continuum with easily executed behaviors at one end and more demanding behaviors (e.g., those behaviors that require more resources, opportunities, specialized skills, etc.) at the other (Conner et al., 1999). According to the TPB, performance of a behavior is a joint function of behavioral intentions and perceived behavioral control. When a behavior or situation affords a person complete control over his or her behavioral performance, intentions alone should be sufficient to predict behavior (as specified in the theory of reasoned action). Perceived behavioral control, however, is useful in helping to predict behavior (Ajzen, 1991). For example, if a parent or child has low self-efficacy in making healthy food choices, he or she may perceive low behavioral control, which could lead to a parent deciding it is too difficult to eat healthier.

Tables 10.4 and 10.5 provide examples of a mother and her attempt to delay the early introduction of solid foods before the AAP recommendation of close to six months of age, and a mother dealing with her picky eater toddler using the theory of planned behavior. The mother's attitudes, subjective norm, and perceptions of control predict the mother's intention to delay the early introduction of solid food to her infant and to serve a fruit or vegetable to her toddler.

Table 10.4
Theory of planned behavior feeding example.

Constructs	Definition of Construct	Example for Infant Feeding Behavior
Attitude	Beliefs about engaging in the behavior	"My baby is bigger than others and needs more food." "The AAP guidelines for infant feeding are important to me."
Subjective Norms	Beliefs about what others think about the behavior	"My sister and friends follow the AAP guidelines and didn't feed their babies solid foods until six months."
Perceptions of Control	Beliefs about own abilities to make change or engage in the behavior	"I worry about what my day care provider feeds my baby when I am not there." "I think I will be able to stick to the AAP recommendation."
Behavioral Intention	Individual's plan of whether or not to perform the behavior	"I am really going to try to only feed my baby breast milk and/or formula for the first six months."
Behavior	Individual's actual engagement of the behavior	Mother adheres to the AAP recommendation and does not introduce solids before six months.

Table 10.5
Theory of planned behavior feeding example.

Constructs	Definition of Construct	Example for Toddler FeedingBehavior
Attitude	Beliefs about engaging in the behavior	"My toddler is a picky eater and will only eat macaroni and cheese." "It is important to me to feed my toddler healthy foods, like fruits and vegetables."
Subjective Norms	Beliefs about what others think about the behavior	"My sister and friends tell me that being a fussy eater is normal for a toddler."
Perceptions of Control	Beliefs about own abilities to make change or engage in the behavior	"I worry about my toddler getting enough to eat if he skips a meal or doesn't eat anything I serve." "I think I will be able to let him have his favorite food but I will also offer a variety of other healthy choices, such as a banana."
Behavioral Intention	Individual's plan of whether or not to perform the behavior	"I am really going to try to serve my toddler at least one fruit or vegetable at every meal and snack."
Behavior	Individual's actual engagement of the behavior	Mother buys light canned fruit and frozen peas and introduces one new food at a time.

Overall, both the TTM and TPB are useful tools for focusing prevention and intervention efforts. We have provided examples of feeding behavior in our explanations of the TTM and the TPB. Now we will now consider an extended example of how the two theories might inform prevention efforts of a local organization that wants to take action against the obesity problem in its community. The TTM will be used to target the community's readiness for change and the TPB will be used as a strategy to identify and target attitudes, norms, and perceptions of control.

The Theories in Action

A community-based nonprofit organization that provides nutrition classes to its community members recognizes its education efforts are not making an impact on the waistlines of community. The organization would like to move beyond nutrition classes and create a community-wide campaign that targets families, with a primary focus on parents. To determine whether their primary audience is interested in making some changes, they develop a survey and disseminate it to the parents of the children who are enrolled in various day care, early childhood programs, church, and educational activities. The survey assesses healthy eating, family habits, perceived barriers to preparing and eating healthy foods, and their readiness to make changes in their diets. The results indicate that parents have been considering making some changes (contemplation and perhaps preparation) and have positive attitudes about eating healthy, but do not really know how to prepare healthy foods. They also perceive that eating healthy is not cost effective on their limited budgets. These survey results provide significant areas for campaign messages that target the community member audience.

First, the survey results reveal that parents are open to making changes. Parents report contemplating and even preparing to make some changes and have an overall positive attitude about eating healthy—even if they currently are not eating healthy. Campaign messages, therefore, designed to address their concerns will be salient to them. Parents are likely to attend to campaign messages that are directly targeted to them. For example, a key campaign message based on nutrition research might include the following recommendation, "A *Golden Rule* for feeding children: *Parent Decides* what food is served and when food is served; *Child Decides* whether to eat and how much to eat" (Satter, 2004). A recommendation like this one provides some general guidelines for parents.

Second, survey results indicated that parents are concerned about proper preparation of healthy foods. Campaign messages would want to provide simple messages about the benefits of baking, grilling, or broiling food rather than frying it or adding heavy sauces and butter to food. Parents would likely be interested to know that a cold meal such as meat and bread with fruit or salad is also healthy and nutritious for the child. Parents should also be encouraged to offer a variety of foods from each of the food groups to their children. It is also essential that campaign messages address the issues that healthy foods and snacks can be affordable as well as easy to prepare.

Finally, campaign messages would want to directly address serving size by providing recommended amounts of food appropriate for infants' and toddlers' digestive systems. Toddlers' appetites fluctuate from day to day depending on many things such as their activity levels, whether or not they are in a growth spurt, how tired or excited they might be, and whether or not they are sick. One to two-year-old toddlers need less to eat than three- to five-year-old preschoolers do. A tablespoon serving of each food, such as meat, potatoes, peas, may be enough for a one year old. Offer more when they finish and ask for more. The message is that it is the child's responsibility to decide how much to eat and to select foods to eat from choices offered; the parent provides nutritious foods, offers a variety of healthy food choices, serves routine meals and snacks, and establishes where meals and snacks are served. This example illustrates how the transtheoretical model and the theory of planned behavior can inform message strategies that aim to address parental concerns over infant and toddler feeding practices.

SUMMARY

Childhood obesity has been and continues to be on a rapid increase in the United States. To reverse this trend, interventions must occur early. Children must learn healthy eating and exercise habits. Parents are critical role models who determine what food is purchased and how it is prepared for children. They are pivotal in setting standards for healthy eating. During their child's infancy, parents make decisions about when to introduce solid foods to children. Parents are clearly primary influencers over the health of their children and set the stage for children's choices and behavior as they grow and take more responsibility for their eating. In other words, parents' decisions about food also influence, in part, adolescent health or adolescent overweight and obesity, which is significantly related to whether or not a child becomes overweight or obese as an adult.

Parents and others who are trying to prevent childhood obesity and promote healthy eating behavior can bolster their attempts by understanding some basic theories that provide insight about human behavior. These theories are very useful in helping us understand how people make decisions and why they choose to perform (or not to perform) a behavior. The TTM identifies a person's stage of readiness to make a behavior change. This stage model articulates 10 processes of change that can inform what should be done to best influence individuals in each of the five stages of readiness. For example, someone who is in the contemplation stage and considering making a change in their toddler's diet would probably benefit from considering stimulus control so they can examine what might cue them to make positive versus negative food choices for their child.

The TPB helps predict behavior based on attitudes, subjective norms, and perceived behavioral control. Parents and interventionists can attempt to change attitudes, reinforce positive norms, and increase perceptions of control to influence behavior. If one considers that people are likely to engage in behaviors for which they have a positive attitude, favorable norm perception, and feelings of control over—it makes the utility of the TPB very evident. A parent, for example, who has a positive attitude about the AAP recommendation to only introduce solid foods to infants at six months and perceives a supportive norm among significant others (e.g., siblings and friends), is more likely to adhere to the guideline than someone who has a negative attitude and norm toward the recommendation. Parents are even more likely to adhere to the guideline if they feel like they have control over their ability to perform the behavior. Overall, the TTM and TPB provide us with some ideas of how to think about and address the problem of overweight and obesity.

DIRECTIONS FOR FUTURE WORK

While there has been a great deal of research about childhood nutrition and feeding behaviors, there is still room for further investigation. Research needs to investigate multi-causal models that account for the many factors that influence obesity. More longitudinal studies need to be conducted that follow families for more than a few months. Longitudinal studies are essential for learning more about how eating and physical activity patterns develop throughout childhood so that more effective obesity prevention strategies can be developed, implemented, and evaluated. With so many Americans eating high-fat, energy-dense foods at earlier and earlier ages, we need to understand how these preferences develop and how they can be modified. More studies investigating the effect of family mealtime environments and parental feeding practices on the permanent dietary practices of children are critical for the development of behavior change strategies. Future research goals should include: (1) identifying the specific nutritional factors necessary for optimal health, growth, and child development; (2) identifying social and cultural factors related to body weight and body composition during infancy and childhood; and (3) identifying childhood dietary habits that contribute to long-term health outcomes. Information learned from these research areas can assist in developing interventions to improve child-feeding practices, which may lead to the development of healthier eating habits throughout the lifespan.

Implications for Health Care Professionals and Others Working with Parents of Young Children

Parents are typically eager to learn what they can do to promote a healthy environment for their infants and toddlers. They seek information from multiple sources and want to do what is best for their children, but behavior change is challenging. Individuals working with parents should make parents more aware of risk factors and AAP guidelines related to infant and toddler feeding. Parents need to be made aware of their role in the prevention of obesity in their children. Parents, themselves, need to be willing to make changes in their own eating behaviors. Health care professionals also need to be aware of the problems associated with childhood obesity. Professionals working with families with young children need to be cognizant of prevention strategies and promotion of healthy eating practices within families and implement them.

Policy Implications Related to the Prevention of Childhood Obesity

Priority attention must be given to the prevention and management of childhood obesity. Family- and community-based campaigns that address parental roles in the prevention of childhood obesity need to be developed, implemented, and evaluated. These campaigns should be based on theory as well as the most recent evidence related to nutrition science, behavior change, and communication research. Educational campaign efforts need to be directed toward policy makers, health care professionals, community leaders, and parents so that the problem is defined at multiple levels rather than simply at the individual level. Public policy is needed to manage the childhood obesity crisis. These efforts can only be achieved though coordinated efforts among policy makers, business and community leaders, schools, parents, and concerned citizens (Hill & Trowbridge, 1998).

The overall diet quality of young children needs to improve dramatically. Early attention to children's diets would provide immediate nutritional benefits, help prevent obesity, and could reduce the risk of related chronic diseases if healthful dietary habits were continued into adulthood. Childhood obesity is best viewed as a societal problem, which reflects the interactive influences of the environment, genetics, and behavior. Healthful dietary and physical activity behaviors need to be established in early childhood to promote a healthy lifestyle and prevent childhood obesity.

NOTE

1. Food groups shown in cup (c.) or ounce (oz-eq.), with number of servings in parentheses when it differs from the other units. Daily amounts of food are based on 1,000 calorie diet level. Half of all grains should be whole grains. The American Academy of Pediatrics recommends that low-fat/reduced fat milk be started before two years of age.

REFERENCES

Adair, L., & Popkin, B. (2005). Are child eating patterns being transformed globally? *Obesity Research, 13,* 1281–1299.

Ajzen, I. (1991). The theory of planned behavior. *Organizational Behavior and Decision Making Processes, 50,* 179–211.

Ajzen, I., & Fishbein, M. (1980). *Understanding attitudes and predicting social behavior.* Upper Saddle River, NJ: Prentice Hall.

American Academy of Pediatrics. (2005). *Pediatric nutrition handbook* (5th ed.). Elk Grove Village, IL: Author.

American Dietetic Association. (2005). Position of the American dietetic association: Promoting and supporting breastfeeding. *Journal of the American Dietetic Association, 105,* 810–818.

Baptist, E., & Castillo, S. (2002). Cow's milk-induced iron deficiency anemia as a cause of childhood stroke. *Clinical Pediatrics, 41*(7), 533–535.

Blass, E., Anderson, D., Kirkorian, H., Pempek, T., Price, I., & Koleini, M. (2006). On the road to obesity: Television viewing increases intake of high-density foods. *Physiological Behavior, 88*(4–5), 597–604.

Chatterjee, N., Blakely, D., & Barton, C. (2005). Perspectives on obesity and barriers to control from workers at a community center serving low-income Hispanic children and families. *Journal of Community Health Nursing, 22*(1), 23–36.

Conner, M., Warren, R., Close, S., & Sparks, P. (1999). Alcohol consumption and the theory of planned behavior: An examination of the cognitive mediation of past behavior. *Journal of Applied Social Science, 29*(8), 1676–1704.

Davison, K., Marshall, S., & Birch, L. (2006). Cross-sectional and longitudinal associations between TV viewing and girls' body mass index, overweight status, and percentage of body fat. *Journal of Pediatrics, 149*(1), 32–37.

Dewey, K. (2003). Is breastfeeding protective against child obesity? *Journal of Human Lactation, 19*(1), 9–18.

Drewnowski, A., & Specter, S. (2004). Poverty and obesity: The role of energy density and energy costs. *American Journal of Clinical Nutrition, 79,* 6–16.

Escott-Stump, S. (2002). *Nutrition and diagnosis-related care* (5th ed.). Baltimore, MD: Lippincott Williams and Wilkins.

Fishbein, M., & Ajzen, I. (1975). *Belief, attitude, intention, and behavior: An introduction to theory and research.* Reading, MA: Addison-Wesley.

Fox, M., Reidy, K., Novak, T., & Ziegler, P. (2006). Sources of energy and nutrients in the diets of infants and toddlers. *Journal of the American Dietetic Association, 106,* S28–S42.

Furst, T., Connors, M., Bisogni, C., Sobal, J., & Falk, L. (1996). Food choice: A conceptual model of the process. *Appetite, 26,* 247–265.

Hill, J., & Trowbridge, F. (1998). Future directions and research priorities. *Pediatrics, 101,* 570–574.

Jackson, P., Romo, M., Castillo, M., & Castillo-Duran, C. (2004). Las golosinas en la alimentacion infantil. *Revista Medica de Chile, 132,* 1235–1242.

Jahns, L., Siega-Riz, A., & Popkin, B. (2001). The increasing prevalence of snacking among us children from 1977 to 1996. *Journal of Pediatrics, 138,* 493–498.

Kumanyika, S., & Grier, S. (2006). Targeting interventions for ethnic minority and low-income populations. *Future Child, 16*(1), 187–207.

National Center for Health Statistics. (2000). *CDC growth charts: United States.* (Advance data from vital and health statistics No. 314). Hyattsville, MD: Author.

North, K., Emmett, P., & the ALSPAC Study Team. (2000). Multivariate analysis of diet among three-year-old children and associations with socio-demographic characteristics. *European Journal of Clinical Nutrition, 54,* 73–80.

Plourde, G. (2006). Preventing and managing pediatric obesity. *Canadian Family Physician, 52,* 322–328.

Prochaska, J., & Diclemente, C. (1983). Stages and processes of self-change of smoking: Toward an integrative model of change. *Journal of Consulting and Clinical Psychology, 51,* 390–395.

Prochaska, J., & Velicier, W. F. (1997). The transtheoretical model of health and behavior change. *American Journal of Health Promotion, 12*(1), 38–48.

Rolfes, S., Whitney, E., & Pinna, K. (2006). *Understanding normal and clinical nutrition* (7th ed.). Baltimore: Lippincott Williams & Wilkins.

Satter, E. (2004). Children, the feeding relationship, and weight. *Maryland Medicine, 5*(3), 26–28.

Sherry, B. (2005). Food behaviors and other strategies to prevent and treat pediatric overweight. *International Journal of Obesity, 29,* S116–S129.

Siega-Riz, A., Kranz, S., Blanchette, D., Haines, P., Guilkey, D., & Popkin, B. (2004). The effect of participation in the WIC program on preschoolers diets. *Journal of Pediatrics, 144,* 229–234.

United States Department of Agriculture (2005). Nutrition and your health: Dieting guidelines for Americans. 6th edition. Washington, DC: Author.

Whitaker, R., Wright, J., Pepe, M., Seidel, K., & Dietz, W. (1997). Predicting obesity in young adulthood from childhood and parental obesity. *New England Journal of Medicine, 337*(13), 869–873.

Chapter 11

SURGICAL TREATMENT OF OBESITY

Jeff M. Gauvin

Evidence reviewed by the North American Association for the Study of Obesity (1998, 2000), indicates that non-surgical approaches to sustained weight loss are relatively ineffective in treating obesity. Surgical treatment is the most effective method for achieving weight loss with significant improvement or complete resolution of comorbidities (Buchwald, 2005). In light of these data it is no wonder that obesity surgery, also known as bariatric surgery (from the Greek *baros,* meaning weight and *iatrike,* meaning treatment) has become such a popular option for patients and healthcare professionals. Although bariatric operations were developed over 50 years ago, there has been a dramatic increase in their frequency over the past decade. Between 1998 and 2002 the number of bariatric procedures performed in the United States increased by more than five fold, from 13,000 to 71,000. Current estimates by the American Association of Bariatric Surgeons (ASBS) are estimated to be 180,000 annually (Kushner & Noble, 2006)

Surgical treatment of obesity is not a cosmetic procedure, nor does it simply involve the removal of fat. Bariatric procedures are major operations that fall into one of three categories: restrictive procedures that limit the amount of food ingested; malabsorptive procedures which limit the amount of nutrients absorbed; and combination procedures that limit both the volume ingested and nutrients absorbed. Eating behavior improves dramatically after the surgery. In order to understand the current surgical practice, one must look at the evolution of bariatric surgery and the many lessons learned over the past 50 years.

HISTORY OF BARIATRIC SURGERY

The first bariatric procedure, the jejunoileal bypass (JIB), was reported by Kremen, Linner & Nelson (1954). This purely malabsorptive operation involves connecting the proximal jejunum to the distal ileum, thus bypassing the vast majority of the nutrient-absorbing small bowel (figure 11.1). JIB was the dominant bariatric procedure for more than 20 years. Although weight loss was excellent, nutritional deficiencies, electrolyte imbalances, and frequent diarrhea were common complications. As patients were followed for longer periods (10–20 years), it became apparent that more serious complications such as hepatic failure, renal failure, cirrhosis, and even death resulted. The majority of these complications

Figure 11.1
Jejunoileal Bypass

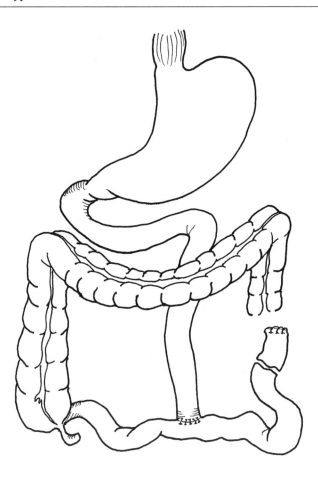

resulted from bacterial overgrowth in the non-functioning limb of small bowel that resulted in such dramatic weight loss. As the serious nature of these complications were recognized some authors recommend surgical reversal in some patients (Joffe, 1981; Thirlby, 1990). Currently, the ASBS (American Society for Bariatric Surgery [ASBS], 2007) strongly recommends long-term follow-up by an experienced bariatric surgeon for all patients who have had JIB. Experience with the JIB taught us the dangers of permanent malabsorption and, perhaps more importantly, the importance of long-term follow-up.

Despite the dismal long-term consequences of the JIB, the need for effective obesity treatment lead to the emergence of numerous modifications. Unlike the JIB, these second generation malabsorptive procedures did not leave a stagnant limb of small bowel, thus eliminating the problematic bacterial overgrowth that was responsible for most of the serious complications of the JIB. Additionally, several of these safer options, such as the biliopancreatic bypass, duodenal switch, and gastric bypass incorporated a restrictive component by also reducing the size of the stomach. Weight loss thus resulted from a combination of malabsorption and a restrictive component that limited the volume of food ingested. It is beyond the scope of this chapter to discuss all the nuances of these various combination procedures, however, the gastric bypass is most noteworthy as it is the precursor to the currently used Roux-en-Y gastric bypass (RYGB).

Dr. Mason and colleagues at the University of Iowa developed the gastric bypass in the mid-1960s. The original procedure consisted of an undivided gastric pouch (stapled, not divided) attached to a loop of jejunum creating both malabsorptive and restrictive components. Over the years, several important modifications have taken place; instead of a loop of jejunum, a Roux limb of jejunum is brought to the gastric pouch, and the intestine is reconfigured to resemble a Y with the two proximal limbs joining to form a common channel (figure 11.2). This configuration, though technically more challenging, eliminates the reflux of bile and other digestives enzymes into the esophagus that was problematic with the original gastric bypass operation. Additionally, a smaller gastric pouch (30cc) is utilized and is completely divided, not merely stapled, from the remainder of the stomach. This eliminates the gastro-gastric fistula that often resulted with a non-divided pouch. Another advantage of the RYGB is that it involves much less malabsorption than the JIB. The degree of malabsorption is determined by the length of the Roux limb; typically 75–150cm. These modifications have resulted in the most effective operation for sustained weight loss. Today, the term *gastric bypass* refers to this Roux-en-Y configuration and is currently the most commonly performed

Figure 11.2
Roux-en-Y Gastric Bypass

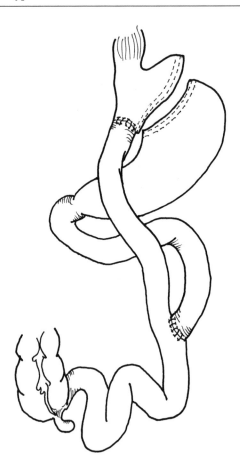

bariatric procedure in the United States and the world (Buchwald, 2005). The RYGB is considered by many, the gold standard of weight loss operations.

In another effort to eliminate the complications associated with the earlier malabsorptive procedures, operations that were purely restrictive, that is, there was no element of malabsorption, were also developed. The gastroplasty, and other purely restrictive procedures were developed in the 1970s. Gastroplasty, often referred to as stomach stapling, involves reducing the gastric reservoir to a small proximal pouch by the placement of a staple line (figure 11.3). This pouch communicates with the remainder of

Figure 11.3
Gastroplasty

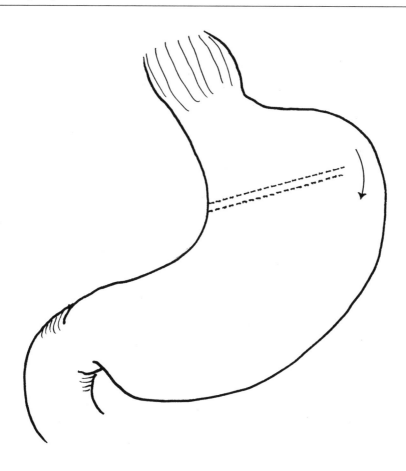

the stomach via a small channel (figure 11.3, arrow). The small pouch and narrow passage would cause early satiety resulting in weight loss without malabsorption.

Though there were many variations, most gastroplasty procedures involved the simple placement of a horizontal staple line in the proximal stomach. These operations were technically much easier to perform, as they require none of the intestinal re-routing of the malabsorptive operations. Because of their technical ease, many were performed by poorly trained surgeons or general practitioners that did not adequately follow long term outcomes (Kelly, Sarr, & Hinder, 2004). We now know that many failed, in part, as a result of the stomach's tendency to stretch, thus enlarging the pouch and widening the conduit between the pouch and the remainder of the stomach. In an attempt to minimize the dilation of this passage, several attempts to band the gastroplasty were developed in the 1980s.

Most banded gastroplasties used a vertical staple line and a synthetic, non-expandable material such as silicone, silastic, or polypropylene to constrict the outlet from the pouch to the remainder of the stomach. The most famous of these is the vertical banded gastroplasty (VBG) also developed by Dr. Mason (figure 11.4). Early results were promising; however long-term failure of the VBG to provide sustained weight loss did occur. One reason for the failed long-term success of any gastroplasty is the disruption of the staple line, thus eliminating the small pouch volume and subsequent early satiety. Additionally, patients found they could ingest

Figure 11.4
Vertical Banded Gastroplasty

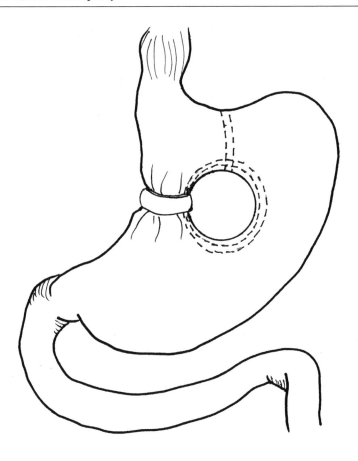

semi-solid, high caloric foods, such as milkshakes, and not experience the unpleasant pain or vomiting that resulted with the overeating of solid foods.

The latest, and least invasive, of the purely restrictive operations is gastric banding. Developed in the 1980s, this procedure involved the placement of a non-adjustable band around the proximal stomach to form a small pouch with a small opening from the pouch to the remainder of the stomach. The stomach is not transected or stapled in any way nor is there any intestinal resection or re-routing. Some years later the band was modified with an adjustable silicone band that is connected to a port placed below the skin. The port is accessed percutaneously via a special needle through which fluid is either injected or removed to change the tension of the adjustable band (figure 11.5). Currently, the devise is

Figure 11.5
Adjustable Gastric Band

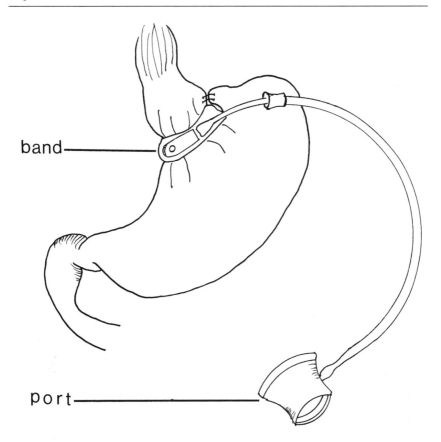

placed almost exclusively via a laparoscopic approach and is referred to as laparoscopic adjustable gastric band (LAGB). The only band approved by the Food and Drug Administration for use in the United States is the LAP BAND system (INAMED Health, Santa Barbara, CA; U.S. Food and Drug Administration, n.d.). Since being approved for use in 2001, it fast became the most common purely restrictive procedure done in the United States and is the most common bariatric procedure performed outside the United States. The LAGB requires multiple adjustments by a trained professional in an outpatient setting. One advantage of the band is that it can be adjusted to minimize undesirable symptoms and maximize weight loss. It also has the advantage to be loosened during pregnancy (Dixon, Dixon, & O'Brien, 2001). Unlike other bariatric procedures, if it becomes necessary, the band can be removed.

The RYGB and the LAGB are by far the two most commonly performed weight-loss operations performed in the United States and world wide. We will limit further discussion to these two procedures.

OPEN AND LAPAROSCOPIC APPROACHES

Both RYGB and the adjustable band surgeries were initially done via a open approach; that is, through a large incision. More recently, the RYGB and the adjustable band have been performed laparoscopically with increasing frequency. In the laparoscopic approach, the operation is performed via multiple small incisions with specially designed instruments and a camera that projects the images of the operation on a video monitor that is viewed by the operative team. The advantages of this approach include less pain, faster recovery period, reduced wound complications, reduced scaring, and shorter hospital stays. Additionally, it eliminates the common complication of large incisional hernias often seen with the open approach.

PRE-OPERATIVE CARE AND PATIENT SELECTION

The National Institutes of Health (NIH, 1991) outlined guidelines for patients considering bariatric surgery. A weight criterion was established using body mass index (BMI). BMI is calculated as a patients weight in kilograms divided by the square of height in meters. Patients with a BMI 40 or greater are considered morbidly obese and are potential candidates for surgery. In some instances patients with a BMI between 35 and 40 may be considered for surgery if they have high-risk, comorbid conditions such as life-threatening cardiopulmonary problems, severe diabetes, or obesity-induced physical limitations interfering with lifestyle.

Patients must be carefully evaluated and followed on an individual basis. This is best done by a multidisciplinary team that should include a surgeon, nurse or nurse practitioner, dietician, office staff, and other specialists as needed. A patient-friendly atmosphere is important in the care of obese patients and should include amenities such easy access to handicap parking, armless chairs, high capacity scales placed in areas that assure privacy, and oversized equipment such as gowns, furniture, and blood pressure cuffs (Collazo-Clavel, Clark, McAlpine, & Jensen, 2006). The multidisciplinary team should try and create an environment of compassion and respect for patients who so often have faced social stigmatization and discrimination because of their weight.

Patients undergo psychological evaluation and are also seen by an internist who specializes in obesity. Inappropriately treated mental illness such as substance abuse, active eating disorders, and some personality disorders may adversely affect postoperative results.

Surgery should only be considered in well-informed patients who are motivated, able to understand and accept the operative risks, and are able to participate in treatment and long-term follow-up. There are few absolute contraindications to bariatric surgery other than the patient being unable to have the cognitive ability to understand the operation and its inherent risks. Additionally, the patient's overall medical condition cannot be so unstable that it renders the risk of surgery unacceptable.

Patients should be instructed that even though they may meet the requirements for surgery, third-party payers often insist on additional requirements before authorizing coverage. Usually one or more documented, medically supervised weight loss attempts are required. These requirements can be extremely varied depending on the third-party payer and is worthy of note. Patients are often very frustrated when they may be required to undergo months of additional medically supervised weight loss attempts while other patients are not. This can results in two patients that start their bariatric surgery evaluation at the same time, but because of different third-party payers, undergo their operation many months apart. Both the patient and medical team should be well informed regarding the criteria that need to be fulfilled before planning surgery. Interestingly, recent work demonstrates that insurance-mandated preoperative dietary counseling, though mandated by many third-party payers, was an obstacle to patient access for surgery and had no impact on weight loss outcome or post-surgical compliance (Buchwald, 2005, Jamal et al., 2006).

Special Considerations of Patient Selection
Pediatric Patients

Though covered in more detail in other chapters, it deserves repeating that pediatric obesity, as in the adult population, has reached epidemic proportions. In fact, childhood obesity has tripled in the past 30 years (Schwimmer, Burwinkle, & Varni, 2003). We know that 50–77 percent of obese children will be obese in adulthood; this number increases if just one parent is also obese (Freedman, Khan, Dietz, Srinivasan, & Berenson, 2001; Guo et al., 2000; Parson, Power, Logan, & Summerbell, 1999; Serdula et al., 1993; Whitaker, Wright, Pepe, Seidel, & Dietz, 1997). Bariatric surgery has been performed in morbidly obese adolescents for over 10 years, yet to some it remains controversial. One of the biggest hurdles in overcoming this controversy is the lack of large studies pertaining to the pediatric population. There are, however, a number of smaller studies that demonstrate considerable improvement or complete resolution of weight-related comorbidities in adolescents who have undergone bariatric operations. Although the results of these studies are similar to that of adult studies, the long-term consequences on such a young population are unknown (Dolan, Creighton, Hopkins, & Fielding, 2003; Horgan et al., 2005; Inge et al., 2004; Rand & MacGregor, 1994; Widhalm, Dietrich, & Prager, 2004).

Also complicating the issue has been the lack of criteria for selection of operative candidates in the pediatric population. To simply adopt adult guidelines would not take in to account the unique needs of the adolescent population. Additionally, behavior therapy to weight loss is more effective in children and adolescents than adults (Epstein, Valoski, Wing, & McCurley, 1990). To help clarify this issue, a group of surgeons and pediatricians specializing in obese children met in 2004 and developed a set of criteria for adolescent bariatric surgery (Inge et al., 2004). They are:

1. Have failed ≥ 6 months of organized attempts at weight management, as determined by their primary care provider
2. Have attained or nearly attained physiologic maturity
3. Be very severely obese (BMI ≥ 40) with serious obesity-related comorbidities or have a BMI of ≥ 50 with less severe comorbidities
4. Demonstrate commitment to comprehensive medical and psychological evaluations both before and after surgery
5. Agree to avoid pregnancy for at least one year postoperatively
6. Be capable of and willing to adhere to nutritional guidelines postoperatively

7. Provide informed assent to surgical treatment
8. Demonstrate decisional capacity
9. Have a supportive family environment

This same group also concluded that adolescent bariatric surgery should only be performed at facilities capable of treating adolescents with complications of severe obesity and where detailed clinical data collection can occur.

Elderly

Although here have been studies that demonstrate the safety of performing bariatric surgery in older patients (Macgregor & Rand, 1993; Murr, Siadati, & Sarr, 1995; Sugerman et al., 2004), other authors argue to the contrary (Livingston, et al., 2002; Mason, Renquist, & Jiang, 1992; Printen & Mason, 1977). Similar to the pediatric population, the reason for the controversy is likely due to the limited studies of older patients. A recent retrospective analysis of over 25,000 bariatric procedures determined that age was an independent risk factor for undesirable results (Livingston & Langert, 2006). Adverse events increased after age 60 years and sharply again after age 65 years. In patients over 65 years, adverse events exceeded 20 percent and mortality was as high as 3.2 percent. The authors conclude that bariatric procedures should be limited to patients younger than 65 years. In our practice we generally limit our patents to younger than 60 years but will very selectively perform surgery on healthy patients between 60 and 65 years.

Pregnancy

Women who have failed to become pregnant prior to bariatric surgery should be advised that fertility may increase with subsequent weight loss. The ASBS (2007) recommends that women of childbearing age who undergo bariatric surgery obtain birth control during times of rapid weight loss as it is feared that maternal malnutrition may lead to impaired fetal development. There has, however, been recent evidence to suggest that outcomes of pregnancy that occur within the first year after weight-loss surgery suffer no significant adverse outcomes or complications (Dao, Kuhn, Ehmer, Fisher, & McCarty, 2006). In our practice, we continue to advise women not to conceive within the first year after surgery as the effects on maternal health are not completely understood nor are the long-term effects on the child.

PERIOPERATIVE CARE

Not only is there a need for a skilled bariatric surgeon to perform the operation and assure adequate coverage, the hospital must also be committed to serving the bariatric patient as well. The anesthesia team must have the skills to deal with the unique demands of the morbidly obese. The operating rooms need to be equipped with the requisite equipment including high capacity operating tables, bariatric retractors, and a variety of specialized surgical instruments. Once the patient is brought to a room there will be demands for larger beds, chairs, wheelchairs, commodes, and specialized lifts to assist in moving the patient. Additionally, the radiology department must be able to perform adequate diagnostic studies. Pre-written orders and protocols can help assure continuity, assist nursing staff, and help assure that nothing is overlooked. Prior to discharge, we have the patient meet again with a dietician to review the dietary instructions and answer any questions though this information is reviewed in great detail well before the day of surgery.

POST-OPERATIVE CARE

Multidisciplinary, lifetime follow-up is recommended for the bariatric patient. In the first year following surgery, at least three visits with the bariatric surgeon is recommended. After the first year, annual visits are recommended. Because of the profound changes in digestive physiology after malabsorptive operations, nutritional deficiencies are common and it is essential that patients are followed by a medical professional that will monitor for any of these deficiencies (Xanthakos & Inge, 2006). The most frequent deficits are protein, iron, calcium, vitamin B12, and vitamin D. Multidisciplinary follow-up will ensure prevention with appropriate vitamin supplementation and treatment of these complications should they be detected (Poitou Bernet, et al., 2007).

Medically supervised support groups should be available and highly recommended to patients. Participation was found to be an important adjunct for patients to achieve and maintain improved weight loss (Elakkary, Elhorr, Aziz, Gazayerli, & Silva, 2006; Marcus & Elkins, 2004).

OUTCOMES

Weight

The long term effectiveness of the RYGB to facilitate sustained weight loss and reduce comorbidities with minimal complications is well established. Excess weight loss is generally rapid and plateaus after one to two years. The amount of weight lost may vary with the length of the Roux limb. A Roux limb fashioned to a length of 75–150 cm in morbidly obese patients results in a loss of 65–70 percent of excess body weight after the first year (Buchwald, 2005). More importantly, weight loss is sustained. In super obese patients (BMI>50) it has been found that a longer Roux limb may be more effective (Choban & Flancbaum, 2002)

Weight loss following LAGB is more varied than with RYGB. Earlier studies demonstrated inferior weight loss compared to the other surgical options. One proposed reason was because of the lack of band adjustment guidelines and the subsequent variety of band adjustment strategies (Jones et al., 2004). Another reason for the discrepancy is likely due to the fact that weight loss following LAGB is more gradual when compared to RYGB; maximal weight loss does not occur until two to three years (Kendrick & Dakin, 2006). Thus, more recent studies, with longer follow-up periods, do indeed report weight loss results similar to that of the RYGB (Jan, Hong, Pereira, & Patterson, 2005).

With better studies and improved techniques, results may become comparable with that of RYGB, but one must exercise caution when predicting long term results of LAGB as long-term studies are lacking (Kendrick & Dakin, 2006; O'Brien & Dixon, 2003).

Resolution of Comorbid Conditions

Numerous studies have documented the improvement or complete resolution of comorbid conditions following bariatric surgery (MacLean, Rhode, Sampalis, & Forse, 1993; Moreno et al., 1998; Mun, Blackburn & Matthews, 2001; Sjöström et al., 2004; Suter, Jayet, & Jayet, 2000). Two studies deserve specific mention. The first, is a large meta-analysis of bariatric patients by Buchwald, et al. (2004). The authors found that in 84 percent of diabetic patients that had RYGB, the diabetes resolved. Hyperlipidemia, hypercholesterolemia, and hypertriglyceridemia also improved in 94, 95, and 94 percent of patients respectively. Hypertension and obstructive sleep apnea resolved or improved in the vast majority of patients as well. The same study found that diabetes resolved in 48 percent of gastric banding patients, and hyperlipidemia, hypercholesterolemia, and hypertriglyceridemia improved in 71, 78, and 77 percent respectively. Hypertension and obstructive sleep apnea also resolved or improved in the majority of patients.

The second study, the Swedish obese subjects trial (SOS), is a well-controlled, prospective study of over 4,000 obese patients that were followed over 10 years (Sjöström, et al., 2004). Half of these patients underwent bariatric surgery and half did not. Results were similar to the Buchwald study; in addition to considerable weight loss, the surgical group also demonstrated significant improvement of comorbidities and an 80 percent decrease in annual mortality when compared to the non-surgical group.

OPERATIVE MORTALITY AND COMPLICATIONS

Operative mortality is defined as mortality at or less than 30 days form the time of surgery. Buchwald et al. (2004) found the operative mortality for gastric bypass, gastric banding, and the purely malabsorptive procedures to be 0.5 percent, 0.1 percent and 1.1 percent respectively.

Interestingly, there is solid data to suggest that postoperative complications are directly related to the experience of the surgeon and hospital volume (Courcoulas, Schuchert, Gatti, & Luketich, 2003; Nguyen et al., 2004; Weller & Hannan, 2006). Risks appear to be lowest when the operation is done by a high volume surgeon at a high volume hospital. Other risk factors that increase adverse events include male gender, and advanced age.

RYGB

Operative complications occur in approximately 5 percent of patients who undergo RYGB and typically include pulmonary embolism, anastomotic leak, bleeding, and wound complications. Compared to the open approach, laparoscopic RYGB have a higher rate of abdominal complications but a shorter length of stay, fewer wound complications, and less pain (Buchwald, 2005).

Long-term complications of RYGB include dumping syndrome, stomal stenosis, marginal ulcers, staple line disruption, and internal and incisional hernias. Incisional hernia rates as high as 39 percent have been reported for cases that are done with an open technique and clearly demonstrate one advantage to the laparoscopic approach. In the same study, the incidence of incisional hernias following laparoscopic RYGB was reported at only 5 percent (Puzziferri et al., 2006). Vitamin and mineral deficiencies can also occur if they are not properly supplemented for the remainder of the patient's life.

Operative revision of RYGB because of complications or failed weight loss is far less likely than with the other surgical options. Although reversing a RYGB is possible, it is rarely done and patients should be counseled that this procedure is non-reversible.

LAGB

Operative complication rates of the LAGB, like the RYGB, are approximately 5 percent. The most common long-term complication is band slippage, or in other words, the herniation of the proximal stomach through the band. Band slippage results in a larger pouch and possible obstruction. Other long-term complications of LAGB include obstruction, proximal dilatation of the esophagus and gastric pouch, erosion, gastric necrosis, perforation, problems related to port access, and infection. In one study of 36 patients with LAGB, 18 (50%) had to be removed for failed weight loss with or without complications and converted to another weight loss operation (Kothari et al., 2002).

There are, however, advantages of the LAGB. Not only is it technically easier to perform than the RYGB but it has the lowest mortality rate of any bariatric procedure. Additional advantages include: shorter operative time, less blood loss, shorter hospital stay, adjustability, and essentially no risk of nutritional deficiency. As previously mentioned, the LAGB can be removed if necessary, and another weight loss procedure can be done should the LAGB technique yield unsatisfactory results.

Although the potential removal of the band is indeed a unique advantage to LAGB, patients should be advised to think of LAGB as a permanent operation as weight will be regained in the event of its removal. Additionally, it seems reasonable to assume a permanent commitment to long term weight loss is likely to be more effective than a temporary one.

CONCLUSION

Non-surgical approaches to sustained weight loss are relatively ineffective in treating obesity. Surgical treatment is the most effective method for achieving sustained weight loss. Although bariatric operations were developed over 50 years ago, there has been a dramatic increase in their frequency over the past decade. Bariatric procedures are major operations that are either restrictive, malabsorptive, or a combination of the two. Eating behavior improves dramatically after the surgery.

Defined guidelines for patient selection are well established, and once met, there are few contraindications to bariatric surgery. Surgery should only be considered in well-informed, motivated patients, who are able to understand and accept the risks and participate in lifetime follow-up. There are few data on the effects of bariatric surgery at the extremes of age, thus bariatric surgery for adolescents and older patients remains controversial.

The RYGB and the LAGB are by far the two most commonly performed weight-loss operations performed in the United States and world wide. Both can be done with minimal risk by a properly experienced surgeon in an appropriate facility. Each operation has unique advantages and disadvantages but the RYGB has clearly withstood the test of time. Both can safely be done via a laparoscopic approach which results in less pain, shorter hospital stays, and fewer incisional hernias. RYGB is currently the most commonly performed bariatric procedure in the United States and is considered by many, the gold standard of weight loss operations.

The comorbidities associated with obesity (diabetes, hyperlipidemia, hypertension, and obstructive sleep apnea) completely resolve or greatly improve following the weight loss resulting from surgery. It follows that quality of life and life expectancy should significantly improve as well.

REFERENCES

American Society for Bariatric Surgery. *Questions*. Retrieved April, 2007, from http://www.asbs.org.

Buchwald, H. (2005). Consensus Conference Statement. Bariatric surgery for morbid obesity: Health implications for patients, health professionals, and third-party payers. *Journal of the American College of Surgeons, 200*, 593–604.

Buchwald, H., Avidor, Y., Braunwald, E., Jensen, M. D., Pories, W. Fahrbach, K., et al. (2004). Bariatric surgery: A systematic review and meta-analysis. *Journal of the American Medical Association, 292*(14), 1724–1737.

Choban, P. S., & Flancbaum L. (2002). The effect of Roux limb lengths on outcome after Roux-en-Y gastric bypass: A prospective, randomized clinical trial. *Obesity Surgery, 12*(4), 540–545.

Collazo-Clavel, M. L., Clark, M. M., McAlpine, D. E., & Jensen, M. D. (2006). Assessment and preparation of patients for Bariatric surgery. *Mayo Clinic Proceedings, 81*(10 Suppl.), S11–S17.

Courcoulas, A., Schuchert, M., Gatti, G., & Luketich, J. (2003). The relationship of surgeon and hospital volume to outcome after gastric bypass surgery in Pennsylvania: A 3 year summary. *Surgery, 134*, 613–621.

Dao, T., Kuhn, J., Ehmer D., Fisher T., & McCarty, T. (2006). Pregnancy outcomes after gastric-bypass surgery. *American Journal of Surgery, 192*(6), 762–766.

Dixon, J. B., Dixon, M. E., & O'Brien, P. E. (2001). Pregnancy after Lap-Band surgery: Management of the band to achieve healthy weight outcomes. *Obesity Surgery, 11*(1), 59–65.

Dolan, K., Creighton, L., Hopkins, G., & Fielding, G. (2003). Laparoscopic gastric banding in morbidly obese adolescents. *Obesity Surgery, 13*, 101–104.

Elakkary, E., Elhorr, A., Aziz, F., Gazayerli, M. M., & Silva, Y. J. (2006). Do support groups play a role in weight loss after laparoscopic adjustable gastric banding? *Obesity Surgery, 16*(3), 331–334.

Epstein, L. H., Valoski, A., Wing, R. R., & McCurley, J. (1990). Ten-year follow-up of behavioral, family-based treatment for obese children. *Journal of the American Medical Association, 264*, 2519–2523.

Freedman, D. S., Khan, L. K., Dietz, W. H., Srinivasan, S. R., & Berenson, G. S. (2001). Relationship of childhood obesity to coronary heart disease risk factors in adulthood: The Bogalusa Heart Study. *Pediatrics, 108*, 712 –718.

Guo, S. S., Huang, C., Maynard, L. M., Demerath, E., Towne B., Chumlea, W. C., et al. (2000). Body mass index during childhood, adolescence and young adulthood in relation to adult overweight and adiposity: The Fels Longitudinal Study. *International Journal of Obesity Related Metabolic Disorders, 24*, 1628–1635.

Horgan, S., Holterman, M. J., Jacobsen, G. R., Browne A. F., Berger, R. A., Moser, F., et al. (2005). Laparoscopic adjustable gastric banding for the treatment of adolescent morbid obesity in the United States: A safe alternative to gastric bypass. *Journal of Pediatric Surgery, 40*, 86–91.

Inge, T. H., Krebs, N. F., Garcia, V. F., Skelton, J. A., Guice, K. S., Strauss, R. S., et al. (2004). Bariatric surgery for severely overweight adolescents: concerns and recommendations. *Pediatrics, 114*, 217–223.

Jamal, M. K., DeMaria, E. J., Johnson, J. M., Carmody, B. J., Wolfe, L. G., Kellum, J. M., et al. (2006). Insurance-mandated preoperative dietary counseling does not improve outcome and increases dropout rates in patients considering gastric bypass surgery for morbid obesity. *Surgery for Obesity and Related Diseases, 2*, 122–127.

Jan, J. C., Hong, D., Pereira, N., & Patterson, E. J. (2005). Laparoscopic adjustable gastric banding versus laparoscopic gastric bypass for morbid obesity: A single-institution comparison study of early results. *Journal of Gastrointestinal Surgery, 9*(1), 30–39.

Joffe, S. N. (1981). Surgical management of morbid obesity. *Gut, 22,* 242.

Jones, D. B., Provost, D. A., DeMaria, E. J., Smith, C. D., Morgenstern, L., & Schirmer, B. (2004). Optimal management of the morbidly obese patient. SAGES appropriateness conference statement. *Surgical Endoscopy, 18*(7), 1029–1037.

Kelly, K. A., Sarr, M. G., & Hinder, R. A. (2004). *Mayo Clinic Gastrointestinal Surgery.* Philadelphia: Elsevier Science Health Science.

Kendrick, M. L., & Dakin, G. F. (2006). Surgical approaches to obesity. *Mayo Clinic Proceedings, 81*(10 Suppl.), S18–24.

Kothari, S. N., DeMaria, E. J., Sugerman, H. J., Kellum, J. M., Meador, J., & Wolfe ,L. (2002). Lap-band failures: Conversion to gastric bypass and their preliminary outcomes. *Surgery, 131*(6), 625–629.

Kremen, A. J., Linner, J. H., & Nelson, C. H. (1954). An experimental evaluation of the nutritional importance of proximal and distal small intestine. *Annals of Surgery, 140,* 439–448.

Kushner, R. F., & Noble, C. A. (2006). Long-term outcome of bariatric surgery: An interim analysis. *Mayo Clinic Proceedings, 81* (Suppl.), S46–51.

Livingston, E. H., Huerta, S., Arthur, D., Lee, S., De Shields, S., & Heber, D. (2002). Male gender is a predictor of morbidity and age a predictor of mortality for patients undergoing gastric bypass surgery. *Annals of Surgery, 236,* 576–582.

Livingston, E. H., & Langert, J. (2006). The impact of age and Medicare status on bariatric surgical outcomes. *Archives of Surgery, 141*(11), 1115–1121.

Macgregor, A. M., & Rand, C. S. (1993). Gastric surgery in morbid obesity: Outcome in patients aged 55 years and older. *Archives of Surgery, 128,* 1153–1157.

MacLean, L. D., Rhode, B. M., Sampalis, J., & Forse, R. A. (1993). Results of the surgical treatment of obesity. *American Journal of Surgery, 165*(1), 155–160.

Marcus, J. D., & Elkins, G. R. (2004). Development of a model for a structured support group for patients following bariatric surgery. *Obesity Surgery, 14*(1), 103–106.

Mason, E. E., Renquist, K. E., & Jiang, D. (1992). Perioperative risks and safety of surgery for severe obesity. *American Journal of Clinical Nutrition, 55*(Suppl.), 573S–576S.

Moreno, P., Alastrué, A., Rull, M., Formiguera, X., Casas, D., Boix, J., et al. (1998). Band erosion in patients who have undergone vertical banded gastroplasty: Incidence and technical solutions. *Archives of Surgery, 133*(2), 189–193.

Mun, E. C., Blackburn, G. L., & Matthews, J. B. (2001). Current status of medical and surgical therapy for obesity. *Gastroenterology, 120*(3), 669–681.

Murr, M. M., Siadati, M. R., & Sarr, M. G. (1995) . Results of bariatric surgery for morbid obesity in patients older than 50 years. *Obesity Surgery, 5,* 399–402.

National Institutes of Health. (1991). Gastrointestinal surgery for severe obesity. *NIH Consensus Statement, 9*(1), 1–20.

National Institutes of Health (1992). Gastrointestinal surgery for severe obesity: National Institutes of Health Consensus Development Conference Statement. *American Journal of Clinical Nutrition, 55*(2 Suppl.), 615S–619S.

Nguyen, N. T., Paya, M., Stevens, C. M., Mayandadi, S., Zainabadi, K., & Wilson, S. E. (2004). The relationship between hospital volume and outcome in bariatric surgery at academic medical centers. *Annals of Surgery, 240,* 586–593.

North American Association for the Study of Obesity (NAASO) and the National Heart, Lung, and Blood Institute (1998). *Clinical guidelines on the identification, evaluation, and treatment of overweight and obesity in adults: The evidence report.* (NIH publication 98–4083). Bethesda, MD: National Institutes of Health.

North American Association for the Study of Obesity (NAASO) and the National Heart, Lung, and Blood Institute (2000). *The practical guide: Identification, evaluation, and treatment of overweight and obesity in adults* (NIH publication 00–4084). Bethesda, MD: National Institutes of Health.

O'Brien, P. E., & Dixon, J. B. (2003). Lap-band: Outcomes and results. *Journal of Laparoendoscopic Advanced Surgical Techniques A, 13*(4), 265–270.

Parsons, T. J., Power, C., Logan, S., & Summerbell, C. D. (1999). Childhood predictors of adult obesity: A systematic review. *International Journal of Obesity Related Metabolic Disorders, 23*(Suppl. 8), S1–S107.

Poitou Bernet, C., Ciangura, C., Coupaye, M., Czernichow, S., Bouillot, J. L., & Basdevant, A. (2007). Nutritional deficiency after gastric bypass: Diagnosis, prevention and treatment. *Diabetes Metabolism, 33*(1), 13–24.

Printen, K. J., & Mason, E. E. (1997). Gastric bypass for morbid obesity in patients more than fifty years of age. *Surgery in Gynecology and Obstetrics, 144*, 192–194.

Puzziferri, N., Iselin, T., Austrheim-Smith, B. S, Wolfe, B. M., Wilson, S. E., & Nguyen, N. T. (2006). Three-year follow-up of a prospective randomized trial comparing laparoscopic versus open gastric bypass. *Annals of Surgery, 243*(2), 181–188.

Rand, C. S., & MacGregor, A. M. (1994). Adolescents having obesity surgery: A 6-year follow-up. *South Medicine Journal, 87*, 1208–1213.

Schwimmer, J. B., Burwinkle, T. M., & Varni, J. W. (2003). Health-related quality of life of severely obese children and adolescents. *Journal of the American Medical Association, 289*, 1813–1819.

Serdula, M. K., Ivery, D., Coates, R. J., Freedman, D. S., Williamson, D. F., & Byers, T. (1993). Do obese children become obese adults? A review of the literature. *Previews of Medicine. 22*, 167–177.

Sjöström, L., Lindroos, A. K., Peltonen, M., Torgerson, J., Bouchard, C., Carlsson, B., et al. (2004). The Swedish obese subjects study scientific group. Lifestyle, diabetes, and cardiovascular risk factors 10 years after bariatric surgery. *New England Journal of Medicine,351*, 2683–2693.

Sugerman, H. J., DeMaria, E. J., Kellum, J. M., Sugerman, E. L., Meador, J. G., & Wolfe, L. G. (2004). Effects of bariatric surgery in older patients. *Annals of Surgery, 240*, 243–247.

Suter, M., Jayet, C., & Jayet, A. (2000). Vertical banded gastroplasty: Long-term results comparing three different techniques. *Obesity Surgery, 10*(1), 41–46.

Thirlby, R. C. (1990). Jejunoileal bypass: Can the mistake be corrected? *Gastroenterology, 98*, 1710–1711.

U.S. Food and Drug Administration, Center for Devices and Radiological Health. LAP-BAND Adjustable Gastric Banding (LAGB) System-P000008. Available at http://www.fda.gov/cdrh/pdf/p000008.html.

Weller, W. E., & Hannan, E. L. (2006). Relationship between provider volume and postoperative complications for bariatric procedures in New York State. *Journal of the American College of Surgery, 202*, 753–761.

Whitaker, R. C., Wright, J. A., Pepe, M. S., Seidel, K. D., & Dietz, W. H. (1997). Predicting obesity in young adulthood from childhood and parental obesity. *New England Journal of Medicine, 337,* 869–873.

Widhalm K., Dietrich S., & Prager G. (2004). Adjustable gastric banding surgery in morbidly obese adolescents: Experiences with eight patients. *International Journal of Obesity Related Metabolic Disorders, 28*(Suppl. 3), S42–S45.

Xanthakos, S. A., & Inge, T. H. (2006). Nutritional consequences of bariatric surgery. *Current Opinion on Clinical Nutrition and Metabolic Care, 9*(4), 489–496.

Chapter 12

ETHICAL CONSIDERATIONS RELATED TO OBESITY INTERVENTION

Leonard M. Fleck and Karen A. Petersmarck

WHY LOOK AT ETHICS?

High Stakes

Obesity[1] in American is a high stakes issue that evokes extreme emotion—for individuals who struggle to achieve lower weight, and for the multitudes of health care and government professionals charged with helping them. The Surgeon General of the United States has described obesity as "the terror within, a threat that is every bit as real to America as the weapons of mass destruction" (Carmona, 2003). Roughly 85 million adults are trying to lose weight, and 45.6 percent of high school students are trying to lose weight (Bish et al., 2005; Centers for Disease Control and Prevention, 2006). A $46 billion dollar weight loss industry has sprung up, providing products and services ranging from diet soda to bariatric surgery (Marketdata Enterprises, 2005). Many jobs and much wealth depend on this industry. For example, hospitals all over the country are creating and advertising profitable obesity surgery facilities (Curtland, 2005). Adults classified as obese have been found to have 36 percent higher medical costs than those classified as having healthy weight (Sturm, 2002). One estimate of annual U.S. obesity-attributable medical expenditures was $75 billion in 2003 dollars, with approximately one-half of these expenditures being financed by Medicare and Medicaid (Finkelstein, Fiebelkorn, & Wang, 2004).

Disagreement

There is tremendous disagreement among people of intelligence and good will—not only as to what should be done about obesity, but also as to what the actual nature of the problem is (Saguy & Riley, 2005). There is significant potential for harming individuals and also for wasting of scarce public resources if inappropriate choices are made. With so much at stake, careful consideration of ethical issues surrounding weight loss treatment is timely.

OVERVIEW OF RELEVANT PERSONAL AND PROFESSIONAL MORAL PRINCIPLES

Principle: Patient Right to Autonomy/Personal Responsibility

How might we initially identify the relevant moral issues? One common moral principle in contemporary medical ethics is respect for patient autonomy (Beauchamp & Childress, 2004). Patients have the right to make decisions about their own medical care (or refusal) in the light of their own goals and values (as opposed to some idealized set of health goals and values endorsed by the medical profession). This includes the right (ultimately) to refuse life-sustaining medical care so long as that patient is competent to make such a choice. One implication of this principle is that patients have the right to be overweight so long as they have chosen this as free and informed persons. So physicians have the professional right to call attention to the medical risks of being overweight and to try to persuade patients to make weight reduction choices, but physicians may not use their professional authority to manipulate or coerce patients into accepting medical interventions aimed at weight loss.

Still, rights are typically paired with responsibilities; and one way of framing the relevant moral issue is to say that individuals who are overweight are morally irresponsible. However, that judgment itself might be a little too quick and morally irresponsible. At least two assumptions would have to be validated for that judgment to be morally justified. One assumption is that being overweight represents a significant increase in risk of harm to self. As we shall see below, however, a large body of medical literature would question the correctness of that assumption, at least in the case of individuals who are not morbidly obese. Another assumption is that individuals are overweight primarily as a result of voluntary choices they have made. Again, substantial medical literature suggests that a number of factors beyond an individual's control may be responsible for determining an individual's normal weight. If this is true (even if only for some percentage of individuals), then judgments of irresponsibility regarding weight management will have to be made with much greater care. What should be noted here is a comparable phenomenon where individuals have been accused of choosing to be gay, when the best medical evidence now would say that sexual orientation is not a matter of voluntary choice at all.

Principle: Do No Harm

Another principle at the core of contemporary health care ethics is the harm principle. This is usually taken to mean that physicians (and other heath professionals) should always seek to offer medical options that are in the best interests of their patients, or, at the very least, offer options that will not harm patients. This principle is very often in danger of being violated in the context of experimental medicine where physicians might be motivated to put their patients at excessive risk for the sake of advancing medical knowledge. However, the harm principle can also be violated in the practice of normal medicine. *In the case of weight loss care, harm can come to a patient in a number of ways* (for further discussion, refer to section "Principle 2: Harm in Weight Loss Treatment").

OVERVIEW OF RELEVANT SOCIAL JUSTICE ISSUES

The ethics issues identified thus far might be regarded as personal and professional ethics issues. There are ethics issues at the social level as well. Most often those are characterized as a matter of justice. There are two major ones that we will identify now and discuss at length later in this essay.

Issue: Unfair Costs to Society

One is the claim that obese individuals have excess health problems (heart disease, diabetes, joint problems, renal failure, etc.) that impose very substantial health costs on the rest of society in the form of either higher insurance premiums or higher taxes for Medicare and Medicaid. In either case, the ethical claim is that this represents an unfair shifting of this cost burden to others who have been more conscientious about caring for their health, and consequently, should not have to bear these excess costs.

Issue: Rationing of Scarce Resources

The other justice issue pertains to the rationing and prioritization problem. In brief, it is widely accepted that we cannot escape the need for health care rationing, that we have only limited social resources for a virtually limitless domain of health care needs (Fleck, 2002; Ubel, 2000; Callahan, 1990). So the question we need to address is what the metric of justice ought to be for determining which health needs get very high priority and which health needs get relatively lower priority. More specifically, how high a priority ought to be given to various weight reduction and weight management interventions? Should Medicare and Medicaid cover these interventions (the whole spectrum from bariatric surgery to dietary supplements)? Or should these interventions be available to individuals entirely on the basis of individual ability to pay? Would it be unjust if the obese wealthy could have unlimited access to all these weight loss interventions while the obese poor had virtually no access to these interventions?

THE SOCIAL CONTEXT OF WEIGHT LOSS TREATMENT

Any consideration of ethics and weight loss must begin with recognition of the social context in which weight loss care occurs. It is quite a peculiarity of American culture that being overweight—a situation in which the majority of adults find themselves—is considered socially unacceptable. At the same time that the shape of the average American is rounding out, the cultural ideal for body shape remains one of extreme slenderness—a shape that most normal adults are not genetically capable of achieving. This is especially true for women, for whose bodies the cultural ideal is "barely distinguishable from the bodies of women with full-blown anorexia nervosa" (Campos, 2005). Those who fail to attain a socially acceptable body shape are often stigmatized.

Puhl and Brownell (2001) documented a clear and consistent scientific literature showing pervasive stigmatization, and in some cases discrimination in employment, education, and health care. Negative attitudes toward obesity run very deep in our culture. As one advocate puts it, "In our time, for women especially, being called fat has eclipsed being called a slut as a major vehicle for put-downs" (Burgard, 2005). It is extremely telling that in one survey, 11 percent of parents agreed that they would consider aborting a child predisposed to fatness (Cowley, 1990).

The social stigma associated with obesity leads many to embrace risky procedures and regimens to control weight. The national 2005 Youth Risk Behavior Survey, has documented dangerous, disordered weight loss practices among high school students of all grades, all ethnicities, and both genders: 12.3 percent of high school students reported going without eating for 24 hours or more, and 4.5 percent admitted to vomiting or taking laxatives to control weight. The figures are higher for female students (17% and 6.2% respectively; Centers for Disease Control and Prevention, 2006).

In considering ethical questions related to obesity treatment, it is noteworthy that very negative attitudes about overweight individuals have been reported in physicians, nurses, and medical students, much the same as in general society. Significant bias has been documented even among health professionals who specialize in the treatment of obese persons (Teachman & Brownell, 2001). In one study, 24 percent of nurses agreed that caring for an obese person "repulsed" them (Bagley, Conklin, Isherwood, Pechiulis, & Watson, 1989). Dread of scolding or humiliation by a physician may engender reluctance on the part of overweight persons to seek medical care, hence screening and treatment for diseases may be delayed (Puhl & Brownell, 2001).

Ironically, socially acceptable rude behavior toward overweight people makes their weight control efforts more difficult. Large persons are often scorned or taunted by patrons in traditional fitness facilities (Bliss, 2006). Large women walking in public places are commonly subjected to ridicule, such as, people rolling down car windows and making pig noises, or yelling things like "Lose weight, Fatso!" Policy efforts to address cruelty and humiliation dished out to overweight individuals are hampered by a fear that promoting "size acceptance" may lead to even greater weight gain in the population. Joann Ikeda, formerly of the University of California Berkeley Center for Weight and Health, dismissed this concern at a 2004 presentation with the sentiment "If feeling bad about our bodies were an effective motivator for weight loss, we would all look like Barbie dolls" (Ikeda, 2004).

PRINCIPLE 1: PATIENT AUTONOMY/PERSONAL RESPONSIBILITY

Is Being Obese a Personal Choice?

Given the high degree of stigmatization and discrimination that is brought on by being obese in mainstream American culture, it is unlikely that the majority of large-bodied individuals have actively chosen to embrace obesity as a personal preference. If people are not actively choosing obesity, what can explain the dramatic increases in prevalence of overweight and obesity—in every age group, every gender, every income group, and every ethnic group in the United States (Flegal, Carroll, Ogden, & Johnson, 2002), as well as in almost every nation in the world (World Health Organization, 2006)—all over a time span of just one generation? Ethical treatment of a condition generally requires at least an educated guess as to the underlying causes of the condition. Three views of underlying causes for obesity are presented below.

View 1: Moral Failure

Weight gain is often cast as a moral failure, as manifestation of the vices of sloth and gluttony. When cast in this light, the widespread bias against overweight individuals seems justified. Attitudes supporting this view have been summarized by Puhl and Brownell (2001) as follows: "First, overweight people are assumed to have multiple negative characteristics, ranging from flaws in personal effort (being lazy), to more core matters such as intelligence and being a good or bad person. Second, overweight individuals are believed to be responsible for their condition and that an imperfect body reflects an imperfect person. Finally, whatever bad comes from the bias and discrimination is acceptable, even merited, based on the common belief that people get what they deserve and deserve what they get."

Thoughtful consideration of the trends in personal behaviors and trends in weight gain in the United States call this view into question. Weight status does not correlate well with physical activity or dietary patterns. Although national surveys find that overweight and obese individuals often fail to meet recommendations for physical activity and dietary intake, the same surveys show that a considerable proportion of lean as well as obese persons have elevated levels of modifiable risk factors (Gregg et al., 2005).

Obese individuals in the general population have essentially normal psychological functioning (Fabricatore & Wadden, 2003). It is implausible that 1.6 billion overweight adults worldwide (World Health Organization, 2006) have all suddenly slipped into sloth and gluttony over the past 20 years.

View 2: Obesogenic Environment

The universal shift toward obesity is more credibly explained by drastic changes in the environment. Widespread weight gain can be seen as a normal and natural response to changes in our culture and in our physical and social environments that negatively impact access to physical activity and health-promoting foods. A few of these changes include:

- Practical elimination of the need for physical activity as part of employment for most people
- Increased time spent behind the wheel of a car, up to an average of 87 minutes per day behind the wheel in 2005 (U.S. Department of Transportation, 2004; Langer, 2005)
- Increased demands on time leading to greater reliance on fast foods and a trend for sleep deprivation
- Reduction in safe places for children and adults to be physically active secondary to sprawl and urban crime
- Universal availability of low-cost, highly-palatable food with high fat content and relatively low nutrient density (Drewnowski & Darmon, 2005)
- Increasing portion sizes in the 1980s and 1990s and increases in available calories in the food supply (Young & Nestle, 2002)
- Increases in screen time (time spent on television, computer use, and video games)
- Increase in major depressive disorders in the population and corresponding use of prescription medications that cause weight gain (Hasin, Goodwin, Stinson, & Grant, 2005; Schwartz, Nihalani, Jindal, Virk, & Jones, 2004)
- Rising consumption of high-caloric sweetened beverages (Bray, Nielsen, & Popkin, 2004)

Changes such as these create an environment that promotes weight gain in the population as a whole. Every person makes choices every day that could influence body weight. However, the range of options available to individuals has shifted such that personal choices that would promote body weight in a lower range are often far more difficult than those promoting weight gain. It is important to note that the same changes that promote weight gain also independently contribute to chronic disease risk. Individuals who fail to get minimal amounts of physical activity, and fruits and vegetables have increase risks for long-term health problems such as osteoporosis, heart disease, stroke, and cancer, whatever their weight status.

View 3: Personal Factors Contributing to Weight Gain

Given the fact that most of the population is exposed to the same obesogenic environment, why is it that some people manage to avoid excessive weight gain? The answer lies in differences in vulnerability. One crucial determinant of vulnerability to obesity is an individual's genetic background. Body weight reflects interaction between genes and the environment. About one-half of the variation in body mass within a population is a result of inherited factors (Lyon & Hirschorn, 2005). Some individuals have such a strong genetically determined propensity for fat storage that that avoiding unwanted weight gain would require superhuman feats of self-denial and unrealistic time commitments to physical activity. Others with a more moderate genetic susceptibility may encounter situations which make weight gain essentially unavoidable, however strong their moral fiber. For example, a person may maintain a healthy weight for many years, but then encounter orthopedic injuries or physical conditions like osteoarthritis that severely limit the ability to exercise. Many medical conditions cause weight gain including hypothyroidism, depression, hypoglycemia, and Cushings syndrome. Weight gain is a recognized side effect of hundreds of commonly used prescription drugs such as steroids, some antihypertensives, insulin, and most psychiatric medications (Adviware Pty Ltd., 2007) The health-promoting decision to quit smoking leads to weight gain in most people (Flegal, Troiano, Pamuk, Kuczmarski, & Campbell, 1995). Another powerful factor leading to unwanted weight gain is uncertain access to food, sometimes called "food insecurity" (Wilde & Peterman, 2006), a condition experienced by 12.6 million households in the United States annually (Nord, Andrews, & Carlson, 2006). The lowest-cost options available to people with very limited incomes are energy-dense foods composed of refined grains, added sugars, or fats (Drewnowski & Specter, 2004).

In today's obesogenic environment, individuals with a genetic predisposition to store fat will easily become overweight or obese, but many others whose weights remain in the normal range are at increased risk of chronic disease due to inadequate physical activity and less than optimal diets.

Moral Choices Affecting Body Weight

Assessments of moral character simply cannot be made based on the size or shape of someone's body. People do make choices every day which can affect body weight. Healthy choices typically require greater investments of time, energy, and money than less healthy choices. Individuals with the fewest resources in time, energy and money may face moral dilemmas as they decide whether to take care of their bodies or address other needs. For example,

- "Should I take a 30-minute walk after work or should I go straight home to relieve my partner who has been caring single-handedly for a handicapped child all day?"
- "Should I buy a pair of good walking shoes for myself, or replace outgrown shoes for my children?"
- "If I stop at the gym on the way home from work, I'll have to grab fast food for the family rather than fix a lower-fat home-cooked dinner."
- "Should I take a bike ride on my lunch hour, or finish this report that is holding up work for 25 people?"

Some Moral Conclusions

Complexity

These hypotheticals demonstrate how obesity is clearly much more of a morally complex phenomenon than many people are willing to allow. Most individuals do not become obese as a result of choices that are indifferent or irresponsible. Holding all obese individuals morally blameworthy for their obesity is far from being a fair or morally justifiable judgment. It may be true that *some* individuals might be open to justified moral criticism for being obese. However, the natural question then is: who should be responsible for investigating the causes of their obesity and then judging their degree of guilt or innocence? Is this a role we would assign to physicians, a role we might dub that of medical prosecutors? Is this a role that physicians should warmly embrace? What would we see as the good that could be accomplished by such a role? And what might be the corresponding harm that might be caused by such a role? Could such a role of moral investigation for physicians ultimately lead to extreme patient reluctance to seek help, even when there was clear medical need for medical assessment? No doubt weight loss is a medically desirable goal for many individuals, but it might be more readily achieved without physicians having to act as medical prosecutors. It might be more achievable through methods of education and persuasion that are respectful of patient autonomy rights.

Dangerous Metaphors

We also need to comment on the very widespread reference to the epidemic of obesity (Campos et al., 2006; Flegal, 2006). This language is morally dangerous and ought not be glossed over as any more than an imaginative metaphor. Epidemics represent public health threats. Governments and medical authorities are clearly justified in constraining a broad range of individual liberties for the sake of protecting the health of the broader public. Confining individuals with TB (in the 1940s) or the Spanish flu (in 1918) to isolated areas would be clearly morally justified as public health responses given the risks of death associated with these infectious diseases. AIDS is a deadly infectious disease (and a public health threat in many respects), but quarantining HIV+ individuals is clearly not morally defensible, given the very limited routes of transmission associated with HIV. No one has suggested quarantining obese individuals. However, what we have seen is broad social tolerance (maybe even acceptance or legitimation) of stigmatizing and discriminatory attitudes toward obese individuals. These attitudes will often translate into behaviors clearly harmful to these individuals (job denial, promotion denial, public humiliation). The term *epidemic* can serve to legitimate these intolerant attitudes, as if these attitudes were a reasonable defensive response to the threat to public health posed by obese individuals.

Paternalism?

But, even if we are critically self-conscious about the use of such language and we recognize that obesity is not a threat in any meaningful sense to the health of the *public,* it can still be viewed as a threat to the health and well-being of an individual. Further, it might be viewed as a very powerful threat that most individuals as individuals are incapable of resisting without outside assistance. If we take this view, then a paternalistic response would appear to be morally justified. Or in other words, this response assumes that individuals lack the autonomous capacity to manage their weight problem on their own. The moral risk in this case is that the paternalism would take the form of tough love, which again could be used to justify stigmatizing and discriminatory behavior as a necessary means of correcting the self-destructive behavior of obese individuals. Again, while an intervention may be necessary and morally justified in the case of an alcoholic under the rubric of tough love, tough love would still not justify broadly stigmatizing and discriminatory behavior regarding an individual with an alcohol problem. The same should hold true for overweight or obese individuals.

PRINCIPLE 2: HARM IN WEIGHT LOSS TREATMENT

Is Weight Loss Safe?

Weight loss treatment holds risks and may have negative side effects. The least risky weight loss methods are those that maintain a balanced diet and use modest caloric reductions accompanied by increased physical activity such that weight is lost gradually over an extended period. The greatest risks are associated with the most drastic treatments—very low calorie regimens and bariatric surgery. Providers can do harm, however, even with more conservative treatment approaches. Some examples of potential harm are offered below.

Very Low Calorie Regimens

The idea that low-calorie diets could be hazardous was not part of the national consciousness until the 1970s, when 55 sudden deaths occurred among individuals consuming several popular over-the-counter very low calorie diet products referred to as liquid protein. Investigators from the Centers for Disease Control and Prevention charged with identifying the cause of death conducted extensive reviews of autopsy reports, pathology studies, and medical records. They tentatively concluded that the chronic caloric deficits had caused the atrophy observed in all organs, and that the atrophy of the heart muscle resulted in fatal cardiac arrhythmias. Essentially, they believed, victims starved to death (Sours et al., 1981). Very low calorie regimens can produce vitamin deficiencies, loss of lean body mass, decrease in bone density, development of gallstones (Villareal et al., 2006; Strychar, 2006), and unpleasant side effects such as cold intolerance, hair loss, and headaches.

Surgery

For bariatric surgery, estimates of mortality rates within the first year after surgery range from less than 1–5 percent depending on the procedure and where it done (Mitka, 2006; Reuters Health Information, 2006). Failure to monitor for and correct nutritional deficiencies that frequently result from obesity surgeries (severe protein-calorie malnutrition, deficiencies in vitamin B12, iron, calcium, vitamin D, thiamine, folate, and fat-soluble vitamins) can result in serious metabolic complications (Malinowski, 2006). In a recent review, Shah, Simha, and Garg (2006) cautioned that significant weight regain occurs over the long term, and the improvement in comorbidities associated with weight loss is lessened in the long term on weight regain. According to a 2005 Cochrane review of the effects of obesity surgery, the evidence was limited and of poor quality, making it difficult to draw any conclusions about comparative safety and effectiveness (Colquitt, Clegg, Loveman, Royle, & Sidhu, 2005).

Psychological Effects

Weight loss can have negative psychological effects. The classic hunger study conducted during World War II (Keys, Brozek, Henschel, Mickelsen, & Taylor, 1950) demonstrated that restricting calories, can produce striking psychological effects. In this study, normal, healthy intelligent men were restricted to 1,800 calories per day for a period of six months. Negative effects observed included fatigue, apathy, extreme weakness, irritability, neurological deficits, relentless craving for and preoccupation with food, overpowering hunger, decreased ability to concentrate on anything but thoughts of food, and food hoarding.

Initiation of Binge Eating

Uncontrollable hunger leading to bingeing is observed with semi-starvation regimens, even in people without emotional problems. This type of over-eating was observed in the classic hunger study mentioned above. When the period of food restriction ended, the subjects entered into a period where they ate more than normal amount to satisfy hunger; in some cases, this period lasted until long after their lost weight was regained. In one study of a self-help weight loss approach, 41 percent of participants reported bulimic episodes (Delinsky, Latner, & Wilson, 2006). Attempts to lose weight in some vulnerable individuals evolve into eating disorders (American Psychiatric Association Work Group on Eating Disorders, 2000).

Emotional Harm

All health care is provided within a social context of fat-phobia, stig-matization, and weight discrimination. Providers can inadvertently add to emotionally debilitating feelings of shame that many overweight indi-viduals hold by using disrespectful or insensitive language or approaches to patients. Emotional harm can also occur if the weight loss treatment is one that is not effective in the long-term; feelings of shame or self-loathing may be worse after a failed weight loss attempt than they were before weight loss occurred.

Complication of Existing Medical Conditions

Serious harm can befall individuals who are placed on weight loss regimens without regard for existing medical conditions. For example, a person taking a prescription drug could experience drug overdoses if the dose is not adjusted to take into account changed eating patterns or reduced kilograms of body weight. A person with compromised renal function could have renal damage exacerbated by a low carbohydrate high protein intake.

Ineffective Treatment

Providing medical care that is not efficacious would not be something an ethical provider would purposely do. It has been well-demonstrated that most people can lose weight, but time and again research shows that the vast majority of people who lose weight regain it during subsequent months and years (Hill, Thompson, & Wyatt, 2005). Anecdotes and testimonials about large, permanent weight losses are plentiful, but large, systematic research studies documenting the state of the art are rare. The most popular structured weight loss programs in the United States have not released data on long-term results. Most clinical studies of weight loss do not collect data past one year. Estimates of the long-term success of weight treatment vary from a low of "almost all weight is regained within five years" (NIH Technology Assessment Conference Panel, 1993) to an optimistic high of approximately 20 percent (Wing & Phelan, 2005).

Part of the variability in estimates is due to differing definitions of success. A National Weight Control Registry (NWCR), created to study the characteristics of successful weight losers, defines success as maintenance of loss of at least 30 pounds for at least one year (Hill, Wyatt, Phelan, & Wing, 2005). One year is a relatively short period to be considered long-term success; studying people after only one year may lead to an overly optimistic picture of weight loss maintenance. Although the NWCR is a worthwhile study of individuals who have kept lost weight off for some time, its 5,000 subjects are volunteers, not representative of the 85 million Americans trying to lose weight (Gaesser, 2006).

Several relatively recent studies (Anderson, Konz, Frederich, & Wood, 2001; McGuire, Wing, & Hill, 1999) support the more optimistic estimates of around 20 percent success, and are interpreted by many as support for continued focus of health improvement for overweight individuals efforts on weight loss. The same findings of 20 percent success are translated to 80 percent failure rates by HAES advocates, who argue that any treatment modality with an 80 percent failure rate should be considered unacceptable.

The effectiveness of weight loss treatment is a critical part of the picture needed to assess ethics and weight treatment because repeated cycles of weight loss and regain may not be innocuous events. Weight regain is often accompanied by deterioration in self-esteem as well as reversion to pre-weight loss status in terms of health risk factors such as blood lipid concentrations and blood pressure (Bacon, Stern, Van Loan, & Keim, 2005). Worse, rebound weight gain is common, where dieters regain all the weight lost plus additional weight (Gaesser, 2002). A number of physiologic mechanisms have been proposed to explain the relentless weight regain experienced by the majority of dieters, including, for example, enhanced appetite due to weight-loss-induced decreases in the hormone leptin (Infanger et al., 2005), and increased efficiency of dietary fat storage after weight loss (Faraj, Jones, Sniderman, & Cianflone, 2001).

Is Weight Loss Actually Necessary to Correct the Health Problems Associated with Higher Weights?

Disagreement

Saying that weight gain is a natural and normal response to an obesogenic environment is not to say that it is a positive phenomenon. There is no disagreement from any quarter that people who are obese are more likely to have health conditions and risk factors such as insulin resistance, diabetes, hypertension, stroke, dyslipidemia, heart disease, and certain kinds of cancers (Bray, 2004). Nor is there disagreement that even modest weight loss (5–10% of body weight) is accompanied by improvements in risk factors (Krauss et al., 2000). There is disagreement, however, as to the actual causes of the health conditions that accompany obesity. Ascertaining the actual cause of health problems associated with obesity is necessary before informed ethical decisions can be made as to how to best address the issue. Given the high failure rate for weight loss treatment and the potential risks from the more extreme weight loss treatments, an important question for providers is whether losing weight is necessary for improving the health of all heavy individuals.

The facts (whatever they turn out to be) will be very important from a moral point of view. But the facts will often not be decisive at the level of the individual patient. That is, the more common clinical scenario will remain one in which there is considerable uncertainty regarding the medically best course of action, all things considered. There will be some level of risk no matter what course of action a patient might choose. This would be a primary reason why respect for patient autonomy is of utmost moral importance in such situations. Patients will have to live with the consequences of their decisions; physicians will not.

Who Decides?

Physicians (individually or collectively) may have a sense in specific clinical circumstances of what counts as a medical harm or a medical benefit from their perspective as physicians. But patients may look at the very same clinical facts and not have a distorted understanding of those facts, but make very different reasonable judgments (from a physician's perspective) as to what they would regard as harmful or beneficial *to them* in those clinical circumstances. The example that should be regarded as a close moral analogue to the obesity issue is that of the appropriate treatment of prostate cancer. Many of those cancers are very slow growing. Under the circumstances, despite the widespread fear typically engendered on hearing a cancer diagnosis, it is not unreasonable for a man to choose the watchful waiting option as opposed to any more aggressive surgical intervention aimed at extricating the cancerous cells (with the relatively high risks of side effects that many men would dread). Of course, this is not to suggest that this is really the right decision for any man to make. On the contrary, there is too much uncertainty and too much variation in the way in which different men might assess the relative risks posed to them by their options.

Physician's Role

Our suggestion in this essay is that the management of obesity should be thought of as being morally analogous to the management of prostate cancer (which is another reason why stigmatization is morally indefensible). What this means in practice is that it would be morally objectionable for a physician to insist on aggressive interventions to achieve weight loss, as if that were the only reasonable outcome, when in fact a more impartial perspective would suggest that a range of reasonable trade-off options were legitimate. The morally appropriate role for a physician is to facilitate a patient in making a more autonomous choice with respect to the different risk trade-offs. That means that risks must not be exaggerated in order to elicit a physician-desired response. Carrying 30 extra pounds might double an individual's risk of a heart attack in any given year; but if that means an increase in absolute terms from 1–2 percent, then that should be presented to the patient as well since that might well elicit a very different response. Likewise, if it were to turn out to be the case that yo-yo dieting represented more of a risk to long term health than carrying 30 extra pounds, then a physician would be morally obligated to convey that information to a patient, especially if a patient already knew himself well enough that he could say it was very unlikely that he could maintain lost weight for any significant period of time. This is what both the harm principle and respect for patient autonomy requires. Among the things patients need to know is that there can be reasonable disagreements among health professionals about weight loss (or gain) relative to significant health consequences.

View 1: Weight Loss Needed for Health

The prevailing paradigm is that excess weight, in and of itself, is responsible for health risks and early mortality. The mechanism proposed for this perspective is that enlarged fat cells produce the clinical problems associated with obesity because of either the mass of the extra fat or because of the increased secretion of free fatty acids and numerous peptides from enlarged fat cells. People in the highest BMI categories, would certainly fall into the previous category, where increased mass of fat itself impairs mobility and directly lead to conditions such as osteoarthritis and sleep apnea (Bray, 2004). Proponents of this view would continue to focus health improvement efforts for overweight and obese people directly on weight loss, calling for more research on weight loss methods and more vigorous encouragement of weight loss.

View 2: Health at Every Size

Another, less commonly held, view is that the association of body weight with excess morbidity and mortality is not a simple cause and effect relationship. This view recognizes that some of the environmental and lifestyle factors that contribute to obesity also contribute independently to the chronic diseases associated with obesity. Proponents of this view, sometimes called the Health at Every Size (HAES) philosophy, propose refocusing health improvement efforts—away from the weight loss as a primary goal, and toward interventions on lifestyle behaviors and the environments that shape those behaviors.

Limits of Population Studies

HAES proponents point out that the vast majority of large-scale population studies that have found obesity to predict early mortality or disease conditions do not adequately account for the effects of factors such as physical activity, physical fitness, diet quality, depression, social support, or weight change over time—all of which may have a bearing on life expectancy and chronic disease risk (Gaesser, 2006). The few epidemiological studies of mortality or disease outcomes that adequately control for BMI, changes in BMI over time, and lifestyle (such as LaMonte & Blair, 2006; Flegal, Graubard, Williamson, & Gail, 2005) find that BMI does not predict disease or death to the same extent as studies without those controls.

Another factor not generally accounted for in population studies of weight and mortality is the pattern of fat distribution. It has been observed that women with the classical pear shape, carrying fat in peripheral subcutaneous depots, tend to have healthy metabolic profiles and may, in fact, have reduced risk of cardiovascular disease (Tankó, Bagger, Alexandersen, Larsen, & Christiansen, 2003). In contrast, men and women with apple shapes, carrying weight in the visceral region have increased cardiovascular risk. Visceral fat deposition is part of the metabolic syndrome (large waist, elevated blood pressure, elevated blood glucose and trigycerides, and low HDL-cholesterol). In the 2004 report from the Women's Ischemia Syndrome Evaluation (WISE) study, the metabolic syndrome was predictive of future cardiovascular risk, but BMI was not (Kip et al., 2004). Weight loss may not offer health advantages for pear-shaped women carrying extra weight.

Health Improvements without Weight Loss

Powerful additional evidence for the HAES perspective comes from several well-designed clinical studies showing improvement in risk factors among overweight individuals who increased their physical activity and improved dietary quality but did not lose weight. (Appel et al., 1997; Bacon, Stern, Van Loan, & Keim, 2005; Diabetes Prevention Program Research Group, 2002) For example, Bacon, et al. (2005) treated obese women who were chronic dieters with training on size acceptance and intuitive healthy eating. The research showed that improvements in disease risk factors such as blood pressure and serum cholesterol in the intuitive eating group were as great as improvements seen in similar women treated with a traditional, conservative weight loss regimen. What is most notable about that study is the finding at two-year follow-up, that the size acceptance group had maintained their risk factor improvements whereas the weight loss group had regained their weight and had returned to their pre-weight loss risk factor status.

A research challenge that must be met in assigning causality to either body fat or lifestyle factors is that of identifying easy, inexpensive ways to reliably and validly document adiposity, physical activity fat distribution, and nutrient consumption in large scale studies (LaMonte & Blair, 2006).

Social Stress

It is ironic that some of the excess chronic disease experienced by over-weight and obese individuals may be caused, at least in part, by the war on obesity," which sometimes spills over into negative attitudes toward people who are fat. Stigmatization, bullying, and systematic discrimina-tion has been shown, in both primates and humans, to lead to negative health effects such as high blood pressure, elevated cholesterol, and increases in waist-to-hip ratios (Kaplan, Adams, Clarkson, Manuck, & Shively, 1991).

Social Justice Issues: Unfair Costs to Society and Rationing

Costs Matter

This portion of our discussion needs to begin with the generally accepted fact that escalating health care costs represent a serious and persistent ethical and policy challenge. To be precise, the United States spent about $26 billion for health care in 1960, roughly 5.2 percent of GDP then. In 2006 we spent about $2.16 trillion on health care, roughly 16.3 percent of our GDP (Catlin, Cowan, Heffler, & Washington, 2007). Projections to 2014 suggest we will be at $4.08 trillion in health spending then, roughly 19.5 percent of predicted GDP (Heffler et al., 2005). Most policy analysts will agree that there are multiple causes for escalating health care costs, but the single most significant driving force would be costly emerging technologies in all areas of medicine (Aaron, Schwartz, & Cox, 2006). Daniel Callahan (1990, chap.2) for one has noted the very close connec-tion between new technologies and what we identify as health care needs. In 1970 there was no need for either coronary bypass surgery or coronary angioplasty, but in 2005 in the United States we performed more than a half million coronary bypass surgeries at $65 thousand each and an addi-tional 1.2 million coronary angioplasties at about $30 thousand each.

Costs matter for a lot of reasons. As health care costs have increased over the past twenty years we have seen the steady erosion among smaller employers of commitment to providing health insurance as an employee benefit. The result has been a steady increase in the number of working uninsured members of our society, estimated in 2006 to be about 46 mil-lion individuals. Many will judge it unjust that so many in our society would be denied assured access to needed health care. One response to this state of affairs would take this form: If we really believe that we can-not afford to provide needed health care for all in our society (and so we are willing to tolerate 46 million uninsured individuals), then we ought to devise an approach for making rationing decisions that is fair to all. That is, we ought to use expert panels and perhaps a process of rational democratic deliberation to identify very expensive marginally beneficial types of health care that we would deny to everyone, at least as a covered insurance benefit. We would do that in order to achieve the savings that were needed to provide an adequate package of health care benefits to all of the currently uninsured. As things are now, those uninsured individuals have mostly become uninsured for morally arbitrary reasons over which they had no control. The practical implication is that they are denied access to *all* needed health care, whether it is costworthy and significantly effective or not.

Rationing: Who Deserves Care?

However, proposals to endorse any form of health care rationing at all are generally seen as politically perilous. Rationing decisions are seen as deliberate choices "against life" or against the "equal respect" due each person in our society (Calabresi & Bobbitt, 1978). The implicit claim is that individuals do not *deserve* to be treated in that way. This then often generates an alternate proposal for controlling health care costs without having to make explicit undeserved rationing decisions. This alternate proposal is that society ought not have to pay the health care costs of persons who have been responsible for their own medical problems. If individuals have lung disease as a result of smoking, if individuals have liver disease as a result of alcoholism, if individuals have AIDS as a result of casual irresponsible sexual encounters, if individuals have diabetes or coronary artery disease as a result of very bad dietary choices leading to obesity, then they should have complete responsibility for covering the health care costs that are attributable to their bad choices. Much of the health care that these individuals will need is likely to be extraordinarily expensive (transplant surgery, ICU care, bypass surgery, etc.), far beyond the financial capacity of most individuals. That might have the practical implication of these individuals being denied costly life-sustaining health care and dying prematurely (sooner than they would have if they had had access to those effective but costly interventions). However, the argument continues, this is precisely what these individuals deserve. They are not being treated unfairly; on the contrary, if they expected the more responsible members of society to absorb these health care costs, *that would be unfair.*

Irresponsible Behavior: Where Is the Line to Be Drawn?

We believe that this latter line of argument ought to be rejected. We believe that this line of argument is seriously morally flawed. It is discriminatory in a morally objectionable sense. The reader will notice the list of irresponsible behaviors to which we called your attention. What they all have in common is that they have very often been the focus of religious condemnation by some number of religious groups. If we are going to be fair in denying individuals access to needed health care at social expense, then we would have to have a much longer list of behaviors that could potentially result in such health care denials. Individuals who engaged in various sports, especially what are called extreme sports where there is significant risk of costly injuries, would also have to absorb health costs for themselves. After all, why should I have to absorb the costs of the consequences of their choices? They can easily lead a satisfying life without making those choices. Likewise, individuals involved in automobile accidents during very short trips when they could just as easily have walked might also be regarded as having made an irresponsible choice. The same would be true for driving longer distances in cities with high quality safer forms of public transportation. The reader can easily expand this list until a substantial majority of our health problems are seen as the product of voluntarily chosen risky health behaviors for which those individuals would be entirely financially responsible. This is not a consequence most in our society would embrace, but it is a morally required consequence of *consistently* following through the implications of the irresponsible health behavior argument, as opposed to relying upon a religious or political ideology to identify irresponsible health behaviors.

Causality Is Complex

Yet another consideration would speak against appealing to the irresponsible health behavior argument to control costs, namely, the complexity of the causal factors that result in the irresponsible behavior. What that argument requires *as a moral argument* needed to properly attribute moral responsibility is that the dominant causal factor that resulted in that irresponsible behavior (and costly health problems) was a free and deliberate choice by that person. However, one of the things we are coming to learn as a result of our rapidly increasing knowledge in genetics is that there will often be genetic factors beyond the morally responsible control of an individual that cause the bad health outcomes for which we are tempted to hold the individual morally responsible.

Many will remember the long distance runner Jim Fixx who died at age 42 from coronary heart disease (as had a number of other family members). He had a genotype that resulted in his having enormously high levels of so-called bad cholesterol that contributed to his heart disease in spite of an ideal diet. Many in our society will be comparably unfortunate in having genotypes that render them *more vulnerable* to a large range of costly chronic illnesses.

We employ the phrase *more vulnerable* as opposed to *completely vulnerable* because in the vast majority of cases these genetic mutations will require some range of other genetic or environmental factors to conspire with one another to yield the phenotypic disease state. Thus, individuals who are genetically predisposed to higher levels of the bad cholesterol might also have parents who established for them early in life dietary habits and tastes (for rich desserts) that will increase the actual risk of heart disease and obesity. (Note that some favorite foods such as chocolate actually increase brain endorphin levels (Benton& Donohoe, 1999); in such cases, foods are in truth forms of self-medication.) Or these same individuals might be vulnerable to depression for genetic reasons and use favorite-food eating habits as a way of modifying the feelings of depression, thereby increasing their risks of heart disease and obesity. Or they might have been raised in socially and economically impoverished circumstances where the costs of better foods were out of reach. Or they might be working in more stressful environments, which, in combination with this or that genetic vulnerability, results in increased risks of heart disease and obesity. Again, the reader can readily expand this list of factors. In theory such individuals could make better, more responsible choices. But if they are lacking effective access to the relevant educational or health care resources for a large range of social and economic reasons, then making more responsible choices is no more than a theoretical possibility.

A Matter of Degree

Another morally relevant consideration, especially with regard to obesity, is that there are degrees of obesity and degrees of bad dietary habits. The causal linkages to very bad health outcomes may be clear and nearly certain at the extremes of these continua. But as we get further away from the extremes we lack the medical evidence to say with great confidence that *this* degree of obesity is very strongly linked with diabetes or heart disease and so forth. There are too many other factors beyond obesity alone that in various degrees can causally contribute to the actual emergence of these disease states. Some of those factors may be poorly understood; others may be largely beyond conscious control of an individual. All of that should take away from the degree of confidence we might reasonably have in attributing *moral* responsibility to individuals for their diseased state. Further, at numerous points judgments will have to be made as to the degree to which an individual might be responsible for their disease state and have to accept the social consequences of that.

Who Assigns Blame?

Presumably the expertise of physicians would be needed to make such judgments. However, if this role were foisted upon physicians, this would alter very dramatically our understanding of the doctor-patient relationship. No one could confidently believe that a physician was a compassionate partner in protecting his or her best health care interests. Instead, physicians would in part have become agents of insurance companies or the state in seeking to identify irresponsible health behavior by patients that would generate financial denials. Few of us would be comfortable thinking of physicians as compassionate prosecutors, trying to elicit from us the information they would need to convict us of irresponsible health choices. But this too would be a likely practical implication of our seeking to control health care costs by limiting the health care we provided to individuals whose behavior was judged responsible for their diseased state.

What Should be Covered?

The next social justice issue we need to consider is the question of whether some range of weight reduction interventions and techniques (education, counseling, diet drugs, bariatric surgery) ought to be a covered benefit in all health insurance plans, including Medicare and Medicaid. We can address this issue from two different policy perspectives: the world as it is now in the United States with health insurance tied to employment and 46 million uninsured individuals, or a reformed health care system that guaranteed a relatively comprehensive package of health benefits to all. A succinct way to pose our basic question would be this: are we morally obligated as a just and caring society to include in a universal health benefit package a broad range of weight management interventions when it is the case that we have limited resources (tax and premium dollars) to meet virtually unlimited health care needs? That is, could individuals who wanted access to one or another weight management intervention at social expense justifiably claim that they were treated unjustly if such interventions were not part of this benefit package?

Setting Priorities

The work of David Eddy, physician and health economist, might be a useful starting point for thinking through this question. What we are addressing is a rationing and priority setting question. How high a priority ought a range of weight management interventions have relative to all the other health needs and corresponding health interventions available in our society? Eddy draws our attention to the relative costs and effectiveness of various interventions as the key to this priority setting process. If a particular intervention has a very low probability of having a significant therapeutic outcome, and if it costs a lot of money for a small chance of achieving that marginal benefit, then that intervention ought to be very low on our priority list. Eddy gives the following example to illustrate the point (1996, chap. 22).

An Example

There are two types of contrast agents used when patients have a CT scan. They are called HOCA and LOCA. The cost of the first is about $10; the other is $180. Some people (who mostly cannot be identified before the fact) will have a severe allergic reaction to HOCA. This can be quickly reversed by prompt medical attention, but it is a very frightening experience. The chance of this happening to anyone is less than one in a thousand. Patients who receive LOCA are spared this risk. However, the cost of that is an extra $170. That is, relatively speaking, a small amount of money. But we do more than 20 million CT scans per year in the United States. If everyone got LOCA, we would add $3.4 billion to the cost of health care to prevent those non-fatal allergic reactions. Those very same dollars could be invested in a cervical cancer screening program as a public health measure and save the lives of about 100 women per year in the United States. Eddy concludes this latter intervention represents a much greater health benefit than spending the money on LOCAs, and hence, should be thought of as having much higher priority.

The moral theory behind Eddy's work is essentially utilitarian. Many philosophers would have a concern about utilitarianism as a general moral theory, namely, that individual rights get trampled to achieve some social benefit. An alternative moral theory would be contractarian. John Rawls (1971) is considered a preeminent proponent of this theory. The general idea behind Rawls' version of contractarianism is that social policies are just if all would agree to the distribution of burdens and benefits of that policy from behind a "veil of ignorance," an imaginary mental state in which we are entirely ignorant of any details about our identity and life history. In the case of Eddy's example, it seems contractarians would give the same answer as Eddy. If we had a million women behind a health-related veil of ignorance (they did not know whether they might need a CT scan in the future or were at risk for cervical cancer), then how would they use that $3.4 billion? It seems clear that the reasonable choice (freely chosen and self-imposed) would be Eddy's choice, and so that choice can be seen as just and caring and prudent. We should add one further point to avoid alienating libertarians. It would not be unjust to permit individuals to pull out a platinum credit card and pay for the more expensive contrast agent. No one is made worse off because someone wants to use his or her own money in this way. That is, no social resources are unjustly diverted from higher priority health needs to lower priority needs.

How High a Priority for Weight Management?

How does this analysis apply to our question about weight management interventions? To avoid arguments about complex empirical data, our best answer might be expressed in a series of hypotheticals. The reader needs to keep in mind that more than 60 million Americans are defined as being obese. That means that even low cost ($500) weight management interventions would quickly translate into aggregated costs of tens of billions of dollars if these interventions were covered as part of a national health insurance package. Still, if such an investment were very effective (permanent weight loss for at least 80% of patients), and if that meant that there were a 50 percent reduction in the incidence of heart disease and diabetes and other such costly chronic illnesses in that treated population, then those gains would clearly offset the front end costs of that intervention. This would again be a just and caring and prudent investment of social resources. However, if the facts are more nearly the precise opposite of this first hypothetical (which seems to be the case), if less than 20 percent of obese individuals who try multiple weight loss interventions are capable of sustaining that loss long term (five years or more), if the incidence of heart disease and diabetes and other chronic illnesses typically thought of as being linked to obesity decline only very slightly, if there are significant adverse health affects associated with yo-yo dieting linked to multiple unsuccessful efforts at weight reduction, then neither justice nor prudence would seem to require that public funding mechanisms underwrite the costs of most of these weight management interventions. The moral correctness of this conclusion would seem to be further reinforced if individuals try multiple weight reduction interventions unsuccessfully, thereby adding substantially to overall social costs, in part because these costs are covered at the social level rather than at the individual level.

How might we test the validity of our latter hypothetical? We can imagine a contractarian mental experiment. Alternatively, we can organize real world rational democratic deliberative conversations about this specific rationing and prioritization issue (see Fleck, 2006, for guidelines regarding such conversations). We will go with this latter alternative. What we recognize with regard to this latter alternative is that individuals are not behind a thick veil of ignorance. More specifically, individuals will know whether or not they are obese and their personal history regarding weight management. Nevertheless, we could still have a fair-minded, unbiased public conversation.

Those with weight management problems may initially feel very strongly that they want the costs of weight management programs as a covered benefit (say, in a national health insurance program, or as part of Medicare). But then they would be reminded that they are vulnerable (like all Americans) to a very wide and costly range of medical problems, among which would be various cancers, various forms of heart disease, arthritis, diabetes, Parkinson's, and so forth. If we invested tens of billions of dollars per year in weight management interventions, then what other health care interventions that we currently cover (and that are very effective) would they be willing to give up in order to generate those resources? Would they give up the Medicare prescription drug benefit? Would they give up expensive drugs that effectively relieved 90 percent of the suffering associated with arthritis? Would they give up very expensive cancer drugs ($50 thousand per course of treatment) if those drugs yielded two or three years of additional satisfactory quality life with the cancer kept at bay?

If enough of these sorts of questions were asked, it would be very likely that most of these weight management interventions would have very low priority in the total scheme of health care interventions (which is what current research seems to show). Most of these weight management interventions show too little sustained benefit for the dollars spent. The practical moral implication of such a deliberative process is that it would not be unjust to deny public coverage for these weight management interventions. Again, individuals would be free to spend their own money on these interventions. Further, this could conceivably have the desirable outcome that individuals would be more motivated to take such interventions seriously since it was clearly *their* money they would be spending. Also, the fairness of this outcome would be further legitimated if obese individuals in the conversation reflectively endorsed this outcome so that it was clear that this outcome did not simply result from prevailing social prejudices.

Denying public coverage for weight loss interventions is not the same as turning society's back on the issue of obesity in the population. What we propose, given the absence of evidence-based population approaches to weight loss, is that government and health care resources be focused not on weight loss, per se, but rather on the root causes of obesity—the factors that make it difficult for our citizens to increase physical activity and improve food choices. Focusing on healthy eating and physical activity rather than weight loss offers several advantages:

- Weight loss is often achieved by individuals who adopt healthier lifestyles.
- Improving diet quality and physical activity will reduce chronic disease risk, even if weight loss is absent or minimal.
- Interventions that focus on positive behaviors that can be maintained are more likely to improve mental health and self-esteem than weight loss interventions, which are likely to end with the perception of personal failure when weight is regained.
- Interventions that improve a community's walkability, bikability, and access to healthy food typically improve the quality of life and economic health of a community.
- Health messages focused on positive behaviors are unlikely to worsen the social pressure for excessive slenderness which contributes to unsafe weight loss practices and eating disorders (Michigan Department of Community Health, 2005).

There are many reasons why an individual may have a specific body size. Since we do not have complete control over our body weight, it seems logical to focus on something over which we have more control. We can affect our actions. Both as individuals and as a society, we can build systems that encourage the actions of healthy eating and fitness activities. We can make our GOAL healthy living rather than choosing a goal of some specific weight.

Kelly Bliss, M.Ed., A.C.E.
Health at Every Size Advocate (2006)

CONCLUSIONS

The problem definition of obesity needs to be expanded beyond the fact that many individuals are gaining weight. The current narrow emphasis on trying to get people to lose weight is causing harm. Efforts to address obesity—by society as a whole and by individual health practitioners—should also address widespread bias and discrimination against heavy individuals, the obesogenic properties of the environment, lack of knowledge on how to adapt medical procedures for people who are heavy, and prevention. Risks associated with weight loss treatments, as well as the long-term failure of current obesity treatments needs to be more widely recognized. Initiatives to help those who are overweight should be those most likely to actually benefit overweight individuals and least likely to cause harm.

Implications for health care practitioners:

1. Primary care: incorporate prevention into routine care for both children and adults.

2. Avoid adding to the burden of shame and self-hatred that overweight individuals often experience. Reign in any personal feelings of disgust to allow respectful behaviors and respectful medical care environments.

3. Avoid knee-jerk assumptions that every person who is carrying extra weight can or should lose it.

4. Do not withhold needed treatment until weight is lost.

5. Given that overweight patients present additional risk for some procedures, learn how to adapt procedures to take the extra weight into account rather than using standard procedures.

6. Given the overall failure of weight loss treatment to effect long-term weight loss, focus intervention on positive eating and physical activity behaviors that will positively affect health risk independent of weight status.

7. Given that obesity is a chronic rather than acute condition, get information about risks associated with specific weight loss regimens over time, and disclose those risks fully to patients. When new treatments become available with no track record of safety, recognize and describe them as experimental.

8. Avoid weight control regimens that place patients at unnecessary risk.

Implications for government:

1. Aggressively pursue remedies to the widespread discrimination and bias shown to overweight individuals.

2. Aggressively pursue reversing national and local polices that have contributed to creating the obesogenic environment in which most American live (i.e., school food service polices, school siting policies that result in

schools being built at locations that preclude walking to school, land use policies encouraging sprawl, etc.)

3. Identify and adopt national and local policies that will make it easier for all residents to be physically active and obtain foods consistent with health.

4. Implement policies that encourage prevention of obesity in primary care such as insurance coverage for dietary and physical activity counseling.

5. Reign in marketing of foods with minimal nutritional value to children.

6. Monitor effectiveness and risks of weight loss treatments and publicize findings; reign in marketing of fraudulent and weight loss services.

7. Given the current failure of most weight loss treatment, refocus some of the obesity research funding to explore ways of enhancing health at higher weights (i.e., physical activity that is safe and beneficial for heavy individuals, special nutritional requirements for heavier people, modifying standard treatments to correct for higher weights). Develop policies to help people with sustainable, appropriate physical activity and dietary improvement. Social investment in that area would be appropriate.

NOTE

1. For this chapter, the terms overweight and obesity are based on the body mass index (BMI) guidelines from the Centers for Disease Control and Prevention (CDC). BMI is defined as weight (in kilograms) divided by height (in meters) squared [weight in kilograms/(height in meters)^2]. CDC classifies adult BMI of 25.0–29.9 as overweight, and 30 and above as obese.

REFERENCES

Aaron, H. J., Schwartz, W. B., & Cox, M. (2006). *Can we say no? The challenge of rationing health care.* Washington, DC: Brookings Institution.

Adviware Pty Ltd. (2007, January 15). *Medications or substances causing weight gain.* Retrieved January 17, 2007, from http://www.wrongdiagnosis.com/symptoms/weight_gain/side-effects.htm.

American Psychiatric Association Work Group on Eating Disorders. (2006). Practice guideline for the treatment of patients with eating disorders (revision). *American Journal of Psychiatry, 157*(1 Suppl.), 1–39.

Anderson, J. W., Konz, E. C., Frederich, R. C., & Wood, C. L. (2001). Long-term weight-loss maintenance: A meta-analysis of U.S. studies. *American Journal of Clinical Nutrition, 74,* 579–584.

Appel, L. J., Moore, T. J., Obarzanek, E., Vollmer, W. M., Svetkey, L. P., Sacks, F. M. et al. (1997). A clinical trial of the effects of dietary patterns on blood pressure. *New England Journal of Medicine, 336,* 1117–1124.

Bacon, L., Stern, J. S., Van Loan, M. D, & Keim, N. L. (2005). Size acceptance and intuitive eating improve health for obese, female chronic dieters. *Journal of the American Dietetic Association, 105,* 929–936.

Bagley, C. R., Conklin, D. N., Isherwood, R. T., Pechiulis, D. R., & Watson, L. A. (1989). Attitudes of nurses toward obesity and obese patients. *Perceptual and Motor Skills, 68,* 954.

Benton, D., & Donohoe, R. T. (1999). The effects of nutrients on mood. *Public Health Nutrition, 2,* 403–409.

Bish, C. L., Blanck, H. M., Serdula, M. K., Marcus, M., Kohl, H. W., III, & Khan, L. K. (2005). Diet and physical activity behaviors among Americans trying to lose weight: 2000 Behavioral Risk Factor Surveillance System. *Obesity Research, 13,* 596–607.

Bliss, K. (2006). Redefine the problem so it has a solution. *Health at Every Size, 20,* 17–18.

Bray, G. A. (2004). Medical consequences of obesity. *Journal of Clinical Endocrinology and Metabolism, 89,* 2583–2589.

Bray, G. A., Nielsen, S. J., & Popkin, B. M. (2004). Consumption of high-fructose corn syrup in beverages may play a role in the epidemic of obesity. *American Journal of Clinical Nutrition, 79,* 537–543.

Burgard, D. (2005). Blinded by BMI. *Health at Every Size, 19,* 45–53.

Calabresi, G., & Bobbitt, P. (1978) *Tragic choices: The conflicts society confronts in the allocation of tragically scarce resources.* New York: W.W. Norton.

Callahan, D. (1990) *What kind of life: The limits of medical progress.* New York: Simon and Schuster.

Campos, P. (2005). Anorexia nation. *Health at Every Size, 19,* 11–17.

Campos, P., Saguy, A., Ernberger, P., Oliver E., & Gaesser, G. (2006). The epidemiology of overweight and obesity: public health crisis or moral panic? *International Journal of Epidemiology, 35,* 55–60.

Carmona, R. (2003, February 28). *"Surgeon general to cops: Put down the donuts." Remarks to the National Sheriff's Association.* Retrieved December 12, 2006, from http://www.cnn.com/2003/HEALTH/02/28/obesity.police/index.html.

Catlin, A., Cowan, C., Heffler, S., & Washington, B. (2007). National health spending in 2005: The slowdown continues. *Health Affairs, 26,* 142–153.

Centers for Disease Control and Prevention (2006). Youth Risk Behavior Surveillance—United States 2005. *Morbidity and Mortality Weekly Report 55*(Suppl. 5), 27–28.

Colquitt J., Clegg, A., Loveman, E., Royle, P., & Sidhu, M. K. (2005, August 15). Surgery for morbid obesity. *The Cochrane Database of Systematic Reviews.* The Cochrane Collaboration. Cochrane review abstract and plain language summary. Retrieved January 19, 2007, from http://www.cochrane.org/reviews/en/ab003641.html.

Cowley, G. (1990). Made to order babies. *Newsweek Special Issue,* Winter/Spring, 98.

Curtland, L. (2005, July 8). Hospitals chasing bariatric surgery business. *Silicone Valley San Jose Business Journal.* Retrieved January 22, 2007, from http://www.bizjournals.com/sanjose/stories/2005/07/11/story4.html.

Delinsky, S. S., Latner, J. D., & Wilson, G. Y. (2006). Binge eating and weight loss in a self-help behavior modification program. *Obesity, 14,* 1244–1249.

Diabetes Prevention Program Research Group (2002). Reduction in the incidence of type 2 diabetes with lifestyle intervention or Metformin. *New England Journal of Medicine, 346,* 393–403.

Drewnowski, A., & Darmon, N. (2005). The economics of obesity: Dietary energy density and energy cost. *American Journal of Clinical Nutrition, 82,* 265S–273S.

Drewnowski, A., & Specter, S. E. (2004). Poverty and obesity: The role of energy density and energy costs. *American Journal of Clinical Nutrition, 79,* 6–16.

Eddy, D. M. (1996). *Clinical decision making: From theory to practice.* Boston: Jones and Bartlett.

Fabricatore, A. N., & Wadden, T. A. (2003). Psychological functioning of obese individuals. *Diabetes Spectrum, 16,* 245–252.

Faraj, M., Jones, P., Sniderman, A.D., & Cianflone, K. (2001) Enhanced dietary fat clearance in postobese women. *Journal of Lipid Research, 42,* 571–580.

Finkelstein E. A., Fiebelkorn, I. C., & Wang, G. (2004). State-level estimates of annual medical expenditures attributable to obesity. *Obesity Research, 12,* 18–24.

Fleck, L. M. (2002). Last chance therapies: can a just and caring society do health care rationing when life itself is at stake? *Yale Journal of Health Policy, Law, and Ethics, 2,* 255–298.

Fleck, L. M. (2006). Creating public conversation about behavioral genetics. In E. Parens, A. Chapman, & N. Press (Eds.), *Wrestling with behavioral genetics: Science, ethics, and public conversation* (pp. 257–285). Baltimore: Johns Hopkins University Press.

Flegal, K. M. (2006). Commentary: The epidemic of obesity—what's in a name? *International Journal of Epidemiology, 35,* 72–74.

Flegal, K. M., Carroll, M. D., Ogden, C. L, & Johnson, C. L. (2002). Prevalence and trends in obesity among U.S. adults, 1999–2000. *Journal of the American Medical Association, 288,* 1723–1727.

Flegal, K. M., Graubard, B. I., Williamson, D. F., & Gail, M. H. (2005). Excess deaths associated with underweight, overweight, and obesity. *Journal of the American Medical Association, 293,* 1861–1867.

Flegal K. M., Troiano, R. P., Pamuk, E. R., Kuczmarski, R. J., & Campbell, S. M. (1995). The influence of smoking cessation on the prevalence of overweight in the United States. *New England Journal of Medicine, 333,* 1165–1170.

Gaesser, G. (2002). *Big fat lies.* Carlsbad, CA: Gurz Books.

Gaesser, G. A. (2006). Is "permanent weight loss" an oxymoron. The stats on weight loss and the National Weight Control Registry. *Health at Every Size, 20,* 91–95.

Gregg, E. W., Cheng, Y. J., Cadwell, B. L., Imperatore, G., Williams, D. E., Flegel, K. M., et al., (2005). Secular trends in cardiovascular disease risk factors according to body mass index in U.S. adults. *Journal of the American Medical Association, 293,* 1868–1874.

Hasin, D. S., Goodwin, R. D., Stinson, F. S., & Grant, B. F. (2005). Epidemiology of major depressive disorder: Results from the National Epidemiologic Survey on Alcoholism and Related Conditions. *Archives of General Psychiatry, 62,* 1097–1106.

Heffler, S., Smith, S., Keehan, S., Borger, C., Clemens, M., & Truffer, C. (2005). U.S. health spending projections for 2004–14. *Health Affairs, 24* (Suppl. 1), W5, 74–85.

Hill, J. O., Thomson, H., & Wyatt, H. (2005). Weight maintenance: What's missing? *Journal of the American Dietetic Association, 105,* S63–S66.

Hill, J. O., Wyatt, H., Phelan, S., & Wing, R. (2005). The National Weight Loss Registry: Is it useful in helping deal with our obesity epidemic? *Journal of Nutrition Education and Behavior, 37,* 206–210.

Ikeda, J. (2004, October). *Connecting the dots: Providers, patients and the fight for health.* Paper presented at the Michigan Department of Community Health conference "Obesity in Michigan: Join the Fight for Health," Novi, MI.

Infanger, D., Baldinger, R., Branson, R., Barbier, T., Steffen, R., & Horber, F. F. (2003). Effect of significant intermediate-term weight loss on serum leptin levels and body composition in severely obese subjects. *Obesity Surgery, 13,* 879–888.

Kaplan, J. R., Adams, M. R., Clarkson, T. B., Manuck, S. B., & Shively, C. A. (1991) Social behavior and gender in biomedical investigations using monkeys: Studies in atherogenesis. *Laboratory Animal Science, 41,* 334–343.

Keys, A., Brozek, J., Henschel, A., Mickelsen, O., & Taylor, H. L. (1950). *The biology of human starvation I–II.* Minneapolis: University of Minnesota Press.

Kip, K. E., Marroquin, O. C., Kelley, D. E., Johnson, D., Kelsey, S. F., Shaw, L. J., et al. (2004) Clinical importance of obesity versus the metabolic syndrome in cardiovascular risk in women. A report from the Women's Ischemia Syndrome Evaluation (WISE) Study. *Circulation, 109,* 706–713.

Krauss R. M., Eckel, R. H., Howard, B., Appel, L. J., Daniels, S. R., Deckelbaum, R. J., et al. (2000). AHA Dietary Guidelines: revision 2000: A statement for healthcare professionals from the nutrition committee of the American Heart Association. *Circulation, 102,* 2284–2299.

LaMonte, M. J, & Blair, S. (2006). Physical activity, cardiorespiratory fitness, and adiposity: Contributions to disease risk. *Current Opinionsin Clinical Nutrition and Metabolic Care, 9,* 540–546.

Langer, Gary. (2005, February 13). *ABC News poll: Traffic in the United States.* Retrieved December 15, 2006, from http://abcnews.go.com/Technology/Traffic/story?id=485098&page=1.

Lyon, H. N, & Hirschorn, J. N. (2005). Genetics of common forms of obesity: A brief review. *American Journal of Clinical Nutrition, 82*(Suppl.), 215S–217S.

Malinowski, M. M. (2006). Nutritional and metabolic complications of bariatric surgery. *The American Journal of the Medical Sciences, 331,* 219–225.

Marketdata Enterprises. (2005). *The U.S. Weight Loss and Diet Control Market* (8th ed.). Tampa, FL: Marketdata Enterprises, Inc.

McGuire, M. T., Wing, R. R., & Hill, J. O. (1999). The prevalence of weight loss maintenance among American adults. *International Journal of Obesity, 23,* 1314–1319.

Michigan Department of Community Health. (2005, June 30). *Preventing obesity and reducing chronic disease: The Michigan healthy eating and physical activity plan. A five-year plan to address the obesity epidemic.* Lansing, MI: Michigan Department of Community Health.

Mitka, M. (2006). Surgery useful for morbid obesity, but safety and efficacy questions linger. *Journal of the American Medical Association, 296,* 1575–1577.

NIH Technology Assessment Conference Panel. (1993). Methods for voluntary weight loss and control. NIH Technology Assessment Conference Panel. Consensus Development Conference, March 30 to April 1, 1992. *Annals of Internal Medicine, 119*(7 Pt. 2), 764–770.

Nord, M., Andrews, M., & Carlson, S. (2006, November). *Household Food Security in the United States, 2005.* Economic Research Report No. ERR-29. United States Department of Agriculture. Retrieved January 17, 2007, from http://www.ers.usda.gov/publications/err29/.

Puhl, R., & Brownell, K. D. (2001). Bias, discrimination, and obesity. *Obesity Research, 1,* 788–805.

Rawls, J. (1971). *A theory of justice.* Cambridge, MA: Harvard University Press.

Reuters Health Information. (2006, November 24). *Complication rates of bariatric surgery vary by hospital experience.* Retrieved January 21, 2007, from http://www.medscape.com/viewarticle/548260.

Saguy, A. C., & Riley, K. W. (2005). Weighing both sides: morality, mortality and framing contests over obesity. *Journal of Health Politics, Policy, and Law, 30,* 869–921.

Schwartz, T. L., Nihalani, N., Jindal, S., Virk, S., & Jones, N. (2004). Psychiatric medication-induced obesity: A review. *Obesity Reviews, 5,* 115–121.

Shah, M., Simha, V., & Garg, A. (2006). Long-term impact of bariatric surgery on body weight, comorbidities, and nutritional status. *Journal of Clinical Endocrinology and Metabolism, 91,* 4223–4231.

Sours, H. E., Frattali, V. P., Brand, C. D., Feldman, R. A., Forbes, A. L., et al. (1981). Sudden death associated with very low calorie weight reduction regimens. *American Journal of Clinical Nutrition, 34,* 453–461.

Strychar, I. (2006, January 3). Diet in the management of weight loss (Review). *Canadian Medical Association Journal.* Retrieved January 21, 2007, from http://www.cmaj.ca/cgi/content/full/174/1/56#R71–21.

Sturm, R. (2002). The effects of obesity, smoking and drinking on medical problems and costs. *Health Affairs (Millwood), 21,* 245–253.

Tankó, L. B., Bagger, Y. Z., Alexandersen, P., Larsen, P. J., & Christiansen, C. (2003) Peripheral adiposity exhibits an independent dominant antiatherogenic effect in elderly women. *Circulation, 107,* 1626.

Teachman, B. A., & Brownell, K. D. (2001). Implicit anti-fat bias among health professionals: Is anyone immune? *International Journal of Obesity and Related Metabolic Disorders, 25,* 1525–1531.

Ubel, P. (2000). *Pricing life: Why it's time for health care rationing.* Cambridge, MA: MIT Press.

U.S. Department of Transportation, Bureau of Transportation Statistics. (2004). *Summary of Travel Trends 2001.* National Household Travel Study. Retrieved November 12, 2006, from http://nhts.ornl.gov/2001/pub/STT.pdf.

Villareal, D. T., Fontana, L., Weiss, E. P., Racette, S. B., Steger-May, K., Schechtman, K. B., et al. (2006). Bone mineral density response to caloric restriction–induced weight loss or exercise-induced weight loss. *Archives of Internal Medicine, 166,* 2502–2510.

Wilde, P. E., & Peterman, J. N. (2006). Individual weight change is associated with household food security status. *Journal of Nutrition, 136,* 1395–1400.

Wing, R. R., & Phelan, S. (2005). Long-term weight loss maintenance. *American Journal of Clinical Nutrition, 82*(1 Suppl.), 222S–225S.

World Health Organization. (2006). *Obesity and Overweight. Fact Sheet No. 311.* Retrieved January 18, 2007, from http://www.who.int/mediacentre/factsheets/fs311/en/index.html.

Young, L. R., & Nestle, M. (2002). The contribution of expanding portion sizes to the U.S. obesity epidemic. *American Journal of Public Health, 92,* 246–249.

ABOUT THE EDITORS
AND CONTRIBUTORS

JAY BELSKY, PhD, is professor of psychology and director of the Institute for the Study of Children, Families and Social Issues, Birkbeck University of London. His reearch interests include parent-child relationships, the effects of day care, the etiology of child maltreatment, and the evolutionary basis of parent and child functioning. He is a founding investigator on the National Institute of Child Health and Development (NICHD) Study of Child Care and Youth Development (U.S.) and that National Evaluation of Sure Start (UK). In 2006 he received the American Psychological Association Urie Bronfenbrenner Award for Lifetime Contribution to Developmental Psychology in the Service of Science and Society.

ROBERT H. BRADLEY, PhD, is professor and director of the Center for Applied Studies in Education at the University of Arkansas at Little Rock and adjunct professor of Pediatrics and Psychiatry at the University of Arkansas for Medical Sciences. His research interests include child care, early education, fathers, and family factors that affect child well-being. He served as associate editor of Child Development and currently serves as associate editor of Early Childhood Research Quarterly. He served as chair of the Biobehavioral and Behavioral Research Committee for NICHD and currently serves on the advisory boards for the Maternal Lifestyle Study, the American Indian/Alaska Native Head Start Research Center, the National Household Education Survey, and the Arkansas Birth Defects Research Center and on the steering committees for the NICHD

Study of Child Care and Youth Development and the Early Head Start National Evaluation Study.

ROBERT CROSNOE, PhD, is associate professor of sociology at the University of Texas at Austin and a fellow at the Texas Population Research Center. His research investigates the connection between social development and education and its role in demographic inequalities. His recent book is Mexican Children, American Schools (Stanford University Press, 2006). Crosnoe is the winner of young scholar awards from the Society for Research in Child Development, American Sociological Association (Children and Youth Section), and the William T. Grant Foundation.

H. DELE DAVIES, MD, MS, is professor and chairperson of pediatrics and human development at Michigan State University. He is also chairman of the university's 45-member Obesity Research Council and a member of the Michigan Quality Improvement Consortium Guidelines Committee that developed a Pediatric Healthy Weight Toolkit for management of obesity. He is an elected member of the Society for Pediatric Research and the American Pediatric Society. Davies is a reviewer for many journals including the New England Journal of Medicine, Pediatrics, Journal of Pediatrics, The Lancet, and the Journal of the American Medical Association.

RANDAL D. DAY, PhD, is a professor in the School of Family Life at Brigham Young University. He is also the associate director of the School of Family Life and the director of the Family Studies Center. His research interests include family processes, father involvement, parent-child interaction, and father re-entry from prison. Day is a Fellow of the National Council on Relations and has served as a section chair and board member for that organization. He is the principal investigator for the "Flourishing Families Project," which is currently interviewing over 400 families in Seattle (parents and children) about their experiences within inner-family life and the transition into young adulthood.

IHUOMA ENELI, MD, is associate professor of pediatrics at the Ohio State University College of Medicine and associate director, Columbus Children's Center for Healthy Weight and Nutrition. She coordinates the clinical programs within the center and has been a board certified general pediatrician practicing primary care for the last 10 years. Eneli has received funding for her work and has led different multidisciplinary obesity projects. Her primary research interest focuses on the health care providers perspective on managing the overweight child. A fellow of the American Academy of Pediatrics (AAP), she is active in the Ambulatory Pediatric Association Obesity Interest Group.

HIRAM E. FITZGERALD, PhD, is associate provost for University Outreach and Engagement and University Distinguished Professor of Psychology at Michigan State University, and adjunct professor of psychiatry at the University of Michigan Medical School. A Fellow of the American Psychological Association and the American Psychological Society, his research interests include the study of biobehavioral organization during infancy and early childhood, father involvement in early child development, community prevention programs for families with very young children, the etiology of alcohol problems, and campus-community engagement. He serves on the steering committee of the American Indian/ Alaska Native Head Start Research Center. Since 1992 he has been executive director of the World Association for Infant Mental Health.

LEONARD M. FLECK, PhD, is professor of philosophy and medical ethics in the Philosophy Department and Center for Ethics and Humanities in the Life Sciences at Michigan State University. His primary areas of academic interest are health care ethics (especially issues related to health care justice, rationing, and resource allocation), ethical and policy issues related to genetics and reproductive decisionmaking, and the role of rational democratic deliberation in addressing all these issues. He is currently completing a book for Oxford University Press titled Just Caring: The Ethical Challenges of Health Care Rationing and Democratic Deliberation. He received a Distinguished Faculty Award from Michigan State University in 2003.

SARA GABLE, PhD, is currently associate professor and State Extension Specialist in Human Development and Family Studies, University of Missouri, Columbia. Her research interests include child care provider workforce development, the socialization of children's nutrition and activity habits, and the developmental correlates and consequences of persistent childhood overweight. For Extension, she designs and delivers educational programs for child care providers on topics such as child observation, making math fun, and socializing healthy habits in young children.

SHEILA GAHAGAN, MD, MPH, is the president of the Michigan chapter of the American Academy of Pediatrics (AAP). She is a developmental-behavioral pediatrician at Mott Children's Hospital and a research scientist at the Center for Human Growth and Development, both at the University of Michigan. Gahagan's work focuses on early life conditions that lead to later poor health outcomes and the role of social factors in health disparities.

JEFFREY M. GAUVIN, MD, is a board certified surgeon and an assistant professor of surgery at the University of California, Davis. He completed fellowship training in gastrointestinal surgery and is currently the Program Director of the University of California, Davis general surgery residency program. His interests include gastrointestinal surgery and surgical education.

MICHELLE HENRY is a graduate student at Case Western Reserve University, pursuing a Master's degree in public health nutrition. She received undergraduate degrees in dietetics and nutritional sciences from Michigan State University, where she worked with professors researching eating behaviors and diet quality in low-income women and children.

MILDRED A. HORODYNSKI, PhD, RNC, is a professor in the College of Nursing at Michigan State University. Her research interests focus on interventions for the prevention of childhood obesity targeting infants and toddlers. She is a member of the National Research Consortium for the longitudinal evaluation of the effectiveness of Early Head Start programs. Her two current research projects are funded by United States Department of Agriculture, Nursing Research Institute—Cooperative State, Research, Education and Extension Service, and by Department of Health and Human Services: Administration for Children, Youth, and Families.

RENATE HOUTS is a senior research psychometrician at RTI International in Research Triangle Park, North Carolina. Her research focuses on how normal children grow and develop in a variety of contexts and the methodologies needed to capture change in individuals and relationships over time. RTI International is a trade name of Research Triangle Institute.

ROBIN JOSEPH, MA, is a limited licensed psychologist and a family therapist in the pediatrics program at Michigan State University, Kalamazoo Center for Medical Studies in Kalamazoo, Michigan. She is also a doctoral candidate in clinical psychology at Walden University, Minneapolis. Joseph's research is in the area of type 2 diabetes and obesity.

MANMOHAN KAMBOJ, MD, is a pediatric endocrinologist, assistant professor in the department of pediatrics at Michigan State University, Kalamazoo Center for Medical Studies in Kalamazoo, Michigan. She is very actively involved in patient care for patients with endocrine disorders and diabetes. She takes great interest in the teaching programs for residents and medical students as well. Prior to coming to Kalamazoo, Kamboj completed her residency and fellowship training at New York University Medical Center in New York.

JENNIFER L. KRULL, PhD, is currently an associate professor of quantitative psychology at the University of Missouri, Columbia. Her research interests focus on the development, application, and extension of random coefficient models (also known as multilevel or hierarchical linear models) in social science data.

KARAH DANIELS MANTINAN, MPH, RD, is a research assistant with the Michigan State University Department of Pediatrics and Human Development. She is also a public health consultant for the Michigan Department of Community Health where she specializes in obesity prevention and treatment and population-based nutrition interventions. Her research interests include the influence of environment, policies, and media on eating and physical activity behaviors and integrated, multisetting approaches to obesity prevention and control across the lifespan.

ELIZABETH S. MOORE, PhD, is associate professor and Notre Dame Chair in Marketing at the University of Notre Dame. Her research interests are in marketing and society, the consumer behavior of households, and marketing to children. Moore has published her work in a number of journals, books, and conference proceedings. She has received recognitions for her teaching and research, including the Best Paper Award from the Journal of Consumer Research and the Kinnear Best Paper Award from the Journal of Public Policy and Marketing. She serves on the editorial boards of the Journal of Public Policy and Marketing and the Journal of Macromarketing. Prior to joining the faculty at Notre Dame, she served on the faculties of Boston College and the University of Illinois.

KELLY MOORE, MD, is a member of the Muscogee (Creek) Nation of Oklahoma, is a clinical consultant with the Indian Health Service Division of Diabetes Treatment and Prevention in Albuquerque, New Mexico. With more than 19 years of experience in the Indian Health Service in American Indian communities in Montana, Utah, Arizona, and Washington, she also serves as the Association of American Indian Physicians liaison to the Committee on Native American Child Health of the American Academy of Pediatrics and as the chair of the Natial Diabetes Education Program's American Indian/Alaska Native Work Group. She is a Fellow of the American Academy of Pediatrics. Her primary research interests are childhood overweight, childhood type 2 diabetes, urban Indian health, and health care disparities.

VASILIKI MOUSOULI, PhD, is a school psychologist currently practicing in Greece at the International School of Athens (ISA) with a student population ranging from 2 to 12 years old. She is also a lecturer in the psychology program of the London Metropolitan University located at the Brethern College Abroad College in Athens. Her research interests are in the areas of developmental psychopathology and prevention and include the study of competence, risk and protective factors in childhood and their link to psychopathology or resilience.

PHILIP R. NADER, MD, has a distinguished career of more than 30 years in community research and education. He has held tenured faculty positions at the University of Rochester, the University of Texas Medical Branch at Galveston, and the University of California at San Diego. He retired in 2003 as the founding chief of the Division of Community Pediatrics, having headed several multidisciplinary research teams investigating both epidemiological and randomized experimental trials dealing with childhood activity and nutrition. He continues his active research career as a co-investigator at the National Institute of Child Health Early Child Care Research Network with a focus on obesity and physical activity.

MARION O'BRIEN, PhD is professor in the Department of Human Development and Family Studies at the University of North Carolina at Greensboro (UNCG) and director of the Family Research Center at UNCG, which conducts research on parent-child relationships and early childhood development. O'Brien is one of the core investigators of the NICHD Study of Early Child Care and Youth Development, a 15-year-long longitudinal multisite study of children and families, and has conducted research on parenting, parent-child relationships, and children's physical, social, and cognitive development. This work includes research on families of children with autism and other developmental disabilities, families of children who are at medical risk, adoptive and foster care families, as well as families of typically developing children.

KAREN A. PETERSMARCK, MPH, PhD, recently retired from the Michigan Department of Community Health, where she served as manager of the Obesity Prevention Program. Throughout her 36-year career, she worked in local, state, and federal public health programs, taught at three Michigan colleges, and ran a successful consulting business. Currently she serves on the editorial board for the Journal of Physical Activity and Health and does limited consulting and public speaking.

JAMES M. PIVARNIK, PhD, is a professor in the departments of kinesiology and epidemiology at Michigan State University and adjunct professor in the Department of Pediatrics and Human Development. He is a vice president and Fellow of the American College of Sports Medicine, and associate editor of the journal, Medicine and Science in Sports and Exercise. Pivarnik's research interests focus on physical activity epidemiology, particularly as it relates to pregnancy, the postpartum period, and children.

HELEN D. PRATT, PhD, received her doctoral degree in clinical psychology from Western Michigan University in 1988 and completed her internship at Kalamazoo Regional Psychiatric Hospital in Kalamazoo, Michigan. She is a licensed psychologist and is the director of behavioral and developmental pediatrics in the pediatrics program at Michigan State University, Kalamazoo Center for Medical Studies. Pratt is also a professor of pediatrics and human development at Michigan State University (Kalamazoo Campus) and as an adjunct professor of psychology at Western Michigan University. Her publications have focused on increasing clinician knowledge about issues that affect the lives of children and adolescence with a focus on correcting myths and stereotypes in the literature regarding minorities.

KAMI J. SILK, PhD, is an assistant professor in the Department of Communication and the director of the Master's program in health communication at Michigan State University. She is a health communication researcher, with a specific interest in developing effective health messages for the lay public and diverse audiences that are sensitive to health literacy issues. Silk currently works with the Breast Cancer and Environment Research Centers, funded by the National Cancer Institute and National Institute for Environmental Health Sciences, as part of the Communication Outreach and Translation Core to develop health messages for mothers and adolescent girls that focus on nutrition and exercise as strategies for breast cancer risk reduction.

PAUL SPICER, PhD, is a cultural anthropologist with expertise in substance abuse and child development in American Indian and Alaska Native communities. Since 1995, he has been on the faculty of the American Indian and Alaska Native Programs at the University of Colorado, where he is now associate professor of psychiatry, with primary responsibilities for multimethod research in early childhood development and intervention. His current research, some of which is reported here, is funded by the National Center for Minority Health and Health Disparities, the National Institute for Child Health and Human Development, the National Institute of Mental Health, and the Robert Wood Johnson Foundation.

ARATHI SRIKANTA, BS, graduated from the University of Missouri, Columbia with a degree in psychological sciences. While there, she conducted research on obesity, adolescent risky behavior, juvenile delinquency and multisystemic therapy, and peer relationships. She is currently a counselor at Castlewood Treatment Center for Eating Disorders in St. Louis, Missouri. She wishes to pursue a doctorate in clinical psychology.

MATHEW P. THORPE, MA, is a pre-doctoral fellow in nutritional sciences at the University of Illinois, Urbana-Champaign Medical Scholars Program. His research interests include the multifactorial etiology of obesity across the lifespan and the nutritional management of obesity-related chronic disease. He is a National Needs Fellow of the United States Department of Agriculture.

KIMBERLYDAWN WISDOM, MD, MPH, is the first ever Surgeon General in Michigan, the first State Surgeon General in the United States, and Vice-President of Community Health for the Henry Ford Health Systems. Prior to her appointment to Surgeon General she served as the founder and director for the Institute on Multicultural Health at Henry Ford Health System. Dr. Wisdom has been a board-certified emergency medicine physician at Henry Ford Health System for more than 20 years and an assistant professor of medical education at the University of Michigan Medical Center. She was also the founder and director of a community-based health screening initiative entitled "AIMHI" (African American Initiative for Male Health Improvement). As Michigan Surgeon General, Dr. Wisdom has focused on the economic and social implications of the lack of preventative measures concerning obesity, physical inactivity, unhealthy eating habits, childhood lead poisoning, tobacco use, chronic disease, infant mortality, unintended pregnancy, coordinated school health, HIV/AIDS, health disparities, and suicide.

JOHN WOROBEY, PhD, is professor and chair of the Department of Nutritional Sciences at Rutgers University. A developmental psychologist by training, he is also an adjunct associate professor of pediatrics at the University of Medicine and Dentistry of New Jersey. His current research focuses on the temperamental correlates of infant excess weight gain, and is funded by the National Institute for Child Health and Human Development.

INDEX

academic difficulties, 50, 51, 52–55; and behavior problems, 50, 52; cross-sectional studies, 52–53; and lack of food, 56; prospective/longitudinal studies, 53–55; relationship to weight status, 53; research base limitations, 55–57; and television viewing, 56–57

ACSM. *See* American College of Sports Medicine (ACSM)

Add Health Study, 123; approach to families using, 130–36; family processes, 133–36; structural risk factors, 130–31

adolescents: assessments of, 179–81, 180*t*; BMI measure of obesity, 168–69; definition of overweight in, 168–69; prevalence of obesity in, 37–39; treatment options for, 181–82

adults, stigma-based expectations of, 51

advergaming: brand reinforcement via, 97–99; defined, 93

Aerobics Center Longitudinal Study, 41

African Americans: high fat intake eating habits of, 172; maternal attitudes to-ward infant weight, 16; mortality rate of males, 174; obesity in, 167–84; overweight in children, 4; overweight in youth (12–19 years of age), 169

African Americans, youth, 167–84; physical activity of, 172; television viewing habits of, 172–73; treatment options, 182, 184

alcohol consumption, 29

American Association of Bariatric Surgeons, 251

American College of Sports Medicine (ACSM), 34, 37

American Indian (AI)/Alaska Native (AN) populations: consequences of obesity, 143–45; obesity prevention for infants/families, 153–56; prevalence of obesity, 145–46; and risk/protective factors, 149–51

American Indian (AI)/Alaska Native (AN) populations, programs/studies: American Indian and Alaska Native Programs, 154; Behavioral Risk Factor Surveillance Study, 32, 34, 150; Indian Health Diabetes Best Practices, 155; Nurse-Family Partnership, 154; Pathways Feasibility Study, 151; SEARCH for Diabetes in Youth Study Group, 145; Special Diabetes Program for Indians, 155, 156; Strong Heart Study, 146, 149; tribal nutrition programs, 146

American Indian and Alaska Native Programs (University of Colorado), 154

Amsterdam Growth and Health study, 35

anthropometric study, of height/weight/ skinfold thickness, 171

appearance-based stigma: in adolescence, 64–66; in middle childhood, 62–63

assessments, of adolescents/children, 179–81, 180*t*; BMI, 181; laboratory testing, 180–81; of physical activity, 180; of television viewing time, 180

asthma, 174

bariatric surgery: banded gastroplasties, 256–58; history of, 252–58; jejunoileal bypass, 252–53; open/laparoscopic approaches, 258; operative mortality/ complications, 264–65; outcomes, 262–64; patient selection, 260–61; perioperative care, 262; post-operative care, 262; pre-operative care, 258–59; Roux-en-Y gastric bypass, 253–55

beauty: media influences on, 179; Western ideal of, 177–78

behavioral approaches, to obesity, 213–15, 219–20; pharmacologic treatment, 215, 219; social cognitive theory, 214; transtheoretical model of change, 214

Behavioral Risk Factor Surveillance Study, 32, 34, 150

behavior problems, 50, 52

binge eating disorder (BED), 193

birth size, and fatness measures, 7

birth weight, and BMI, 7–8

blood glucose levels, 28

Blount's disease, 196

BMI. *See* body mass index (BMI)

body fat: distribution of, 175, 177; physiological role of, 123

body mass index (BMI): and birth weight, 7–8; CDC age and sex growth chart, 119*f*–120*f*; description/guidelines for use, 39–41; heritability estimates of, 123; as measure of obesity, 4, 55, 168–69; and physical activity, 35; of pre-pregnant women, and infant body weight, 10; and rapid growth, 8. *See*

also National Institute of Child Health and Human Development (NICHD) Study of Early Child Care and Youth Development

body size, Western ideal of, 177–78

breastfeeding behaviors: human vs. cow's milk, 13; of overweight/obese women, 10–11; by race/ethnicity/ socioeconomics, 15–16

Bronfenbrenner, Urie, 7, 50–51

calories: caloric expenditure (indirect calorimetry), 31–32; caloric restriction, 172

CARDIA study. *See* Coronary Artery Risk Development in Young Adults (CARDIA) study

cardiovascular disease, 121–22, 194–95

CATCH study, 152

Caucasian adolescent girls: body fat distribution of, 175, 177; body mass index of, 175; dietary habits of, 175

causes, of obesity, 26, 50, 171–73; Cushing's syndrome, 181; genetic predisposition, 123–24, 171; high-fat diets, 172; hormonal imbalances, 26, 29, 171; sleep apnea, 181, 195–96. *See also* physical activity; television viewing

CDC. *See* Centers for Disease Control and Prevention (CDC)

Center for Science in the Public Interest (CSPI), 94

Centers for Disease Control and Prevention (CDC), 4; BMI growth chart for age and sex, 119*f*–120*f*; fruit/ vegetable indicators of health, 175; physical activity recommendations, 34, 37, 39

children: assessments of, 179–81, 180*t*; BMI measure of obesity, 4, 168–69; definition of overweight in, 168–69; difficulty resisting commercial messages, 95; management of, 191–221; obesity-related diseases of, 121–22, 167; prevalence of obesity in, 37–39; psychosocial illnesses of, 122; stigmatization of, 60–61; treatment options, 181–82; television advertising aimed at, 103–4; weight status/

academic difficulty relationship, 53. *See also* infants/early childhood

children, Web sites aimed at: design of, 94, 95, 96; incentives for product purchase, 106

children, Web site protections for, 106–8; ad-break reminders, 107–8; information for parents, 107; privacy protections/age blocks, 107

Children Are Our Messengers: Changing the Health study, 173–74

Children's Online Privacy Protection Act, 105

cholelithiasis, 167

Clinical Guidelines on the Identification, Evaluation and Treatment of Overweight and Obesity in Adults report (NIH), 121

commercials, and message resistance difficulties, 95

Competitive Media Reports (CMR) data, 96

consequences, of obesity, 143–45, 173–74; medical, 192*t*; psychological, 192*t*; social/economic, 193–94. *See also* diseases, related to obesity

Coronary Artery Risk Development in Young Adults (CARDIA) study, 30, 35, 36

cross-sectional studies, of academic difficulties, 52–53; females/males, 7th/9th/11th grade, 52–53; 3rd/4th graders, 52

cultural attitudes, toward infant weight, 16

depression, 73, 122, 174

developmental risk factors, of obesity, 3–18; academic difficulties, 49–50; behavior problems, 49; energy balance equation, 5–6; of low-birth-weight, 7–8; metabolic syndrome, 8; psychosocial functioning difficulties, 49; social isolation, 49; type 2 diabetes, 8

diabetes/pre-diabetes, 8, 121, 167, 195

dietary approaches, to obesity, 209–12; altered macronutrient diets, 210–12; balanced macronutrient diet, 210

diseases, related to obesity, 121–22, 167; asthma, 174; Blount's disease, 196; cholelithiasis, 167, 181; diabetes/pre-diabetes, 121, 181; hyperlipidemia, 167; hypertension, childhood, 167; metabolic syndrome, 7, 8, 167, 181; non-alcoholic steatohepatitis, 167, 195; type 2 diabetes, 8, 167

do no harm principle, of obesity intervention, 280–96; necessity of weight loss decision, 284–88; safety of weight loss concern, 280–84

doubly labeled water (DLW) method, of energy expenditure measurement, 5–6

early childhood. *See* infants/early childhood

ecological model of excess weight gain, 6–7; microsystem/exosystem/obesigenic environment, 7

ecological model of excess weight gain (macrosystem, mother-infant dyad), 15–18; breastfeeding patterns by race/ethnicity, 15–16; cultural/maternal attitudes toward infant weight, 16; obesigenic environment, modern, 7, 16–18

ecological model of excess weight gain (microsystem, infant factors), 7–10; birth weight/later BMI, 7–8; rapid growth/later BMI, 8; temperament/early weight gain, 8–10

ecological model of excess weight gain (microsystem, maternal factors), 10–13; feeding method/subsequent fatness, 11–13; maternal BMI/infant overweight, 10–11

energy balance: defined, 28; and DLW measure, 5–6; intake and expenditure, 171–72; and metabolism, 28–30; modulation of, 29–30; normal weight vs. overweight/obesity, 30

energy cost, of physical activity, 33–35; moderate activity/METS, 33–34; vigorous activity/METS, 34

energy dense foods, 27

energy expenditure, resting, 31–33; caloric expenditure (indirect calorimetry),

31–32; *MET* measure, 32; NEAT value, 33; and spontaneous physical activity, 32; thermic effect of food, 32
ethical considerations, of interventions, 271–96; disagreement about obesity, 27; high stakes considerations, 271; weight loss treatment, social context, 274–75
ethical considerations, of interventions (moral principles/personal/professional), 272–73; do no harm principle, 273, 280–96; patient right of autonomy/personal responsibility, 272–73, 275–80
ethical considerations, of interventions (social justice issues), 273–74; rationing of resources, 274; societal costs, 273
exercise: non-exercise activity thermogenesis, 33; vs. physical activity, 30

families, approach to, using Add Health, 130–36; family processes, 133–36; structural risk factors, 130–31
families, processes, in obesity literature, 127–29; activity, 128–29; influence of energy balance, 127–28; sociodemographic influences, 129
Feeding Infants and Toddlers Study (FITS), 17
feeding methods. *See* infant feeding, dynamics; infant feeding, methods
findings: of NICHD Study, 82–86; of online food marketing assessment, 96–108
foods: energy density of, 27; lack of, and academic difficulty, 56; thermic effects of, 32
Food Standards Agency (FSA), 93

GEMS Pilot Study (Stanford), 213
genetic predisposition, to obesity, 123–24, 171; inheritance risk factor/Add Health study, 135–36; mechanism of body weight regulation, 124; and phenotypes, 123; thrifty genotypes, 124
girls, adolescent: Caucasians vs. African Americans: BMI, 175; dietary habits, 175

Harvard Alumni Health Study, 41
Health and Human Services, Dept. of (USDHHS), 25
health costs, of obesity, 121–22
health indicators, 25–26
Health Professionals study (U.S.), 36
health-related fitness components: body composition, 31; cardiorespiratory fitness, 31; musculoskeletal strength, 31
Healthy People 2010, 25
Hispanic infants: breastfeeding patterns, 15; maternal attitudes toward infant weight, 16; and overweight, 4
hormonal imbalances, 26, 29, 171
hospitalizations, obesity-related, 191
hyperlipidemia, 167
hypertension, childhood, 167

Indian Health Diabetes Best Practices, 155
Indian Health Service Division, of Diabetes Treatment and Prevention, 154
indirect calorimetry (caloric expenditure), 31–32
infant feeding, dynamics, 13–15; formula and overfeeding, 13–14; solid food introduction, 14
infant feeding, methods: formula fed infants, 13–14; solid food introduction, 14; and subsequent fatness, 11–13; of white, non-Hispanic infants, 13
infant obesity: contributing factors, 5, 7–8; differential patterns of, 5
infants/early childhood: difficult, defined, 9; DLW measure of energy expenditure, 5–6; ecological model of excess weight gain, 6–7; feeding dynamics/methods, 13–14; formula-fed/activity levels, 9; length/weight measure of obesity, 4; and media screening, 59–60; microsystem/exosystem/obesigenic environment, 7; motor development of, 58–59; nutrition guidelines/ recommendations, 232–33; stigmatization of, 60–61; and television viewing, 59
Institute of Medicine (IOM), 25, 34–35, 93, 94, 123, 152

insulin resistance, 121
International Society on Hypertension in Blacks, 173–74
Internet access, of families, 94
interventions, 196, 209–15, 219–20; behavioral approaches, 213–15; ethical considerations of, 271–96; pharmacologic treatment, 215, 219; physical activity approaches, 213; surgical treatment, 219–20
interventions, dietary approaches, 209–12; altered macronutrient diets, 210–12; balanced macronutrient diet, 210; trust model, 212
IOM. *See* Institute of Medicine (IOM)

juicyfruit.com (Wrigleys), 95

Latino American youth, 167–84; body fat distribution, 175, 177; high fat intake eating habits of, 172; physical activity of, 172; television viewing habits of, 172–73; treatment options, 182, 184

management, of overweight children, 191–221; psychological sequelae, 192–94
management, of overweight children, interventions, 196, 209–15, 219–20; behavioral approaches, 213–15; dietary approaches, 209–12; pharmacologic treatment, 215, 219; physical activity approaches, 213; surgical treatment, 219–20
management, of overweight children, medical sequelae: Blount's disease, 196; cardiovascular disease, 194–95; early maturation, 194; fatty liver/non-alcoholic steatohepatitis, 167, 195; sleep apnea, 195–96; type 2 diabetes, 195
Masai infants, 9
measurement tools: actometers, 9; DLW method, 5–6; triceps skinfold thickness, 52
media, influences on beauty ideal, 179
media screening, of infants/early childhood, 59–60

Medical Expenditures Survey, 26
metabolic syndrome, 7, 8, 167
metabolism, and energy balance, 28–30
MET (one metabolic equivalent), 32; moderate activity, 33–34; vigorous activity, 34
middle childhood, 61–63; appearance-based stigmatization, 62–63; social stigma/stereotype threat, 61–62
minority youth: body fat distribution, 175, 177; physical activity levels of, 172; television viewing habits of, 172–73
mood disorders, 73
moral principles, of obesity interventions, conclusions, 279–80; complexity, 279; dangerous metaphors, 279–80; paternalism, 280
moral principles, of obesity interventions, personal/professional, 272–73; do no harm principle, 273, 280–96; patient right to autonomy/personal responsibility, 272–73, 275–80
mother-infant dyad, in macrosystem, 15–18; attitudes toward infant weight, 16; breastfeeding patterns by race/ethnicity, 15–16; cultural/maternal attitudes toward infant weight, 16; obesigenic environment, modern, 16–18
mothers: breastfeeding behaviors of, 10–11; control during feeding, 14–15; feeding methods/subsequent fatness, 11–13; obese vs. lean, and DLW method, 6; perception of difficult child, 9; pre-pregnant BMI/infant birth weight, 10
motor development, of infants/early childhood, 58

National Academy of Sciences, 25
National Advertising Review Council (NARC), 94
National Health and Nutrition Examination Survey, 35, 50
National Health Interview Survey, 26
National Institute of Child Health and Human Development, Early Care Research Network, 18

National Institute of Child Health and Human Development (NICHD) Study of Early Child Care and Youth Development: families participating in, 74, 76–77; statistical methods/analysis of data, 81–82

National Institute of Child Health and Human Development (NICHD) Study of Early Child Care and Youth Development (findings), 82–86; BMI and internalizing problems, 84*t*; BMI-internalizing problems correlation, 84*t*; characteristics/descriptive statistics, 83*t*; interpretation of, 86–88; refining baseline model, 84–85; stability of internalizing problems, 84*t*; testing moderators, 86

National Institute of Child Health and Human Development (NICHD) Study of Early Child Care and Youth Development (longitudinal procedures), 77–81; BMI, height, weight, 78; changes in household composition, 80; changes in residence, 80; changes in schools within school year, 81; changes in type/amount of child care, 80; gender, 79; internalizing behavior problems, 79; life instability, 79; maternal/paternal employment status changes, 80; negative emotionality, 79

National Institutes of Health (NIH), 121

National Longitudinal Study of Adolescent Health, 193

National Medical Expenditures Panel Survey, 26

Native Americans. *See* American Indian (AI)/Alaska Native (AN) populations

NEAT. *See* non-exercise activity thermogenesis (NEAT)

Neopets.com, 96

Nick.com, 96

Nielsen/Net rating reports, 94

non-alcoholic steatohepatitis (NASH), 167, 195

non-exercise activity thermogenesis (NEAT), 33

Nurse-Family Partnership, 154

nutrition: infants/early childhood recommendations, 232–33; interventions for obesity, 233–36; National Health and Nutrition Examination Survey, 35, 50; online food marketing, findings, 100–101; Pediatric Nutrition Surveillance System, 10; Pregnancy Nutrition Surveillance System, 10; prevention efforts, 235–36; role of parents, 235; Third National Health and Nutrition Examination Survey, 191; tribal nutrition programs, 146

obesigenic environment: description of, 7; modern, 16–18; precipitating changes in environments, 276–77

obesity: in African Americans, 167–84; assessment parameters, 227–32; BMI as determination of, 4, 119*f*–120*f*; causes of, 171; combined with physical fitness, 41; concerns regarding, 121–22; consequences of, 143–45, 173–74, 192*t*, 193–94; definitions/overview of, 121, 168, 227–28, 231–32; early developmental risk factors, 3–18; etiology of, 228, 231–32; family processes related to, 124–27; future work, directions for, 246–47; history of, 228, 231–32; individual developmental factors of, 123–25; interventions for, 196, 209–15, 219–20; in Latino Americans, 167–84; medical consequences of, 192*t*; nutrition interventions for, 233–36; partial causes of, 26; prevalence of, 145–46; preventive approaches to, 214, 236–45; psychological consequences of, 192*t*; surgical treatment of, 219–20, 251–65

obesity, risk/protective factors for, 146–51; early life experiences/parental influences, 147–48; energy gap, 147; for general population, 147–49; parental perceptions of obesity risks, 149; parental perceptions of weight, 148–49

obesity prevention: in American Indian infants and families, 153–56; in children/adolescents, 151–53

obesity-related diseases, 121–22, 167
online food marketing study, background,
    94–95; call for, 94; data analysis, 96;
    on kid's Web site, key features, 98*t*;
    research method, 95–96; selection of
    brands/Web sites, 96–97
online food marketing study, findings,
    96–108; advergames brand
    reinforcement, 97–99; explicit brand
    benefit claims, 100; exposure to
    advertising claims, 99–100; extending
    online advertising to offline, 105–6;
    incentives for product purchase/
    consumption, 106; marketing
    partnerships, promotions/sponsorships,
    102–3; nutritional information
    availability, 100–101; overview,
    96–97; study Web sites, list of,
    109–11; television characters'
    promotion of food brands, 103–4;
    television commercials online, 99–100;
    viral marketing efforts, 102; Web site
    membership offers, 104–5. *See also*
    Web sites, for children
overweight: bio-ecological framework,
    50–51; causes of, 50; definitions
    of, in adolescents/children, 168–69;
    importance of onset of, 57; variance in
    measurement, 55

parents: influences on obesity, 147–48;
    perceptions of obesity risks, 149;
    perceptions of weight, 148–49
Pathways Feasibility Study, 151, 153
patients, right of autonomy/personal
    responsibility, 272–73, 275–80
Pediatric Nutrition Surveillance System, 10
pharmacologic treatment, for obesity,
    215, 219
physical activity: ACSM/CDC
    recommendations, 34, 37, 39; and
    BMI, 35; definition, 30; energy
    cost of, 33–35; exercise vs., 30; as
    interventional approach, 213; IOM
    recommendations, 34–35; of minority
    youth, 172; in physical education
    classes, 170; physical fitness vs., 30–31;

role of, in obesity prevention, 25–42;
    spontaneous, and energy expenditure,
    32–33; vs. physical inactivity, 26–27,
    134–35, 228; vs. television viewing,
    123, 134–35; and weight gain, 35–36,
    123; weight loss intervention, 36–37
physical fitness: cardiorespiratory fitness,
    31; combined with overweight/obesity,
    41; genetic components of, 31;
    health-related fitness components, body
    composition, 31; musculoskeletal
    strength, 31; vs. physical activity,
    30–31, 134–35
physical inactivity, costs of, 26–27
planned behavior theory, of obesity
    prevention, 240–43; attitudes, 240–41;
    feeding examples, 242*t,* 243*t*; perceived
    behavioral control, 241–43; subjective
    norms, 241
poverty, influence on obesity, 173
Pregnancy Nutrition Surveillance
    System, 10
*Preventing Child Obesity: Health in the
    Balance* report, 123
preventive approaches, 236–45; results
    of actions, 243–45; role of physical
    activity, 25–42; transtheoretical model
    of change (TTM), 214, 236–39
preventive approaches, planned behavior
    theory, 240–43; attitudes, 240–41;
    perceived behavioral control, 241–43;
    subjective norms, 241
Program for Women, Infants, and
    Children (WIC), 148
prospective/longitudinal study, of
    academic difficulty, 53–55; kinder-
    garten entry, 53–54; kindergarten–3rd
    grade, 54–55; 7th–12th graders, 53
protective factors, in AI/AN populations,
    149–51; activity levels, 149–50;
    attitudes, 150–51; early life
    experiences, 150
protective factors, in general population,
    147–49; early life experiences/
    parental influences, 147–48; parental
    perceptions of obesity risks, 149;
    parental perceptions of weight, 148–49

protein intake, 28
protein sparing modified fast (PSMF),
    211–12
psychosocial costs, of obesity, 122,
    167, 174
psychosocial functioning difficulties, 49
Pygmalion in the Classroom (Rosenthal &
    Jacobson), 62

race/ethnicity, and breastfeeding
    behaviors, 15–16
research, on online food marketing,
    95–96; brand/Web site selection,
    95–96; data analysis, 96; findings,
    96–108
research, on school performance, 55–57
risk factors: Behavioral Risk Factor
    Surveillance System, 34; Behavioral
    Risk Factor Survey, 32; CARDIA
    study, 30, 35, 36; developmental, of
    obesity, 3–18; resources, of families,
    131–33; structural, of families, 130–31
risk factors, in AI/AN populations,
    149–51; activity levels, 149–50;
    attitudes, 150–51; early life
    experiences, 150
risk factors, in early development: energy
    balance equation, 5–6; of low-birth-
    weight, 7–8; metabolic syndrome, 8;
    type 2 diabetes, 8
risk factors, in general population,
    147–49; early life experiences/
    parental influences, 147–48; parental
    perceptions of obesity risks, 149;
    parental perceptions of weight, 148–49

safety of weight loss concern, 280–84;
    emotional harm, 282; existing medical
    conditions, 282–83; ineffective
    treatments, 283–84; initiation of binge
    eating, 282; psychological effects,
    282; surgery, 281; very low calorie
    regimens, 281
self-esteem issues, 73, 122
skittles.com (Master Foods), 95
sleep apnea, 181, 195–96
social cognitive theory (SCT), 214
social isolation, 49

social stigmatization, in middle
    childhood, 61–62
socio-behavioral consequences, of
    obesity, 167
socioeconomic status (SES), links with
    obesity, 174
Special Diabetes Program for Indians
    (SDPI), 154, 155–56
statistics, on obesity: African American
    male mortality, 174; African American
    youth, 169; CDC, of BMI, 4; Europe/
    U.S., 4; families below poverty line,
    173; Latino American youth, 170;
    obesity-related hospitalizations, 191;
    physical activity in classes, 170t
stigmatization, of being overweight:
    in adolescence, 63–66; of adults, 51;
    appearance-based stigma, 62–63,
    64–66; in middle childhood, 62–63;
    social stigma/stereotype threat, 61–62;
    of young children, 60–61
Strong Heart Study, 149–50
studies/surveys: academic difficulties
    52–55; Add Health Study, 123, 130–36;
    Aerobics Center Longitudinal Study,
    41; Amsterdam Growth and Health
    study, 35; anthropometric study (of
    height/weight/skinfold thickness), 171;
    Behavioral Risk Factor Surveillance
    Study, 32, 34, 150; CARDIA study,
    30, 35, 36; CATCH study, 152;
    Children Are Our Messengers:
    Changing the Health study, 173–74;
    Feeding Infants and Toddlers Study
    (FITS), 17; GEMS Pilot Study
    (Stanford), 213; Harvard Alumni
    Health Study, 41; Health Professionals
    study (U.S.), 36; National Health and
    Nutrition Examination Survey, 35,
    50; National Health Interview Survey,
    26; National Longitudinal Study of
    Adolescent Health, 193; National
    Medical Expenditures Panel Survey,
    26; Pathways Feasibility Study, 151;
    SEARCH for Diabetes in Youth Study
    Group, 145; Strong Heart Study, 146,
    149–50; Third National Health and
    Nutrition Examination Survey, 191. *See*

also National Institute of Child Health and Human Development (NICHD) Study of Early Child Care and Youth Development

surgical treatment, of obesity, 219–20, 251–65; banded gastroplasties, 256–58; history of, 252–58; jejunoileal bypass, 252–53; open/laparoscopic approaches, 258, 265; operative mortality/ complications, 264–65; outcomes of, 262–64; patient selection, 260–61; perioperative care, 262; post-operative care, 262; pre-operative care, 258–59; Roux-en-Y gastric bypass, 253–55, 264–65

teasing, weight-based, 122
television viewing: and academic difficulty, 56–57; by infants, 59; Nielsen/Net rating reports, 94; vs. physical activity, 123, 134–35; of poor minority youth, 172–73; television characters' food brand promotion, 103–4. *See also* online food marketing; Web sites, for children
temperament, and early weight gain, 8–10
Third National Health and Nutrition Examination Survey (NHANES III), 191
thrifty genotypes, 124
transtheoretical model of change (TTM), 214, 236–39; process of change in, 239*t*; stages of, 237*t*
treatment options: for adolescents, 181–82; for African American youth, 182, 184; for children, 181–82; for Latino American youth, 182, 184
triglycerides, 29
type 2 diabetes, 8, 167, 195

Web sites, for children, 93; ad-break reminders, 107–8; design of, 94, 95, 96; extending online offers to offline, 105–6; information for parents, 107; interactivity of, 103–4; offer of membership/ online marketing, 104–5; online food marketing study list of, 109–11; privacy protections/age blocks, 107; protections for children, 106–8; sponsoring of, by food manufacturers, 96, 98*t*
weight gain: appropriate growth and, 232; contributing personal factors to, 277–78; as moral failure, 276; and physical activity, 35–36; and temperament, 8–10
weight loss: factors of success, 29–30; physical activity interventions, 36–37; positive factors associated with, 121; treatment for, social context, 274–75
weight loss, safety issues, 280–84; emotional harm, 282; existing medical conditions, 282–83; ineffective treatments, 283–84; initiation of binge eating, 282; psychological effects, 282; surgery, 281; very low calorie regimens, 281
weight loss, social justice issues, 288–96; assignment of blame, 292; causal factors, complexity of, 290–91; coverage determination, 292; degrees of obesity, 291–92; health care costs, 288–89; irresponsible behavior, 290; rationing of health care, 289; setting priorities, 293; weight management priorities, 294–96
Western ideals, of beauty/body size, 177–78
White, non-Hispanics: feeding methods of, 13; maternal attitudes towards infant weight, 16; overweight in children, 4